Textbook of Head and Neck Pathology

Margaret S. Brandwein

Textbook of Head and Neck Pathology

Volume 1: Nose, Paranasal Sinuses, and Nasopharynx

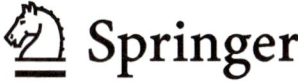

Margaret S. Brandwein
Erie County Medical Center
State University of New York at Buffalo
Buffalo
NY
USA

ISBN 978-3-319-81484-1   ISBN 978-3-319-33323-6   (eBook)
DOI 10.1007/978-3-319-33323-6

Printed on acid-free paper

This Springer imprint is published by Springer Nature
The registered company is Springer International Publishing AG Switzerland

To my children and grandchildren, the light of my eyes

Preface

Each world contains a myriad of smaller worlds.

We choose the scale in which we dwell; perhaps, it selects us before we choose it. We pathologists are among a tiny cadre who can hear the whispering of glass slides. Hold a glass slide up to the air, you see a name, an institution, numbers, and tissue pieces. Put the glass on a micro-scope stage, and magic unfolds. The tissue holds worlds of stories, time lines of disease processes, symptoms, suffering, treatments, both successful and unsuccessful, and predictions. Imagine the worlds of information we glean from slides; now imagine the worlds we have yet to discover. This is our world. We only have to sit quietly, look, and listen to the whispering of slides.

Acknowledgment

Special thanks to Dr. Nestor Rigual for helpful review and feedback

Contents

Sinonasal Tract – Anatomy and Histology

© Springer International Publishing Switzerland 2016
M.S. Brandwein, *Textbook of Head and Neck Pathology*,
DOI 10.1007/978-3-319-33323-6_1

Abstract

One needs constant anatomic confirmation to correctly navigate "the head and neck"; perhaps the idea that "anatomy is destiny" rings truest here. A differential diagnosis can vary according to the anatomic subsite. Tumor staging for sinonasal and nasopharyngeal malignancies differs. Get to know how to recognize the different histologies in the external nose and sinonasal tract.

Keywords

Nasal cavity · Antrum · Septum · Turbinates · Schneiderian mucosa · Seromucinous glands

- Nasal erectile vessels are present in the turbinates and nasal swell body.
- Scroll-like bones confirm the site as turbinates.
- Thin, straight boney plates confirm the site as ethmoid.
- Helpful findings for orienting gross resection specimens:
  1. The turbinates attach to the lateral nasal wall anteriorly, the free edge points posteriorly
  2. The crista gallae points superiorly

Glossary

Vestibule Skin-lined region posterior to the nares, anterior to the anterior choanae

Limen nasi Also known as pyriform aperture, is the posterior lateral ridge that separates the vestibule from the nasal cavity

Anterior choana Separates vestibule from nasal cavity

Posterior choana Separates nasal cavity from nasaopharynx

Nasal septal swell body Thickened area of superior nasal septum containing nasal erectile vessels

Olfactory cleft Narrow vertical aspect of superior nasal cavity

Party wall Comprised of the lateral nasal wall and medial antral wall

Schneiderian mucosa Sinonasal mucosa derived from involuting nasal placodes

Crista galli Bony ridge which projects superiorly from cribriform plate

Seromucinous glands - Sinonasal seromucinous glands with fewer terminal acini

Key Points

- Incorporate important anatomic landmarks in your surgical report to build trust with your audience.
- Get your anatomic bearings by histologically examining not only overlying mucosa but deep tissues for clues.
- The paranasal sinus lamina propria is loose and distensible compared to the nasal septum.

One needs constant anatomic confirmation to correctly navigate "the head and neck"; perhaps the idea that "anatomy is destiny" rings truest in this place. In the sinonasal tract, for example, inverted papillomas commonly arise from the lateral nasal wall, while nasal septal inverted papillomas are a disputable entity. Nasal septal polyps are extremely uncommon, and evoke a specific differential diagnosis (respiratory epithelial adenomatoid hamartoma, sinonasal seromucinous hamartoma, pleomorphic adenoma, mucoepidermoid carcinoma, primary nasal melanoma, metastatic disease). Along the same line, although the nasopharynx and oropharynx are anatomically contiguous, staging schemes for nasopharyngeal and oropharyngeal carcinomas are very different. Likewise, the oropharynx and oral cavity are contiguous subsites, but initial treatment approaches to these two cancers are very different.

A surgical pathology report which incorporates the significant anatomic landscape of the head and neck assists in clinicopathological correlation and goes far in building "the economy of trust." The best way to get your bearings, histologically, is not to limit histologic examination to the overlying mucosa, but examine all associated tissues for important clues.

Table 1.1 provides an overview of the anatomic components of the sinonasal tract. Resections of the external nose may be oriented by the shape of the cartilages and type of overlying tissue (Fig. 1.1). The nasal vestibule is the internal skin-lined region posterior to the nares. The limen nasi (piriform aperture) is a posterior lateral ridge the separates

> ▪ **Table 1.1** Anatomic definitions for the sinonasal tract

Nasal vestibule:

　Anterior boundary: nares

　Posterior boundary: line dropped perpendicular from the frontonasal suture through the anterior aspect of the inferior turbinate

Nasal cavities:

　Anterior boundary: continuous with the vestibule

　Posterior boundary: posterior choanae

　Superior boundary: cribriform plate

　Inferior boundary: Hard palate

　Medial boundary: nasal septum

　Lateral boundary: lateral nasal wall with maxillary and ethmoid ostia and turbinates.

Turbinates:

　Scroll-like projections of bone and vascular soft tissue

　The superior turbinate is smallest, the inferior turbinate is largest

　Attaches to the lateral nasal wall anteriorly, with a free edge, posteriorly

Schneiderian mucosa:

　Pseudostratified columnar ciliated epithelium with goblet cells

　The lamina propria is loose and well vascularized with seromucinous glands

Olfactory mucosa:

　Bipolar olfactory nerve fibers cross through the cribriform plate and terminate in the olfactory mucosa forming olfactory cilia

　Bowman's glands or olfactory glands, appear similar to serous minor salivary glands

Frontal sinus

　Paired sinuses between the interior and external cranial tables

Ethmoid complex

　Paired sinus complex composed of 3–18 cells that are grouped as anterior, middle, or posterior, according to the location of their ostia

　Medial boundary: upper nasal fossa

> ▪ **Table 1.1** (continued)

　Lateral boundary: lamina papyracea, of the orbit

　Superior boundary: fovea ethmoidalis which is the medial extension of the orbital plate of the frontal bone

Sphenoid sinus

　Posterior to the ethmoid sinuses

　Superior boundary: floor of the anterior cranial fossa, anteriorly

　Posterior boundary: optic chiasm and the sella turcica, posteriorly

　Lateral boundary: orbital apex, the optic canal, the optic nerve, and cavernous sinus

　Inferior boundary: nasopharynx

　Anterior boundary: nasal fossa

Maxillary sinus

　Medial boundary: lateral wall of the nasal cavity ("party wall")

　The curved posterolateral wall separates the sinus from the infratemporal fossa.

　The anterior sinus wall is the facial surface of the maxilla

　Inferior boundary: hard palate

　Superior boundary: orbital rim and orbital apex

the nasal vestibule from the nasal cavity (▪ Fig. 1.2). The skin of the nostrils and nasal dome contain abundant large sebaceous glands, whereas vestibular skin is thinner, contains hair follicles, but has fewer, smaller sebaceous glands (▪ Fig. 1.1). The upper lateral nasal cartilages are long and straight, whereas greater and lesser alar cartilages (also known as lower lateral cartilages) have curved ends. The nostrils have no supporting cartilage.

The term "Schneiderian mucosa" is frequently used in the context of the sinonasal tract; this refers to the embryologic nasal placodes, which invaginate to form the sinonasal mucosa (▪ Fig. 1.3). The nasal cavities are bordered medially by the nasal septum and laterally by the lateral nasal wall (party wall). The cartilaginous septum is present in the anterior nasal cavity, articulating anterior inferiorly with the maxilla, posterior inferiorly with the vomer, and posterior superiorly with the perpendicular ethmoid plate. The

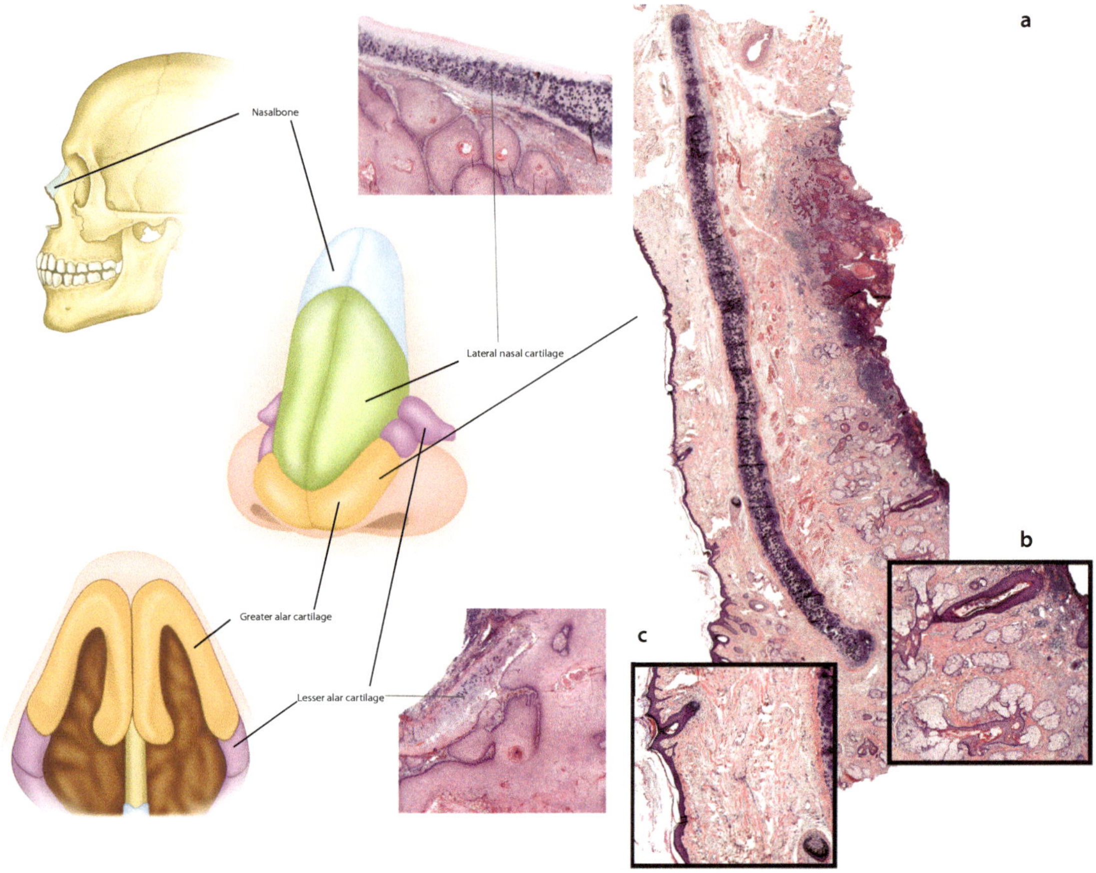

◘ Fig. 1.1   Orienting facial resection specimens can be daunting; knowledge of anatomy helps you to deal. The upper bony external nose (*blue*) articulates with the frontal and maxillary bones. The lower nose is cartilaginous and composed of the flat lateral nasal cartilages (*green*) and two sets of curved cartilages, the greater and lower lateral alar cartilages (*orange* and *pink*). The far right (**a**) depicts squamous carcinoma of the nasal dome skin. The underlying cartilage, 1.5 cm long and curved at one end, is the greater alar cartilage. Compare the skin of the dome (*inset* **b**) which normally contains abundant sebaceous glands, to that of the vestibule (*inset* **c**) which has hair follicles

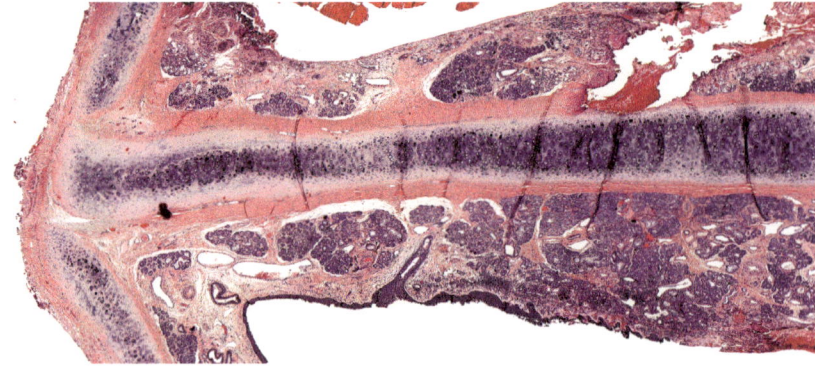

◘ Fig. 1.2   Nasal septum as it relates to the lateral nasal cartilages, which are both straight cartilaginous structures. The lamina propria of the nasal septum has greater amounts of fibroconnective tissue than the paranasal sinuses. Thus, fluids do not accumulate to form respiratory polyps in the nasal septum

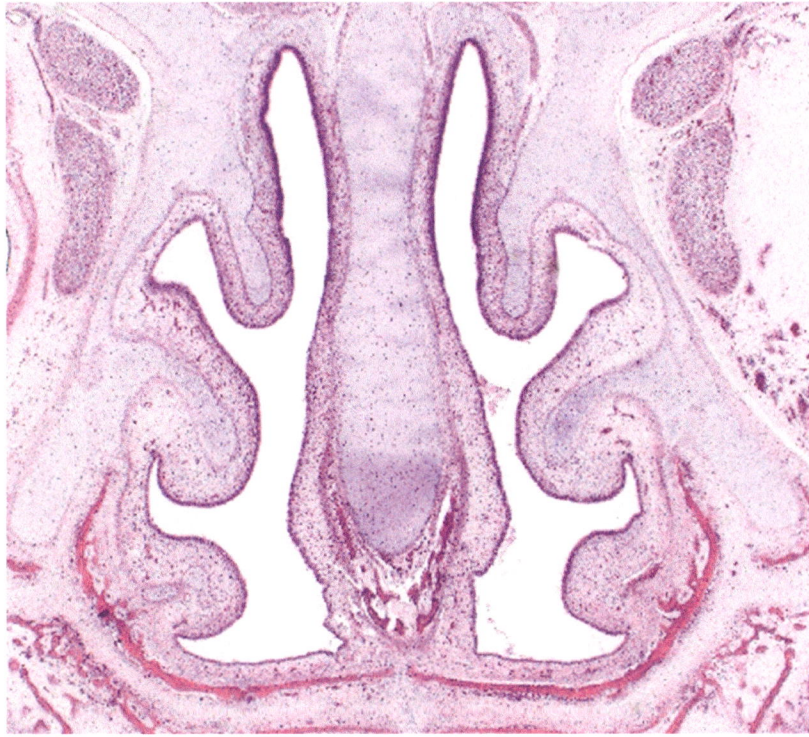

Fig. 1.3 Developing nasal cavity, 13 weeks, which is lined by columnar ciliated respiratory mucosa (Schneiderian mucosa) (Courtesy Dr Rafal Kozielski, Children's Hospital, Buffalo)

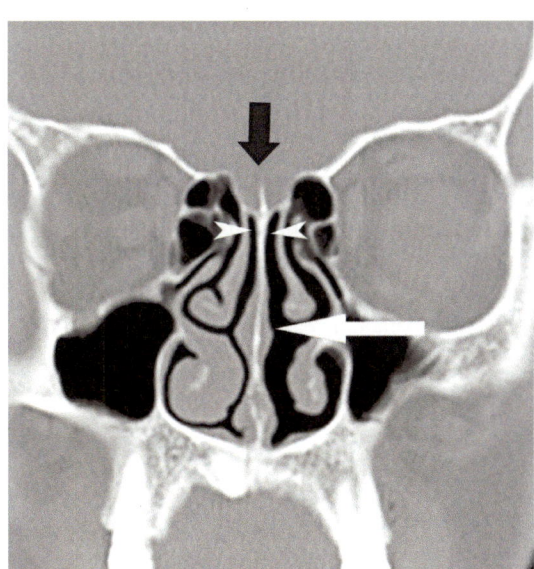

Fig. 1.4 Nasal septal swell body (*white arrow*). Its vascularity is similar to that of the turbinates. The *black arrow* points to the crista galli. The *white arrowheads* point to the olfactory clefts. The muscular vessels of the nasal turbinates and septum comprise the nasal erectile tissue, which is an element of the normal nasal pulmonary cycle. Here, the right inferior turbinate is engorged, while airflow is greater in the left nasal cavity (Courtesy of Dr. Peter Som, The Mount Sinai Hospital, NY, NY)

nasal septal cartilage is long and has a well-defined perichondrium. The nasal septal swell body (also referred to as nasal septal turbinate) appears as a distinct radiographic swelling of the superior septum (Fig. 1.4, **white arrow**) and histologically is distinguished by thick muscular vessels [1, 2]. The inferior nasal septum has thinner submucosa and is usually lined by transitional squamous epithelium (stratified cuboidal epithelium), or occasionally respiratory mucosa (pseudostratified ciliated columnar epithelium with admixed goblet cells) (Fig. 1.5).

The olfactory cleft is the narrow, vertical aspect of the superior nasal cavity, which is bound medially by the perpendicular ethmoid plate, and laterally by the medial aspect of the middle turbinate. It is connected to the anterior cranial fossa by the olfactory groove through the cribriform plate and opens inferiorly into the respiratory nasal fossa (Fig. 1.4). The roof of the olfactory cleft is lined by olfactory epithelium, which may also extend to the nasal septum and superior turbinates [3]. This specialized olfactory epithelium is composed of ciliated olfactory receptors, sensory brush (microvillar) cells, supporting

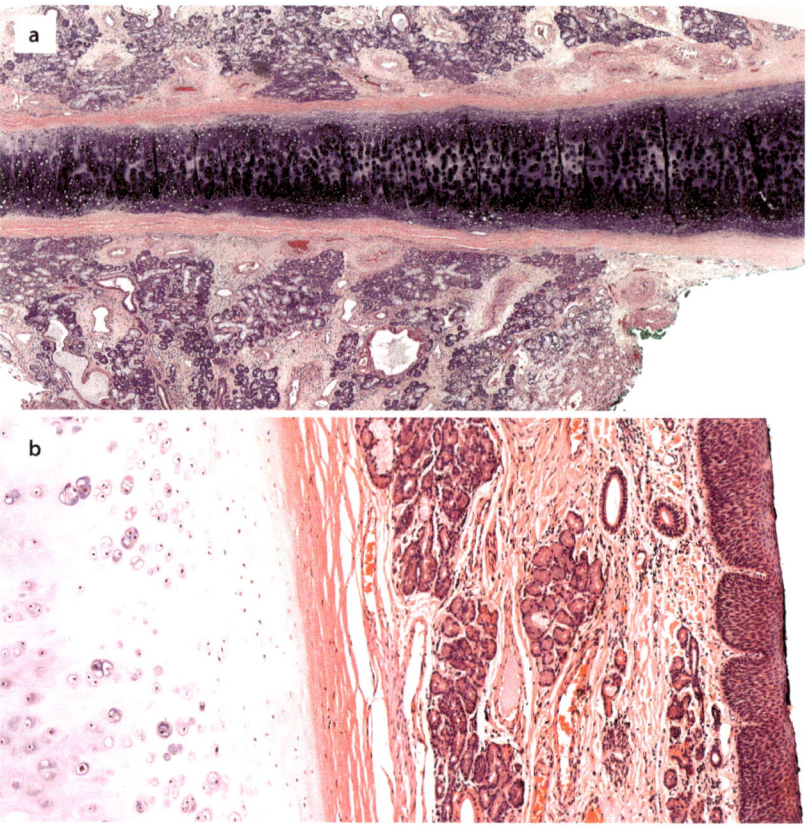

◘ Fig. 1.5 Nasal septum: (**a**) the superior nasal septum has thick muscular vessels, similar to the turbinates. (**b**) The inferior nasal septum is usually lined with stratified squamous epithelium

cells, and basal cells which sit atop a highly cellular lamina propria containing Bowman's glands and the axon bundles from the ciliated olfactory receptors [3]. Olfactory cells are bipolar neurons with apical ciliated chemoreceptors that detect ambient odorants and nerve processes which pass through the cribriform plate to synapse in the olfactory bulb. The brush cells are columnar sensory cells with apical microvilli; basally they make contact with the terminal nerve fibers of the trigeminal nerve. The role of brush cells is still controversial [3, 4]. Sensory cells are maintained

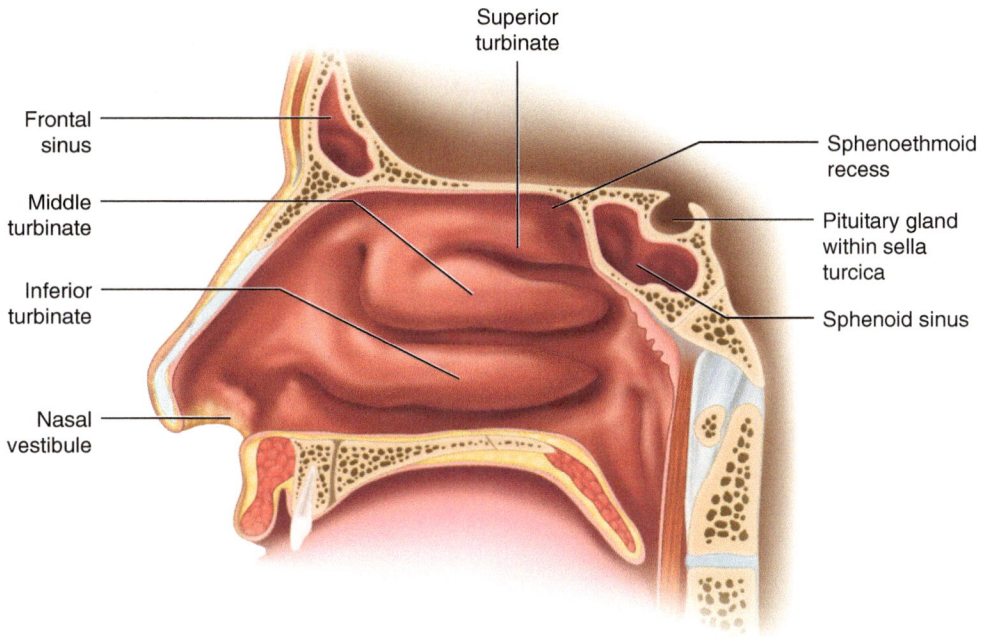

Fig. 1.6 The nasal cavity and paranasal sinuses demonstrated in this cross section are highlighted in *pink*; the anterior boundary between the nasal cavity and the vestibule (*yellow*) is the anterior choana. The posterior boundary separating nasal cavity from nasopharynx (*blue*) is the posterior choana. The lateral nasal wall is also referred to as the "party wall", it represents the medial wall of the maxillary antrum. The maxillary sinus drains upward through the middle ostium, which is underneath the middle turbinate

by supporting cells (sustentacular cells), which are pseudostratified ciliated columnar cells. The basal cells are stem cells that renew both sensory and supporting cell populations. Bowman's glands are tubuloalveolar glands that secrete mucous onto the olfactory mucosal surface; this aids olfaction by fixing and dissolving odorants.

The crista galli (cock's crest) is an anterior bony ridge that points superiorly from the cribriform plate (Fig. 1.4). It can be identified in superior nasal cavity resections (e.g., olfactory neuroblastoma) assisting in specimen orientation.

The nasal turbinates arise from the lateral nasal wall (Fig. 1.6) and can be distinguished

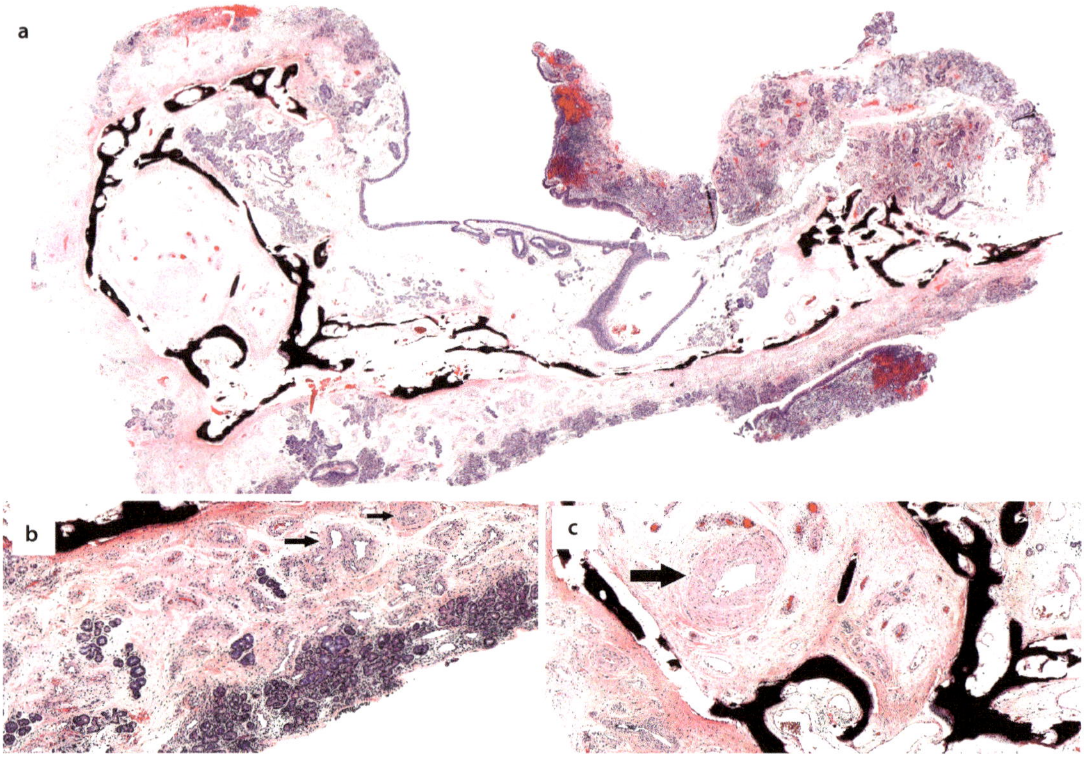

Fig. 1.7   Nasal turbinates can be distinguished from other sinonasal tissues by scroll-like bone (**a**) and vessels with thick muscular walls (**b**, **c**: nasal erectile tissue, *arrows*)

histologically by their scroll-like bones and thick muscular vessels (nasal erectile tissue) (■ Fig. 1.7) [5]. Blood flow to the turbinates cyclically alternate (nasal cycling), and ipsilaterally impede airflow. The decongested side has the dominant airflow per cycle, which is associated with greater ipsilateral pulmonary aeration. The inferior nasal turbinates are the largest set. The maxillary antra drain upward through the middle meatuses which open under the middle turbinates. Resection specimens that include the lateral wall can be oriented by recognizing that the free end of the turbinate points posteriorly (■ Fig. 1.6).

The ethmoid air cells can be likened to small communicating rooms in a shot gun house. The ethmoid sinus is divided into anterior and posterior cells by the basal lamella. The roof of the ethmoid sinuses is the sphenoid bone. The ethmoid air cells can be appreciated in resection specimens by their paper-thin, straight bony walls.

The paranasal sinuses are lined by respiratory mucosa with loose, distensible submucosa containing branched tubulo-alveolar seromucinous glands (■ Fig. 1.8). Seromucinous glands differ from minor salivary glands in their overall

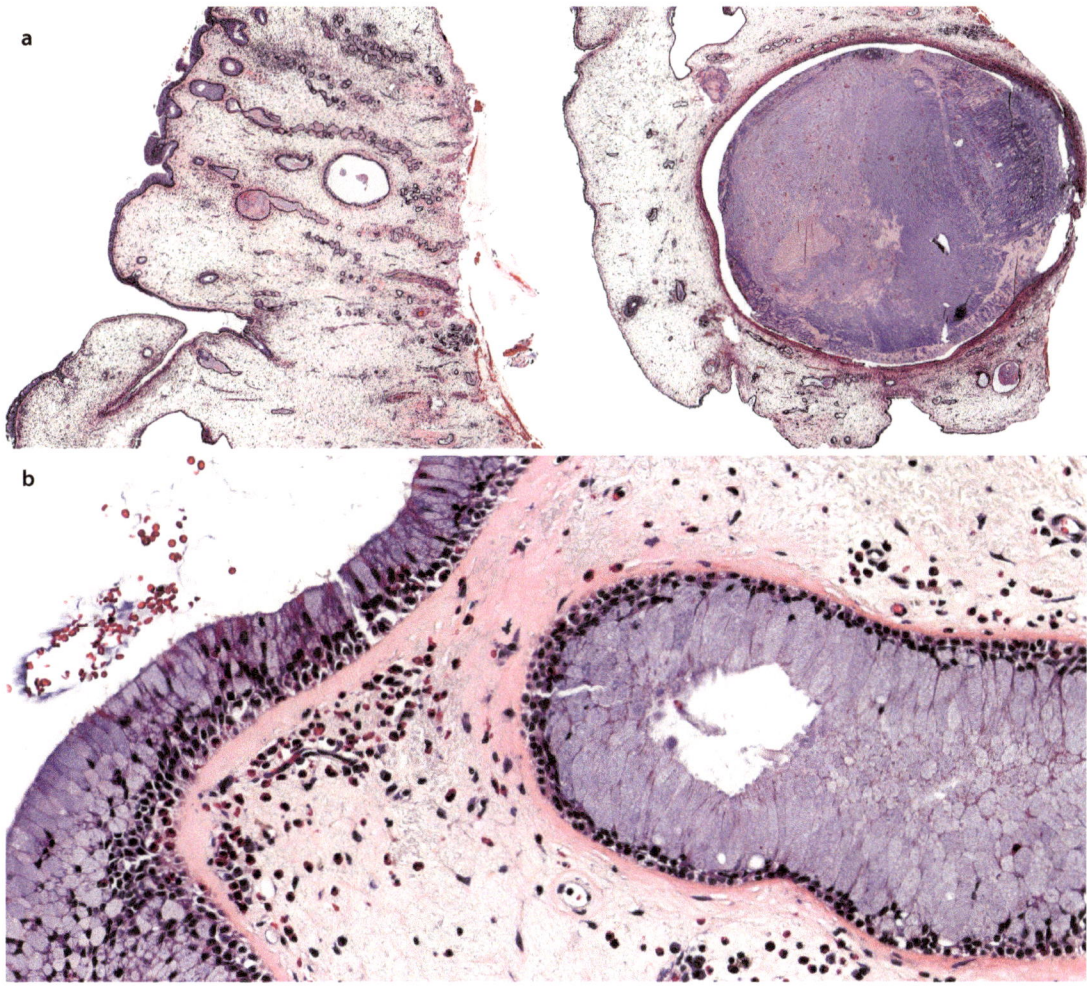

◻ Fig. 1.8 Paranasal sinus – the submucosa is loose and distensible, which allows fluids and inflammation to accumulate. (**a**) Tubular seromucinous glands. *Unlike minor salivary glands, they do not terminate in clusters of acini.* (**b**) Cystic dilation of seromucinous duct. (**c**) Pseudostratified respiratory epithelium: Goblet cell hyperplasia, thickened basement membrane, and eosinophils in the lamina propria signify chronic allergic sinusitis

shape; seromucinous glands have fewer terminal acini compared with minor salivary glands.

Self Study

1. Contains nasal erectile tissue:
    (a) The nasal septal swell body
    (b) Olfactory cleft
    (c) Limen nasi
    (d) Crista galli

2. Which statement is true:
    (a) There is a contralateral relationship between nasal cavity and lung aeration which is termed the pulmonary cycle.
    (b) Nasal septum and turbinate are histologically identical.
    (c) The loose, distensible nasal septal lamina propria is responsible for a predisposition for septal polyps.
    (d) Sinonasal seromucinous glands have fewer acini than minor salivary glands.

Answers

1. Contains nasal erectile tissue:
   (a) The nasal septal swell body – **CORRECT**.
   (b) Olfactory cleft represents the narrow vertical aspect of superior nasal cavity
   (c) Limen nasi separates the nasal vestibule from the nasal cavity
   (d) Crista galli projects superiorly from cribriform plate and is the attachment point of the falx cerebri
2. Which statement is true:
   (a) The relationship between nasal cavity and lung aeration is ipsilateral during the pulmonary cycle.
   (b) The turbinates contain thick-walled nasal erectile tissue and are is usually covered by respiratory mucosa. The nasal septum has less distensible lamina propria compared to the turbinate. The lower septum has a stratified squamous epithelial lining. The vascularity of the septum is less than that of the turbinates, which exception of the nasal septal swell body.
   (c) The nasal septal lamina propria is tethered to the perichondrium, and not predisposed to polyps.
   (d) Sinonasal seromucinous glands have fewer acini than minor salivary glands. – **CORRECT**.

References

1. Wexler D, Braverman I, Amar M. Histology of the nasal septal swell body (septal turbinate). Otolaryngol Head Neck Surg. 2006;134:596–600.
2. Sişman AS, Acıoğlu E, Yiğit O, Akakın D, Cilingir OT. Nasal septal turbinate: cadaveric study. Am J Rhinol Allergy. 2014;28:173–7.
3. Moran DT, Rowley 3rd JC, Jafek BW, Lovell MA. The fine structure of the olfactory mucosa in man. J Neurocytol. 1982;11:721–46.
4. Elsaesser R, Paysan J. The sense of smell, its signalling pathways, and the dichotomy of cilia and microvilli in olfactory sensory cells. BMC Neurosci. 2007;8 Suppl 3:S1.
5. Kiroglu AF, Bayrakli H, Yuca K, Cankaya H, Kiris M. Nasal obstruction as a common side-effect of sildenafil citrate. Tohoku J Exp Med. 2006;208:251–4.

Sinonasal Tract: Nonneoplastic

© Springer International Publishing Switzerland 2016
M.S. Brandwein, *Textbook of Head and Neck Pathology*,
DOI 10.1007/978-3-319-33323-6_2

Abstract

If it appears strange that that one etiologic agent gives rise to such a diversity of disease, then consider the three major components of any infectious process: (1) the inherent virulence of the agent, (2) the infectious dose, and (3) the patient status. Allergic fungal sinusitis represents the most common form of sinonasal fungal disease. Invasive fungal sinusitis {acute, (<4 weeks) and chronic (>12 weeks)} represents the most serious sinonasal fungal disease, which develops in the setting of neutropenia, or neutrophil dysfunction. Other more rare and exotic sinonasal infectious conditions, or infectious mimickers are also discussed in this chapter.

Keywords

Allergic fungal sinusitis · Invasive fungal sinusitis · Granulomatosis with polyangiitis

---

Glossary

Sinusitis ossificans Chronic sinusitis accompanied by heterotopic ossification.

Fungus ball Noninvasive accumulation of fungal hyphae within paranasal sinuses.

Allergic mucin Evidence of eosinophil degranulation and an allergic phenomenon

Rhinoscleroma Caused by *K. rhinoscleromatis* (von Frisch bacilli)

Rhinosporidiosis Caused by *Rhinosporidium seeberi*, a Mesomycetozoea, (eukaryotic aquatic microbe)

Myospherulosis Non-infectious inflammatory condition due to erythrocytes reacting with exogenous lipids, vitamin E, or traumatized fat

Granulomatosis with polyangiitis Systemic vasculitis characteristically involving sinonasal tract, lungs, and kidneys

---

Key Points

- If you see allergic mucin, consider allergic fungal sinusitis and order GMS stains.
- Invasive sinonasal fungal disease is a true emergency, alert clinicians.
- Initial diagnosis of invasive fungal sinusitis can be made at frozen section with H+E stains. After systemic therapy hyphae no longer detectable on H+E, and require GMS stains.

- Mucorales: broad hyphae (7–20 um), "empty bent-cellophane tubes", hyphal walls with uneven thickness, septations are absent or erratic, branching with variable angles (45°–90°).
- Aspergillus: thin hyphae, even wall thickness, regular septations, uniform acute angle hyphal branching.
- Fruiting heads only seen with fungus ball
- The nature of the encysted erythrocytes in myospherulosis can be confirmed by Okajima's hemoglobin stain; Gomori methanamine silver, iron, and periodic acid Schiff stains are negative.

2.1   Polyps and Sinusitis

Sinonasal polyps result from the expansion of the Schneiderian submucosa with fluids and proteins due to myriads of causes, e.g., chronic allergy, vasomotor rhinitis, infectious rhinosinusitis, diabetes mellitus, cystic fibrosis, Kartagener's syndrome, aspirin intolerance, Churg Strauss disease, and nickel exposure (◻ Figs. 2.1 and 2.2). About 20 % of patients with nasal polyps have asthma; conversely about 30 % of asthmatic patients have polyps, more commonly of allergic origin [1]. Aspirin-exacerbated respiratory disease (AERD, also known as Samter's triad) refers to the syndrome of allergic nasal polyps with eosinophils, aspirin intolerance, and bronchial asthma, which affects 4–10 % of asthmatics [2–4]. AERD is the result of inhibiting the cyclooxygenase pathway in sensitive individuals; this shunts metabolism of arachidonic acid to the 5-lipooxygenase pathway leading to increased pro-inflammatory leukotrienes and decreased PGE2, a protective prostaglandin [4, 5].

Polyps: Gross Examination

- Sinonasal polyps may be single, or multiple and bilateral
- Normally, they are translucent and soft
- *If dark, putty-like, think allergic fungal sinusitis*
- *If white, grey, hard, think inverted papilloma or other process*
- *If red and ragged, think oncocytic Schneiderian papilloma*

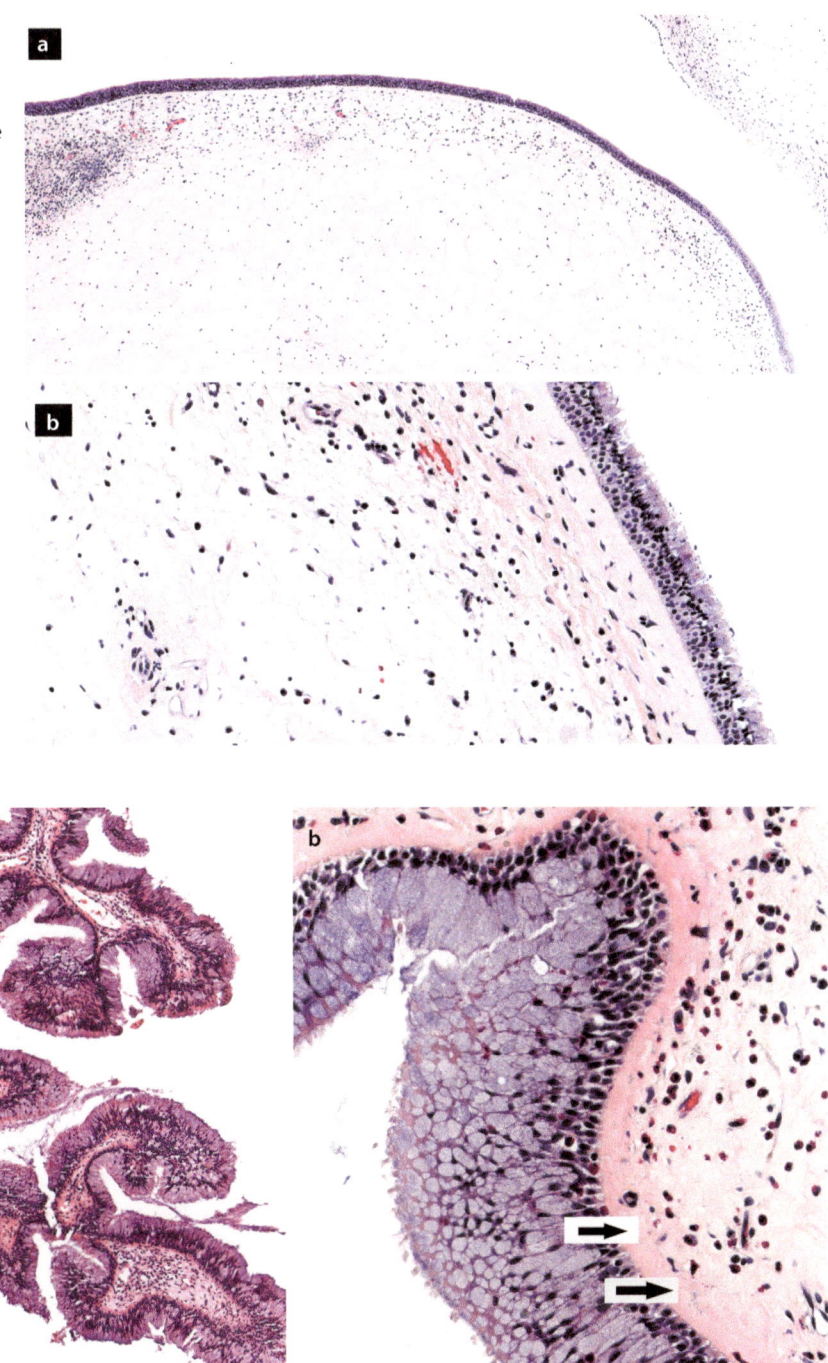

☐ Fig. 2.1 (**a, b**) Low and high-power views of respiratory polyps. These polyps result from accumulation of fluids in the lamina propria, displacing seromucinous glands

☐ Fig. 2.2 (**a**) Chronic sinusitis may lead to papillary hyperplasia. (**b**) The "fat" papillae reveal thickened basement membrane (*arrows*), hyperplastic goblet cells, and chronic inflamation. In contrast, well-differentiated intestinal type adenocarcinoma is composed of thin, simple to complex papillae lined by simple columnar epithelium

■ Histopathology

The minimal criteria for the diagnosis of chronic sinusitis is a thickened basement membrane directly beneath respiratory mucosa and around seromucinous glandular tubuli; this speaks for remote episodes of sinusitis even if no active inflammation is present. Usually, chronic sinusitis is characterized by increased lymphoplasmacytic

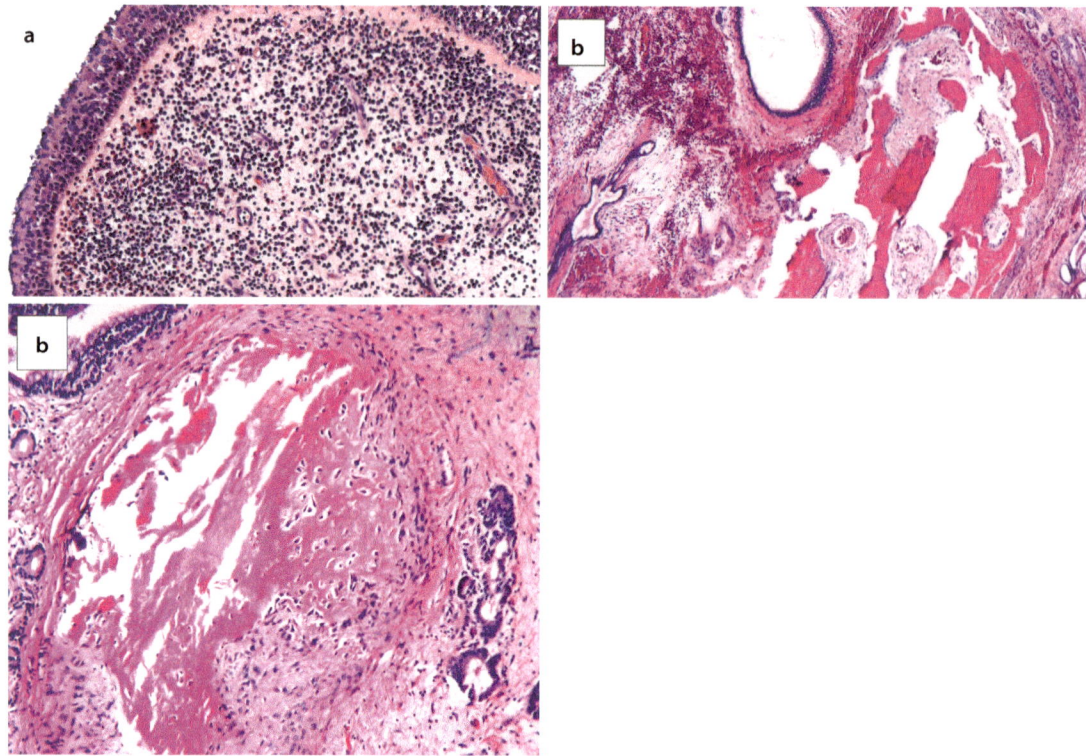

Fig. 2.3 (**a**) Allergic sinusitis is characterized by an eosinophilic infiltrate. (**b, c**) Unusual heterotopic ossification with chronic sinusitis, "sinusitis ossificans"

infiltrate. Severe sinusitis may also demonstrate marked mucosal papillary hyperplasia, goblet cell hyperplasia (■ Fig. 2.2), and squamous metaplasia; the latter is exacerbated by cigarette exposure [6]. Eosinophils denotes allergic etiology (■ Fig. 2.3). Uncommonly, hemorrhage with resorption (cholesterol clefts) can be seen (■ Fig. 2.4) [7]. Rarely, heterotopic ossification ("sinusitis ossificans") can be observed within Schneiderian submucosa (■ Fig. 2.3) [8, 9]. Interestingly, human Schneiderian mucosa contains osteoprogenitor cells, which can be induced to form bone, as demonstrated by *in-vitro* and *in-vivo* experiments [10].

Chronic allergic sinusitis is characterized by tissue eosinophilia. A number of studies demonstrate that tissue eosinophilia correlates directly with recurrent polyposis; predictive cut-offs for eosinophil density have ranged from 20 to 120 eosinophils/HPF [11]. Allergic mucin characteristically contains "blue ripples" appreciated at low-power. At higher power, you can appreciate the eosinophil component and Charcot Leydin

crystals. The presence of allergic mucin requires the next step of ruling out allergic fungal sinusitis (▶ See below Sect. 2.4.1). By contract, nonallergic mucin appears has polymorphonuclear cells and shed goblet and columnar respiratory cells.

Sinonasal polyps most commonly arise from the middle meatus and ethmoid sinuses; they form distinct masses with three contiguous surfaces. Most commonly, sinonasal polyps have edematous stroma. Stromal seromucinous glands may be absent. If the polyp is devoid of glands, has fibrotic stroma and prominent vessels, consider antrochoanal polyp (▶ see below, Sect. 2.3). Stromal atypia ("Polyp with atypical or bizarre stromal cells") either focal or diffuse, may be seen. These atypical stromal cells represent reactive fibroblasts; they are enlarged, have hyperchromatic nuclei and are mitotic inactive.

A timely question is whether or not routine histopathology is indicated for nasal polyps? It has been demonstrated that histopathology on routine bilateral nasal polyposis is unnecessary, from a "missed diagnosis" point of view [12].

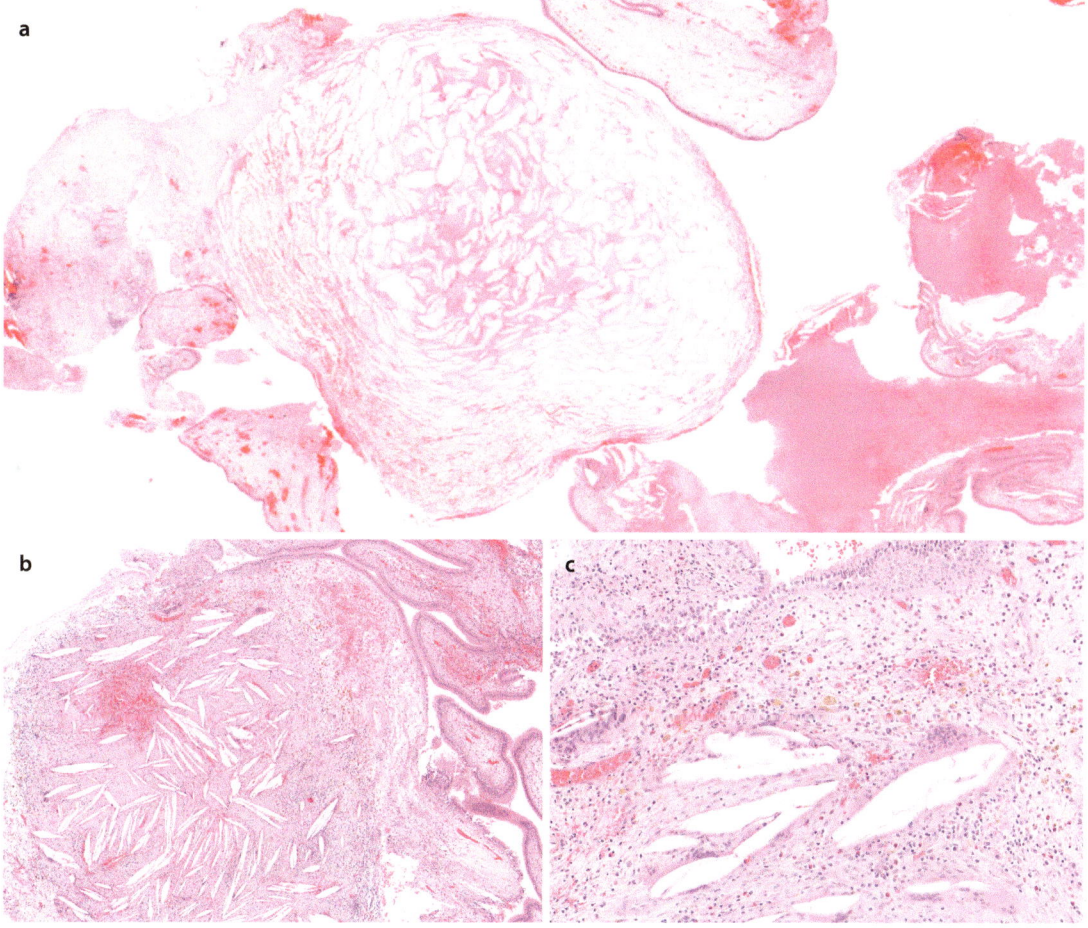

Fig. 2.4 Sinusitis with "cholesterol granuloma": (**a**) Hemorrhage. (**b**) Cholesterol clefts. (**c**) Foreign body granuloma

- *If a fibrotic stalk and prominent vessels seen, consider **antrochoanal polyp***
- *If squamous metaplasia/hyperplasia seen, consider **inverted papilloma***
- *If pierced microglandular cribriform pattern seen, consider **Oncocytic Schneiderian papilloma***
- *If ductoglandular adenosis seen, consider **respiratory epithelial adenomatoid hamartoma**, or **sinonasal seromucinous hamartoma***

2.2   Cystic Fibrosis

Pediatric nasal polyps are generally uncommon; 29 % of such polyps in children are associated with cystic fibrosis (Fig. 2.5). Conversely, between 10 % and 20 % of children with cystic fibrosis have nasal polyps. Histologically, nasal polyps in cystic fibrosis are associated with significantly more seromucinous glands, with dilated glandular tubuli, compared to pediatric chronic polypoid sinusitis [13, 14].

2.3   Antrochoanal Polyps

Antrochoanal polyps represent 4–6 % of all nasal polyps [15]. They arise in the maxillary antrum and prolapse through middle meatus. The polyp can extend posteriorly and prolapse further through the posterior choanae into the nasopharynx (Fig. 2.6). Thus, a long stalk is characteristic of this entity; stalk torsion can give rise to bizarre submucosal reactive fibroblasts. Clinically, they can become quite large, mimicking neoplasia.

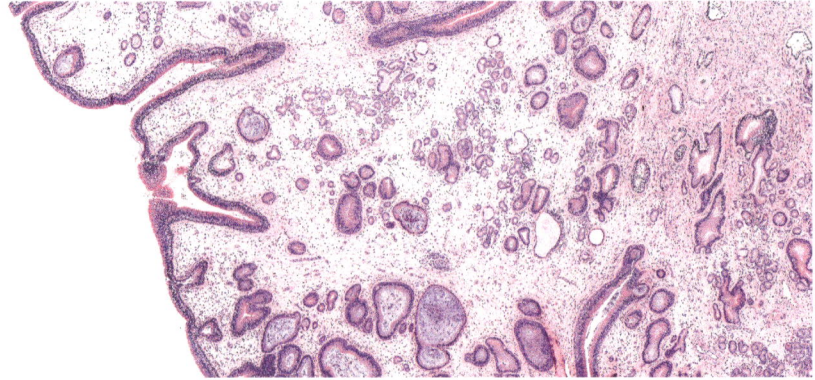

🔲 **Fig. 2.5**   Cystic fibrosis – chronic hyperplastic sinusitis with cystic dilation of seromucinous ducts

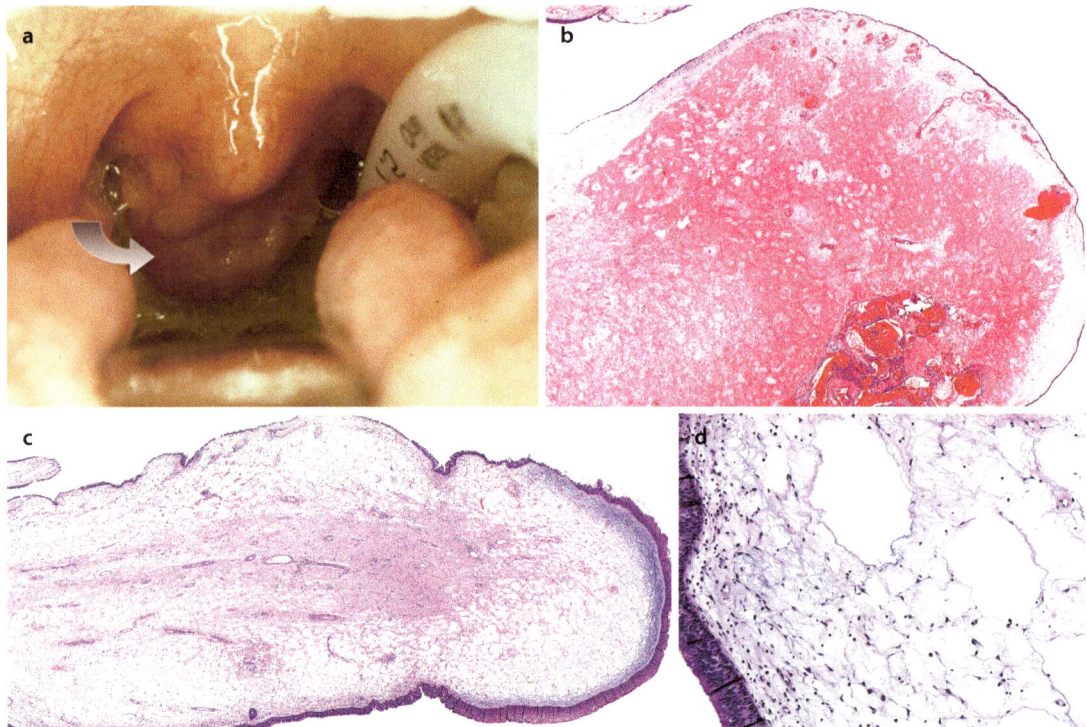

🔲 **Fig. 2.6**   Antrochoanal polyp – (**a**) the polyp is seen behind the uvula (*grey arrow*), originating in the maxilla (antrum) and protruding through the middle meatus and posterior choanae, to fill the nasopharynx. (**b**, **c**) Stalk torsion leads to stromal fibrosis and reactive changes. (**d**) Dilated lymphatic spaces (Courtesy of Dr. Rong Li)

■ **Histopathology**

A strange "emptiness" can be appreciated at low-power view of this polyp. This is the result of diminished seromucinous glands and variable fibrosis. Neovascularization, thick-walled vessels, and increased lymphatic spaces are also seen. On higher power, one sees lymphoplasmacytic infiltrate with Russell bodies. Atypical (bizarre) reactive fibroblasts can be observed, either focal or confluent.

2.4   The Spectrum of Sinonasal Fungal Disease

If it appears strange that that one etiologic agent gives rise to such a diversity of disease [16, 17], then consider the three major components of any infectious process: (1) the inherent virulence of the agent, (2) the infectious dose, and (3) the patient status. For example, granulocytopenia renders patients vulnerable to *A. flavus* fulminant invasive sinusitis, despite the low virulence of this ubiquitous agent [18]. On the other hand, immune competent individuals in Sudan can develop chronic granulomatous sinusitis after prolonged exposure to high concentrations of A. flavus [19, 20].

2.4.1 Allergic Fungal Sinusitis

Allergic fungal sinusitis is the most common form of sinonasal fungal disease, representing 6–9% of all chronic sinus disease requiring surgery. Many cases are associated with A. fumigatus, A. flavus or demateaceous fungi. The controversy continues as to whether environmental fungi are actually etiologic initiators or bystanders of this process. The fungal hypothesis states that allergic fungal sinusitis results from extreme eosinophil-driven hypersensitivity to fungi in susceptible individuals. Allergic fungal sinusitis is a T_H2-like lymphocyte-mediated response; T_H2 cells regulate IgE production and allergic response. The data supporting the fungal hypothesis are at best circumstantial [21, 22].

Fungal hyphae are not always detected in allergic mucin, leading to the question of whether "eosinophilic mucin rhinosinusitis" (EMRS) represents an entity distinct from allergic fungal sinusitis (AFS). Aspirin sensitivity and bilateral sinus disease are more common EMRS compared with AFS, consistent with the idea that ERMS represents a distinct clinical entity [23]. However, the sensitivity for fungal detection by the gold standard Gomori methanamine silver (GMS) stain is dramatically improved by trypsin predigestion which speaks against EMRS as a distinct entity; this issue remains unresolved [24, 25].

Gross examination of allergic mucin characteristically reveals thick, dark, and putty-like mucin.

■ Histopathology

Low-power examination reveals red and blue ripples, or laminations composed of cellular debris, epithelium, polymorphonuclear cells, degranulated eosinophils and Charcot Leyden crystals. (■ Fig. 2.7) The Schneiderian mucosa reveals chronic allergic sinusitis. Charcot Leyden crystals are pink/red refractile, and form long needle-like structures. They do not staining on GMS and should not be confused with hyphae. The thicker and more abundant the allergic mucin, the more likely you will find fungal hyphae. If multiple slides contain allergic mucin, select the slide with the densest allergic mucin for GMS staining. When reading GMS, you need only to concentrate on the mucin, not the tissue (■ Fig. 2.8). AFS can reveal different fungal hyphal morphologies, with respect to hyphal size, branching, septations, and budding. Be aware that tissue artifact can mimic hyphae, but are "out of plane of focus". Occasionally one can see mixed tissue reactions such as allergic fungal sinusitis plus chronic granulomatous fungal sinusitis [17].

2.4.2 Fungus Ball

The term fungus ball is preferred over "mycetoma" which implies a soft tissue infection. Fungus ball is defined as a noninvasive accumulation of fungal hyphae; A fumigatus and A flavus are the most common isolates. The maxilla is most commonly affected [26]. It is the only context in which fungal sexual reproduction (fruiting heads) may be observed.

Radiographically, a fungus ball usually appears as an expansile process with bony remodeling; MR/CT signaling reflects the iron, manganese, and calcium content of fungal hyphae ("iron-like signalling") [27]. Some patients with fungus balls have a history of prior endodontic treatment, which is thought to contribute to the process [28, 29]. Progressive loss of the fungistatic effect of eugenol, a component of endodontic sealer, allows for the zinc oxide, another sealer component, to promote Aspergillus spore germination [27].

■ Histopathology

A fungus ball may present as a large, expansile mass on imaging, or an incidental microscopic finding. A large fungus balls appears, low-power, as serpiginous laminations of refractile hyphae, acute inflammatory exudate, and cellular debris (■ Fig. 2.9). If pigmented hyphae are seen, the fungus ball may be due to dematiaceous group of fungi (■ Fig. 2.10). The presence of characteristic fruiting heads are diagnostic for Aspergillus sp. Dark brown conidia specifically indicate Aspergillus niger (■ Fig. 2.11). Fungal invasion of tissue is usually not seen, although it has been reported [17, 29].

> • If invasive hyphae seen, then consider acute or chronic invasive fungal sinusitis. Notify clinicians.

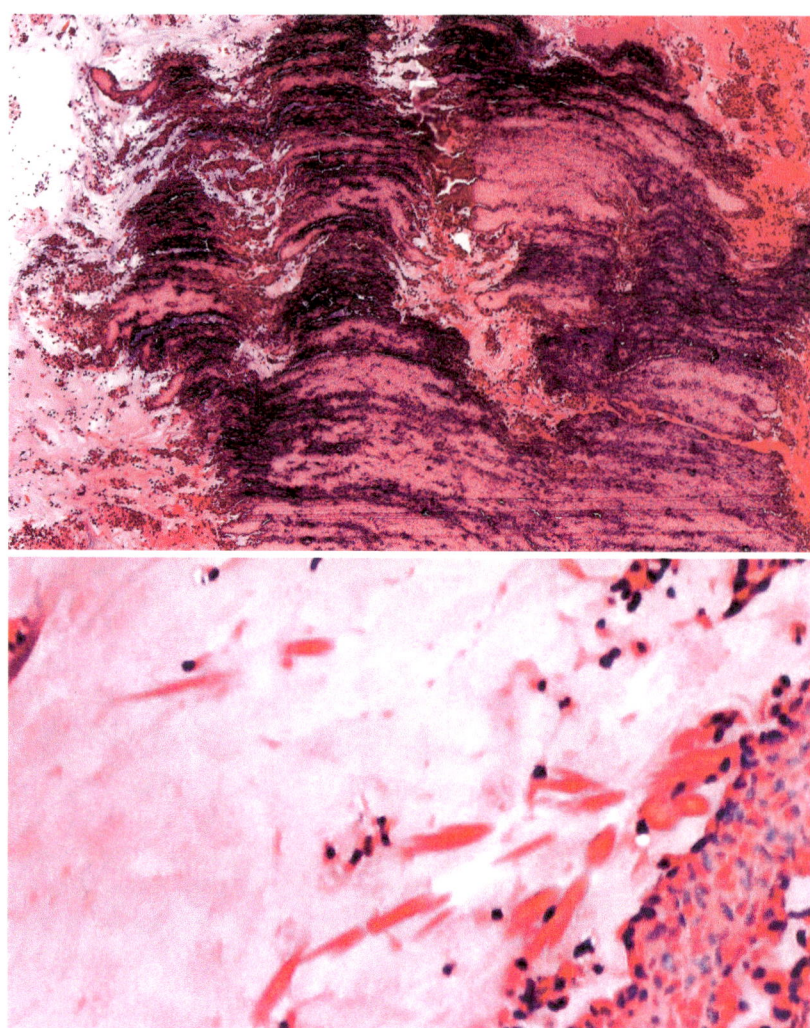

Fig. 2.7 Allergic mucin – (**a**) Lamellar waves of eosinophils (*blue*) and mucin (*pink*). (**b**) Needle-like Charcot Leydin crystals

2.4.3 Acute Invasive Fungal Sinusitis

Acute invasive fungal sinusitis (fulminant fungal sinusitis) represents an aggressive rapidly evolving process (<4 weeks) in patients who are either neutropenic (e.g., leukemia, aplastic anemia, chemotherapy) or have dysfunctional neutrophils (uncontrolled diabetes, post-transplantation corticosteroids). **Chronic invasive fungal disease** is also a destructive infection which develops over longer time (>12 weeks). Patients also have neutrophil dysfunction, but are not neutropenic. The most common pathogens for either disease process are *Aspergillus* sp and zygomycetes. Vascular invasion by *Aspergillus* is potentiated by fungal elastases and proteases [30]. The acidic, high glucose environment of uncontrolled diabetes enhances vulnerability to Mucorales

due to fungal ketone reductase activity [31]. Increased serum iron, present in diabetic ketoacidosis and hemochromatosis, also enhances Mucorales growth.

Patients present with fever, headache, nasal discharge, pain, and periorbital and maxillary swelling. The nasal and palatal mucosa appear pale, then become progressively erythematous, violaceous, then black and necrotic. Intraorbital or intracranial extension is a feared complication. Invasive fungal sinusitis is a true medical emergency. The initial diagnosis is often made on frozen section; hyphae can be seen on H + E frozen slides in untreated patients (Fig. 2.12). After initiation of systemic therapy, further debridements might be necessary and subsequent frozen sections may be requested. However, hyphae can no longer be detected on H + E frozen slides after initiation of systemic therapy.

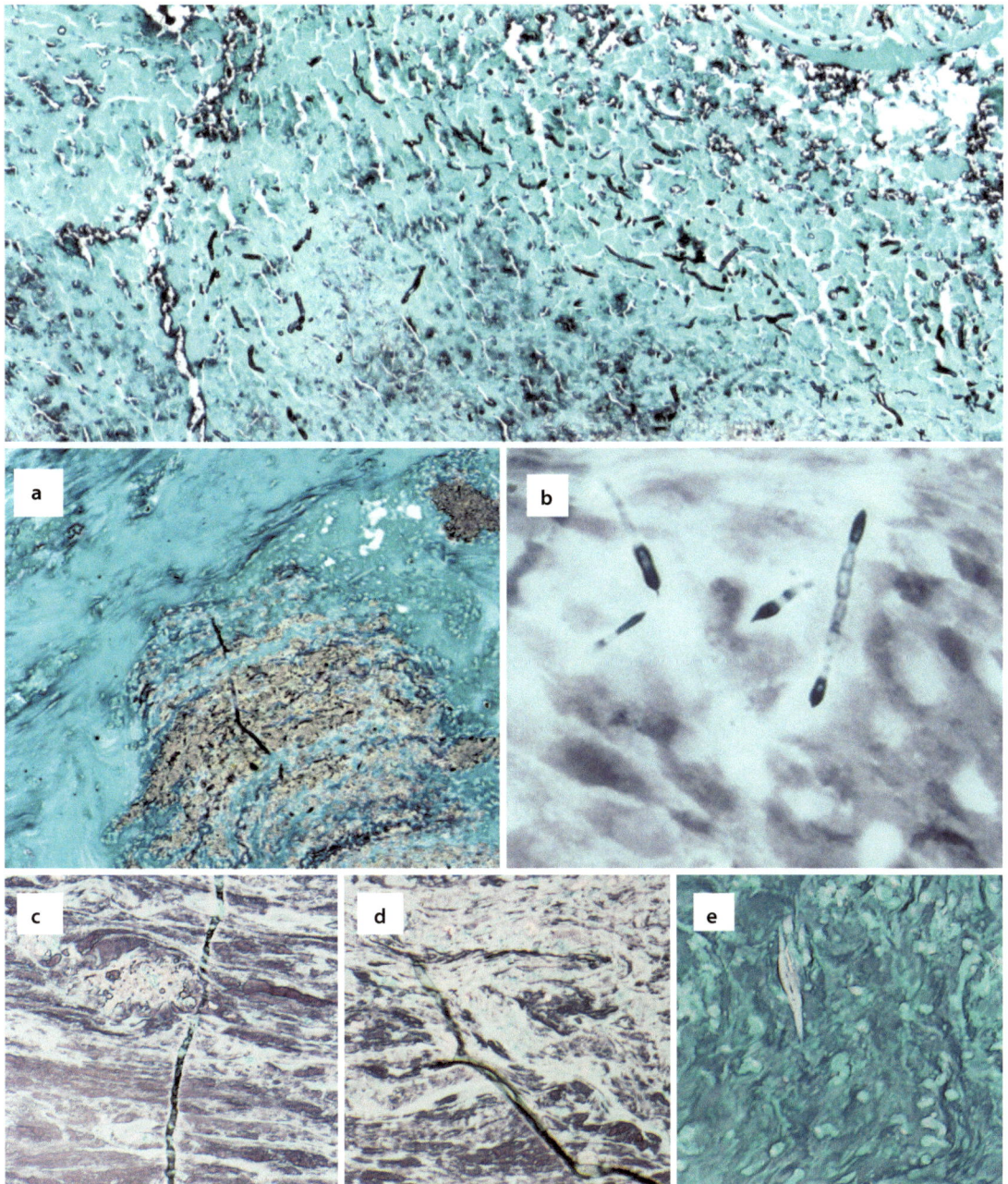

◘ Fig. 2.8 Allergic fungal sinusitis, GMS stain – (**a**) low-power view – search only within the allergic mucin. Here you can see numerous fungal hyphal fragments in the plane of focus. (**b, c**) Hyphal branching and septations confirm the presence of fungus. (**d, e**) Tissue artifact mimickers are "out of plane of focus". (**f**) Charcot Leydin crystals "exclude" GMS and may also mimic hyphae

■ **Histopathology**

The early changes in invasive fungal disease include tissue hemorrhage, perivascular inflammation and fibrin thrombi. Basophilic, refractile fungal hyphae can be seen within vessels, associated with thrombotic infarction. As the process advances, so does the degree of soft tissue and bony necrosis. Intraneural fungal invasion may also be seen (◘ Fig. 2.12). Tissue inflammation is limited in granulocytopenic patients. Invasive fungal disease in patients with dysfunctional granulocytes will demon-

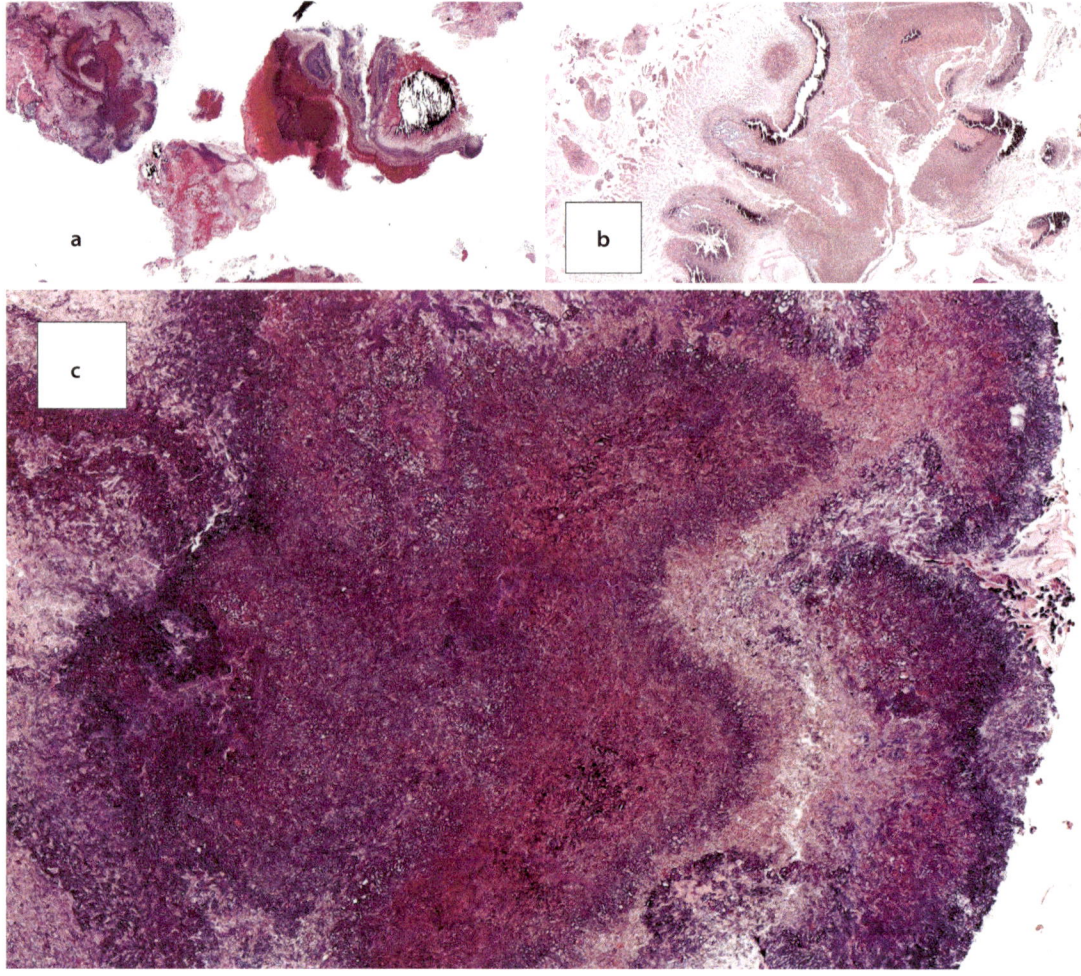

◘ Fig. 2.9 (**a, b**) Low power view of fungus balls. Note the multicolored serpiginous laminations. (**c**) Appreciate the refractile hyphae at low power, which is better appreciated after flipping down the condenser

strate more of the expected inflammatory response. The degree of tissue repair seen will be congruent with duration of the process, e.g., granulation tissue, neovascularization.

Infection with Mucorales demonstrates broad fungal hyphae (7–20 um) which are "floppy" and twisting, thus resembling "empty bent-cellophane tubes". Their outer hyphal walls are slightly refractile with uneven thickness ("pleomorphic hyphae"). Hyphal septations are either absent or erratic; hyphal folding can mimic septations. Hyphal branching appears variable with angles ranging from 45° to 90° due to hyphal "floppiness". Aspergillus infection demonstrates thin hyphae with even wall thickness and regular septations. The hyphal branching occurs at acute angles, and demonstrates greater uniformity.

2.4.4 Granulomatous Invasive Fungal Disease

Granulomatous invasive fungal disease refers to an infectious process in which fungal elements are present within the sinonasal tissue, but tissue "invasive" is limited and host response is robust. It is the rarest form of sinonasal fungal disease encountered, and characteristically geographically associated in regions with high exposure doses such as Sudan, India, Pakistan and Saudi Arabia.

■ Histopathology

Granulomatous invasive fungal disease is characterized by a robust inflammatory response, mixed acute and chronic inflammatory infiltrate, and foreign body type granulomata. Fungal elements

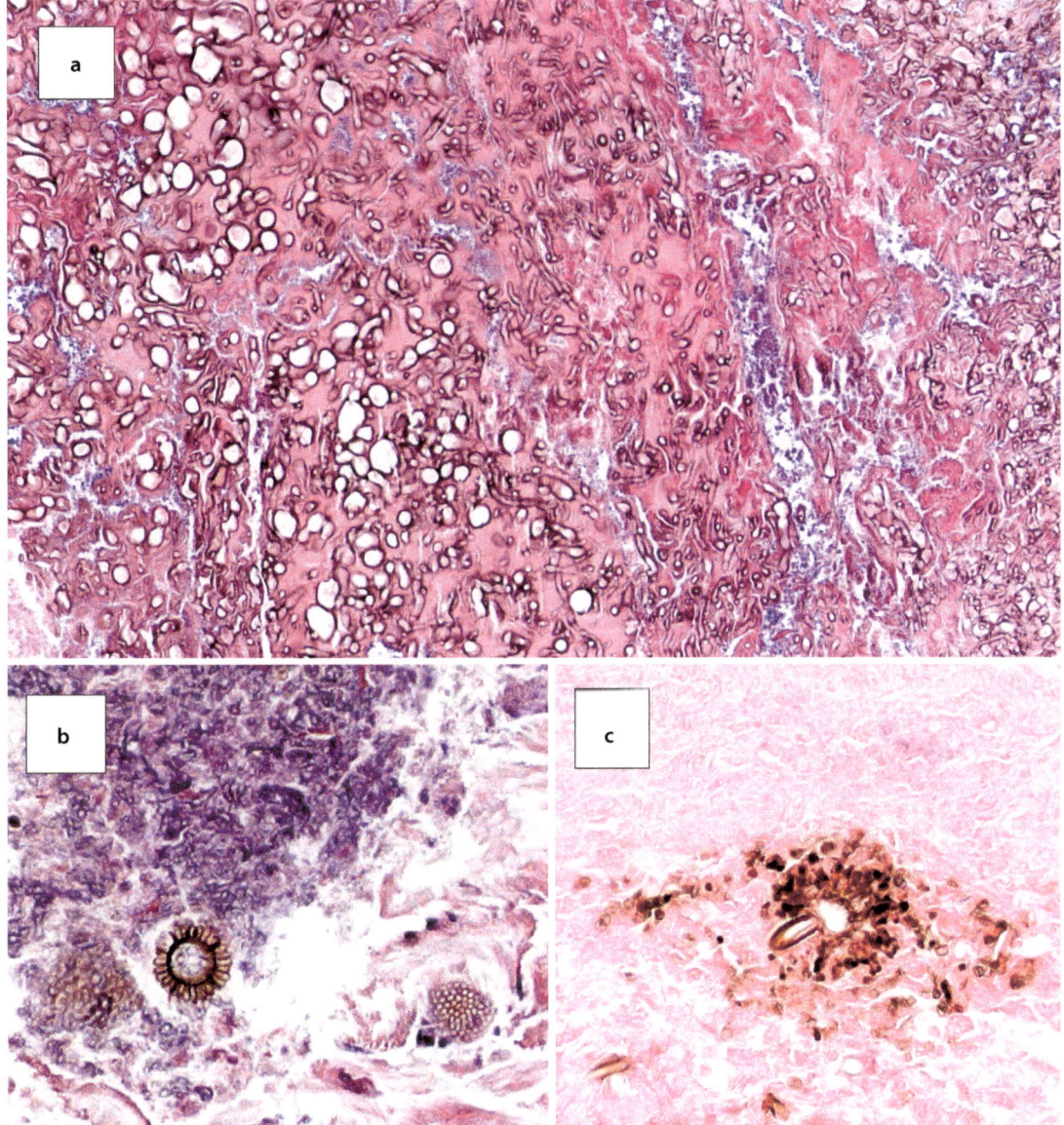

◘ Fig. 2.10 Fungus ball – (**a**) pigmented hyphae suggest dematiaceous fungi. (**b, c**) Pigmented fruiting heads of *Aspergillus niger*

are seen within multinucleated giant cells (◘ Fig. 2.12). Tissue necrosis and vascular invasion is either limited or entirely absent.

2.5   Rhinoscleroma

Rhinoscleroma is endemic to the tropics (Central America, Chile, Central Africa), subtropics (India, Indonesia, Egypt, Algeria, Morroco), and temperate latitudes (Eastern and Central Europe, Russia) and has been reported in emigrants to nonendemic regions [32–36]. The infectious agent, *K. rhinoscleromatis* (von Frisch bacilli) is noncommensural with low infectivity; transmission between humans is assumed to occur after prolonged exposure. Increased incidence among family members and household contacts has been reported [36]. Defective cell-mediated immunity has been long suspected to increase susceptibility to infection, but there is no strong supporting data. Patients usually present in their

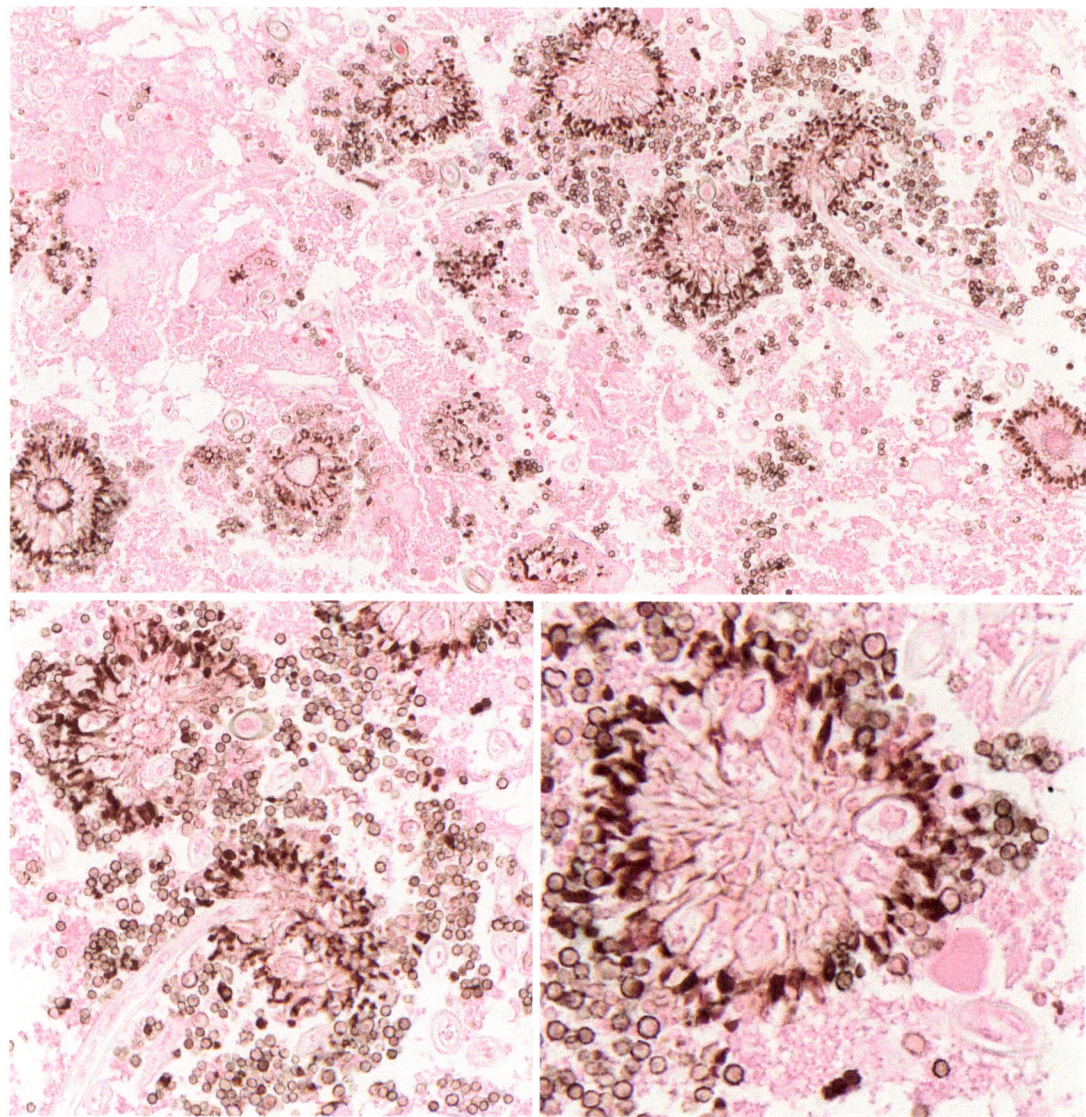

Fig. 2.11   Fungus ball, *Aspergillus niger.* - Pigmented fruiting heads of *Aspergillus niger*

second and third decades; there is a female predominance. Rhinoscleroma affects the entire upper aerodigestive tract, most commonly the sinonasal cavity (95–100 %), and pharynx (50 %). Laryngotracheal involvement occurs in 15–80 % of cases, but is rarely seen in the absence of sinonasal disease.

Initial Catarral Phase ("Rhinitic/catarrhal") – The upper airway mucosa is red, atrophic, with foul purulent discharge and crusting. The clinical differential diagnosis in this early stage includes infection with *K ozena*.

Second Proliferative Phase (**Florid proliferative granulomatous**) – This can develop months to years after the initial catarral phase. Nasal obstruction and epistaxis is common. Patients can present with polypoid masses protruding through the external nares. The inflammatory masses may distort the midface resulting in a "rhinoceros-like" appearance. Clinical remissions and relapses are frequent. The clinical differential diagnosis at this time includes leprosy and syphilis. A tissue biopsy during this phase is most likely to be diagnostic.

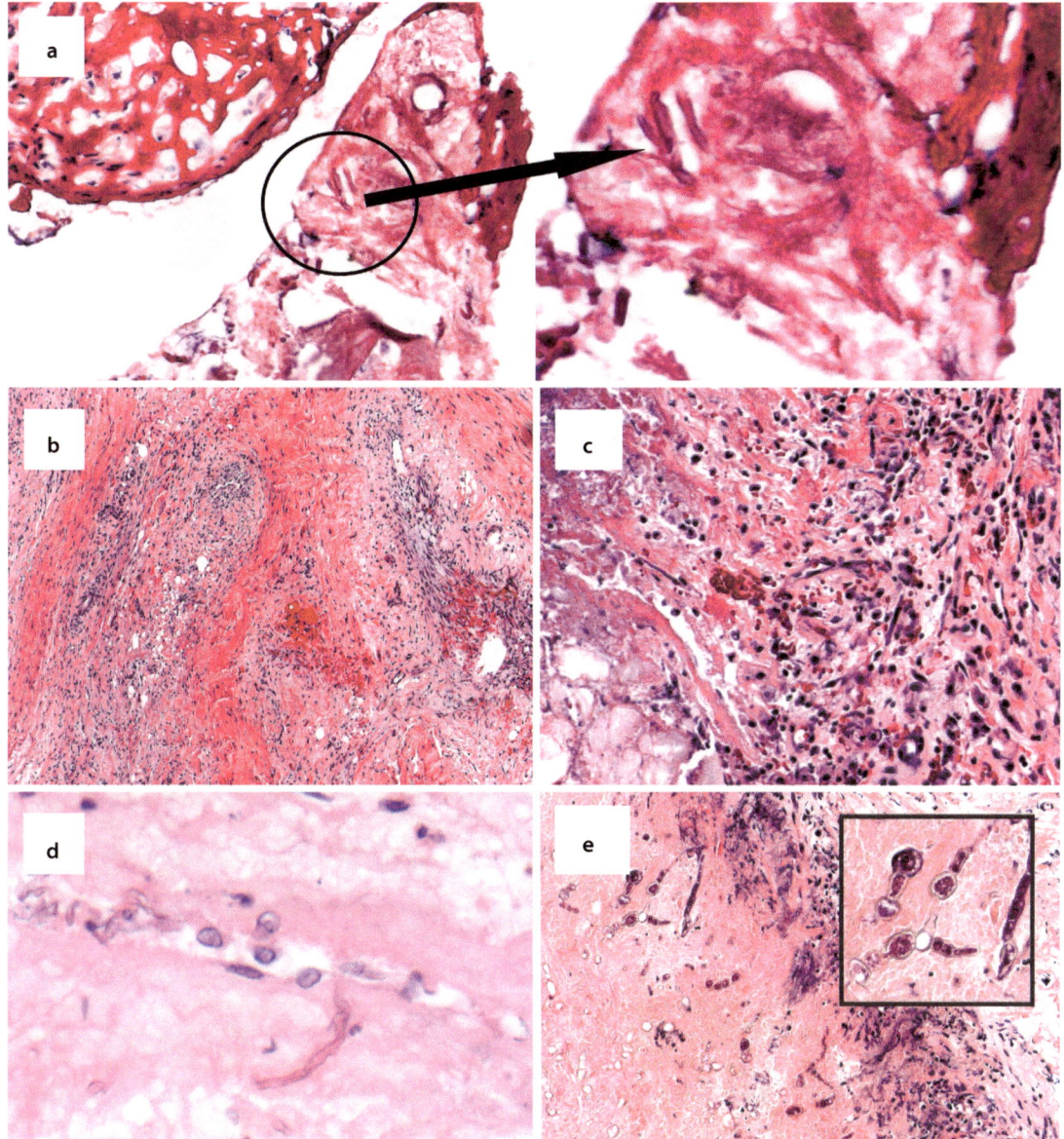

Fig. 2.12 (**a, b**) Invasive fungal sinusitis is a true medical emergency. The initial diagnosis is often made on frozen section; hyphae can be seen on H + E frozen slides in untreated patients. (**c, d**) Tissue hemorrhage and perivascular inflammation are early findings. (**e**) Fungal hypha transgressing a vessel. (**f**) Chronic invasive sinusitis in a renal transplant patient. Septated branching hyphae are seen with intercalated globose bodies (*inset*), suggest *P boydii*

Third Sclerotic Phase – The final stage is characterized by fibrosis and inflammation, culminating in disfigurement, stenosis, and loss of function.

■ **Histopathology**

The initial catarrhal stage reveals nonspecific lymphoplasmacytic inflammation; diagnostic Mikulicz cells are sparse. The second stage, the florid proliferative granulomatous stage, is most likely to yield diagnostic tissue. Mikulicz cells are most abundant and intracellular bacilli are best seen on Warthin-Starry stain. Plasma cells with Russell bodies are also abundant (**Fig. 2.13**). Despite the appellation, granulomas are absent. The final sclerotic stage reveals predominantly fibrotic tissue with limited inflammation and sparse Mikulicz cells.

Fig. 2.13 Chronic invasive fungal sinusitis – this diabetic patient presented with "a really bad headache". Indeed. (**a**) Intraneural fungal invasion is seen on H + E. (**b**) GMS stain demonstrating fungal hyphae in the perineurium. *Candida tropicalis* was confirmed by mycology

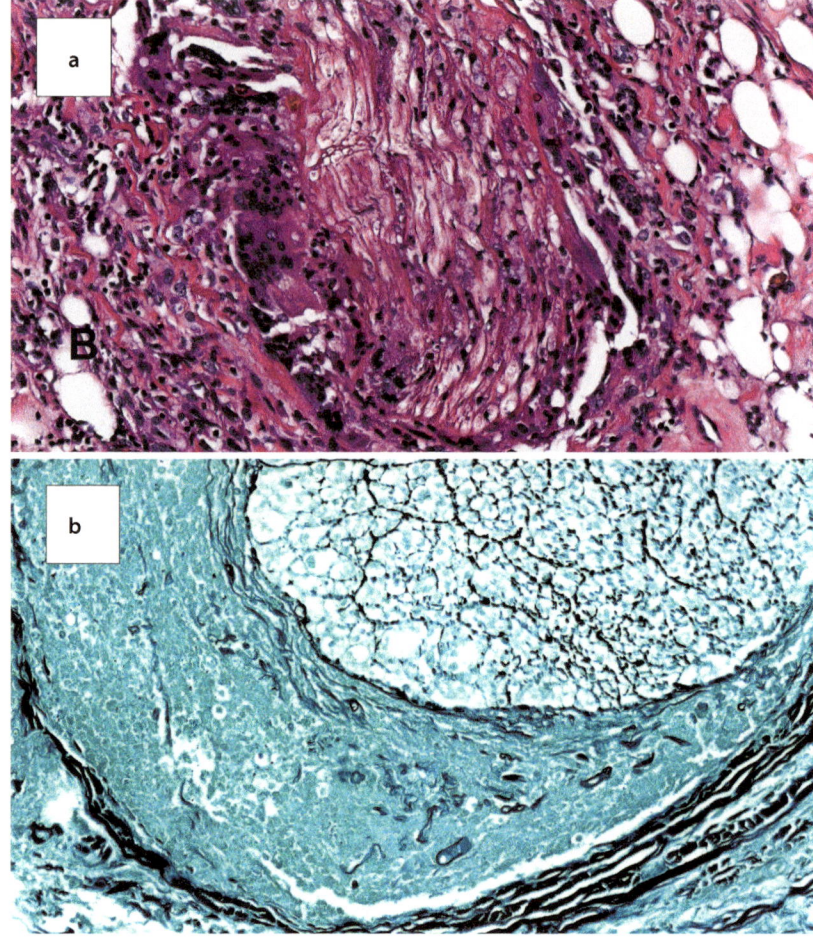

- *If abundant foamy macrophages seen, consider* **atypical mycobacteria** *and* **lepromatous leprosy**
- *If abundant plasma cells present, then consider* **syphilis.**

2.6   Rhinosporidiosis

Rhinosporidium seeberi is a worldwide pathogen, endemic to India, Sri Lanka, Malaysia, Brazil, and Argentina [37–42]. Infections have also been reported in the Southern and Western United States [43–45]. Rhinosporidiosis is a rare infectious disease associated with a robust inflammatory response (■ Fig. 2.14). Rhinosporidium most commonly infects the conjunctiva and nasal cavity causing inflammatory polyps that are friable, lobulated, and red/pink. Other mucosal sites, e.g.,

larynx, genitourinary tract, may also become infected [46]. Nasal and urethral infections have a male predominance whereas female predominance is seen in conjunctival infections. Mucosal trauma is necessary to establish infection. Subcutaneous infection, and disseminated rhinosporidiosis are very rare.

The nature of Rhinosporidiosis has long been elusive and aggravated by its resistance to *in-vitro* culture. Originally, it was considered a fungus, then a prokaryotic cyanobacterium. More recently, molecular data from 18S SSU ribosomal DNA support its classification as Mesomycetozoea, a eukaryotic aquatic microbe related to spherical fish [47, 48].

■ **Histopathology**

Rhinosporidium forms large spherules, up to 300 um in diameter. The largest cysts are seen closest to the mucosal surface. The cyst wall is birefringent and stains with hematoxylin and eosin, Gomori methanamine silver, digested-periodic

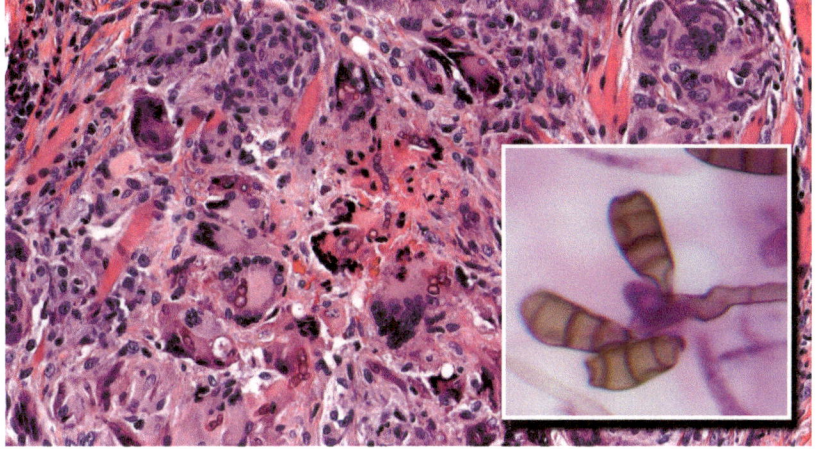

■ **Fig. 2.14** Granulomatous invasive fungal sinusitis: recurrent *Curvularia* infection – Multinucleated giant cells contain "chains" of budding hyphae with bulbous protrusions. *Inset*: Example of *Curvularia* growth in culture conditions

acid Schiff, and mucicarmine stains. The cysts are filled with small endospores (2–5 um); tiny nuclei may be seen within the endospores. A dense lymphoplasmacytic infiltrate is characteristic.

> • *If spherules are smaller, 80 um, then consider Coccicidiodomyces*

2.7 Myospherulosis

Myospherulosis represents a non-infectious inflammatory reaction to agents such as exogenous lipids (e.g., petroleum, lanolin), vitamin E, or traumatized adipose tissue; it is histologically characterized by the hallmark "spherules" which mimic fungal infection [49–51]. Myospherulosis was originally described as the development of painful soft tissue masses in Africans [50]. A "Swiss cheese" pattern of microscopic cysts ("bags of spherules", bags of marbles) is characteristic, hence the name "myospherulosis" or intramuscular spherules. Rosai demonstrated that these puzzling spherules were actually red blood cells [51]. (■ Fig. 2.15) Sinonasal myospherulosis may develop after the use of antibiotic/lipid-based sinus packing gauze (bacitracin-zinc, hydrocortisone, neomycin-polymyxin, tetracycline) [51–57]. (■ Fig. 2.16)

■ Histopathology
Myospherulosis of soft tissue is characterized by lipogranulomas forming "pseudocysts" with a "Swiss cheese" appearance. Large sac-like

structures (parent bodies) (100 um) are seen, with thin, nonrefractile membranes (1 um). The sacs contain numerous dark brown spherules, 5–7 um (endo bodies) which have an irregular "bags of marbles"-type appearance. The surrounding tissue demonstrates fibrosis and chronic inflammation. The nature of the encysted erythrocytes in myospherulosis can be confirmed by Okajima's hemoglobin stain; Gomori methanamine silver, iron, and periodic acid Schiff stains are negative.

> • *If cyst walls are thick, double-walled, birefringent, then consider Coccidioidomyces, Rhinosporidium, which are Gomori methanamine silver positive*
> • *If periodic acid Schiff stain positive, then also consider inhaled pollen*

2.8 Granulomatosis with Polyangiitis

Granulomatosis with polyangiitis represents the entity formerly known as Wegener's granulomatosis. The eponym "Wegener's Granulomatosis" was proposed by Jacob Churg and Gabriel Godman [58] for the disorder described by Heinz Klinger [59] and Friedrich Wegener [60, 61]. Uncovering Friedrich Wegener's association with the Nazi Party and his role in experiments performed on Jewish victims of Lodz ghetto lead to the rescindment of his "Master Clinician" prize awarded in 1989 by the American College of Chest Physicians, and the appropriate

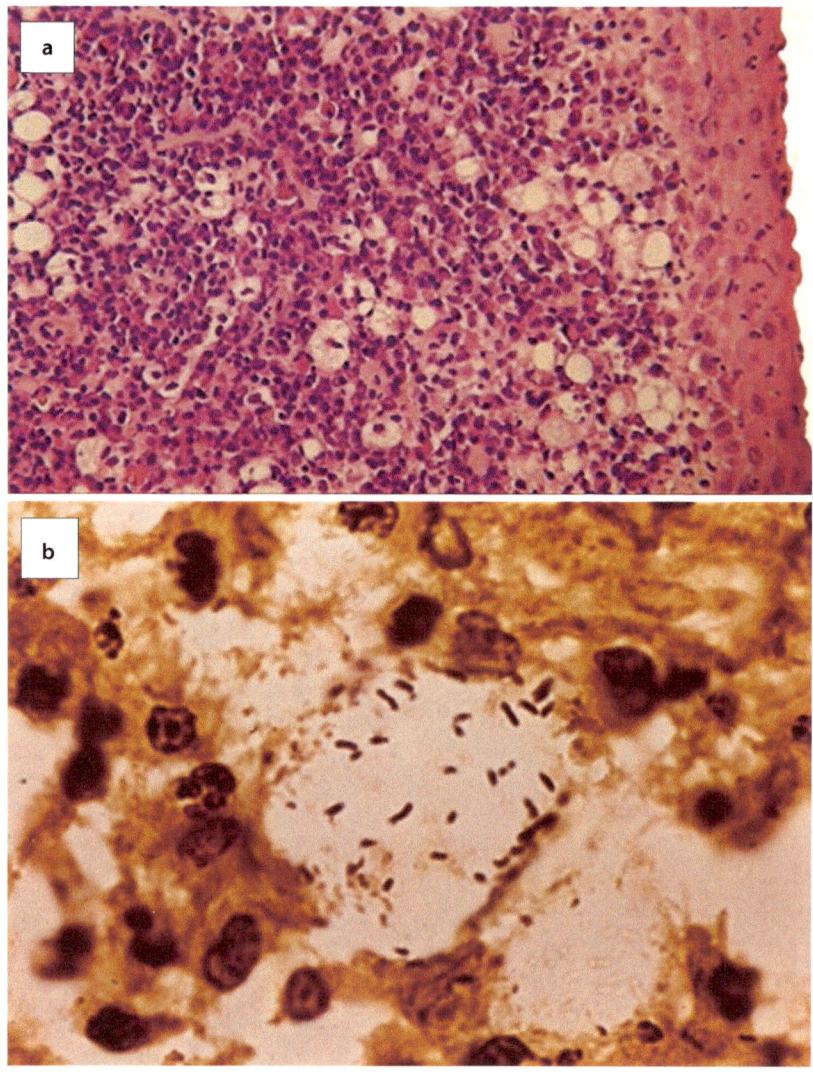

○ **Fig. 2.15**   Rhinoscleroma – (**a**) lymphoplasmacytic infiltrate with abundant foamy macrophages (Mikulicz cells). (**b**) Warthin Starry stain highlights the curved bacilli of *Klebsiella rhinoscleromatis*

renaming of this entity to "Granulomatosis with polyangiitis" (GPA) [62–64]. This is a multi-organ disease which can be fatal if untreated; immediate action is usually required if GPA is suspected. The classic triad of involved organs is (1) sinonasal tract, (2) lungs, and (3) kidneys; disease limited to the sinonasal tract has been described. Other involved sites include spleen, orbit, periorbital soft tissues, ear, subglottis, and skin [58, 65–69].

The histopathologic diagnostic triad consists of (1) **vasculitis**, (2) **necrosis**, and (3) **granulomas** (○ Fig. 2.17). The presence of two of the three findings can be interpreted as "suggestive" for GPA; 21–70 % of biopsies in GPA patients were interpreted as either "suggestive" or "diagnostic" [69–71]. Biopsies from head and neck sites can be less invasive, therefore, preferable to lung biopsies. Anti-neutrophil cytoplasmic autoantibodies specific for myeloperoxidase (MPO-ANCA) or proteinase-3 (PR3-ANCA) are etiologically implicated, and diagnostic in most cases. The absence of serum anti-neutrophil cytoplasmic autoantibodies does not exclude the possibility of GPA, but increases the importance of biopsies (○ Figs. 2.18 and 2.19).

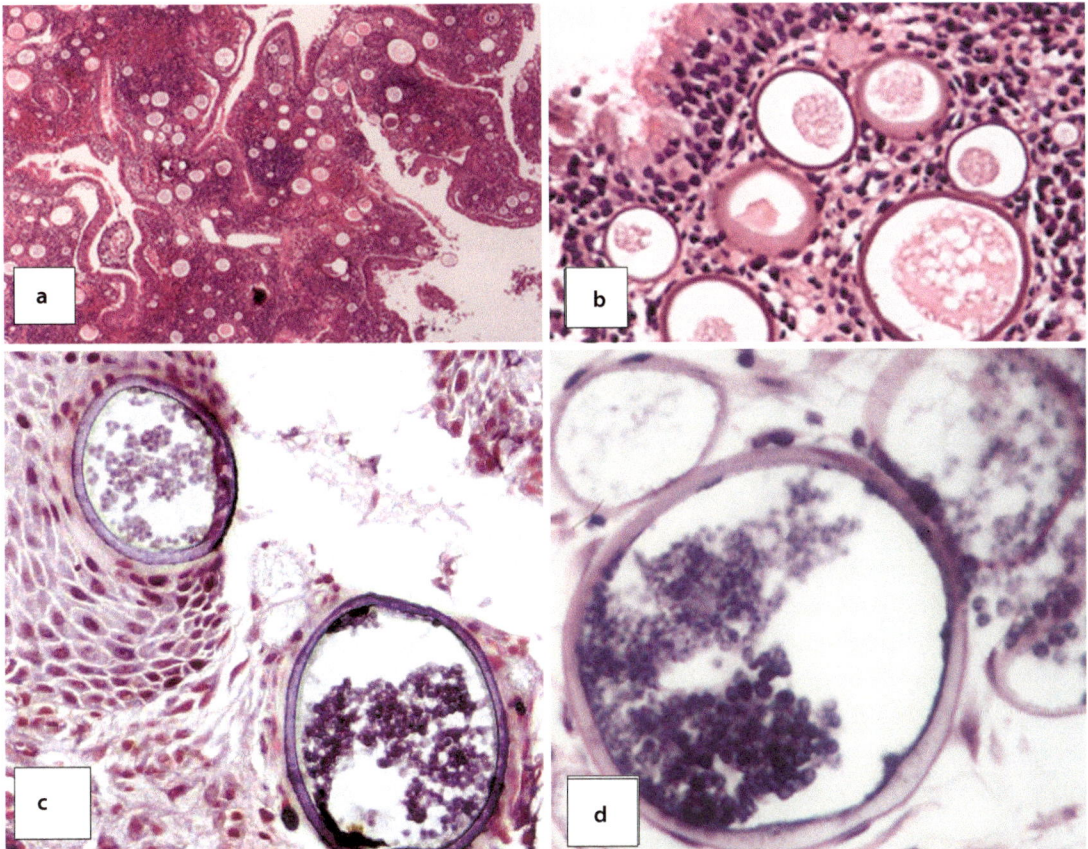

◨ Fig. 2.16 **(a–d)** Rhinosporidiosis – thick-walled spherules of varying size, the largest, most mature spherules are close to the mucosal surface

▪ Histopathology

Characteristically, the vasculitis of GPA is of varying age. Active vasculitis may take the form of arteritis, venulitis, capillaritis, and/or microvasculitis. Healed vasculitis can appear as cicatricial concentric fibrosis or extensive fibrosis with a storiform – like pattern. Elastic Van Gieson stain (EVG) has the potential to confirm that the fibrotic areas of interests conceal arteries. Findings of a lesser vasculitis include intimal hyperplasia, mural fibrosis, and medial hypertrophy. Lastly, thrombophlebitis may be seen.

The characteristic necrosis of GPA follows the distribution of vessels, resulting in large, "geographic" (non-rounded) zones of necrosis (◨ Fig. 2.20). The finding of extravascular necrosis (necrosis adjacent to recognizable vessels) is confirmatory. Perivascular fibrinoid necrosis [72], a degenerative necrosis associated with bright pink fibrin-like material, can also be seen.

Granulomas represent the third diagnostic pillar of GPA. The noncompact granulomas are composed of intense acute and chronic inflammation, microabsesses with nuclear debris, eosinophils, plasma cells, and histiocytes. Multinucleated foreign body giant cells, Langerhans type giant cells, and palisading histiocytes can be present. Phagocytized neutrophils have been described as a specific finding of GPA [73].

- *If plasma cells, eosinophils, and fibrolamellar fibrosis are pronounced, then consider IgG4-related disease. However increased IgG4+ cells, and IgG+/IgG ratio can be seen in GPA [74].*

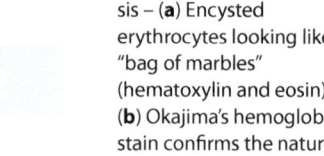

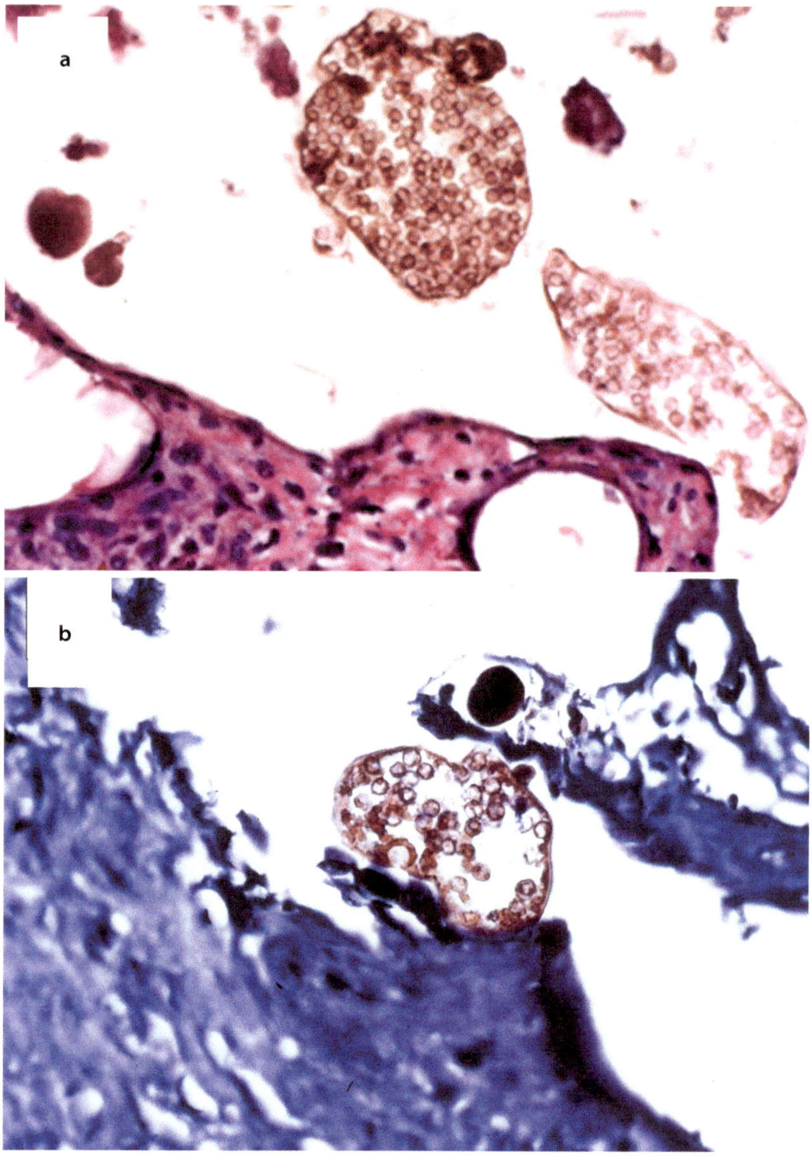

Fig. 2.17 Myospherulosis – (**a**) Encysted
erythrocytes looking like a
"bag of marbles"
(hematoxylin and eosin).
(**b**) Okajima's hemoglobin
stain confirms the nature of
these round bodies
(Courtesy of Dr. Juan Rosai)

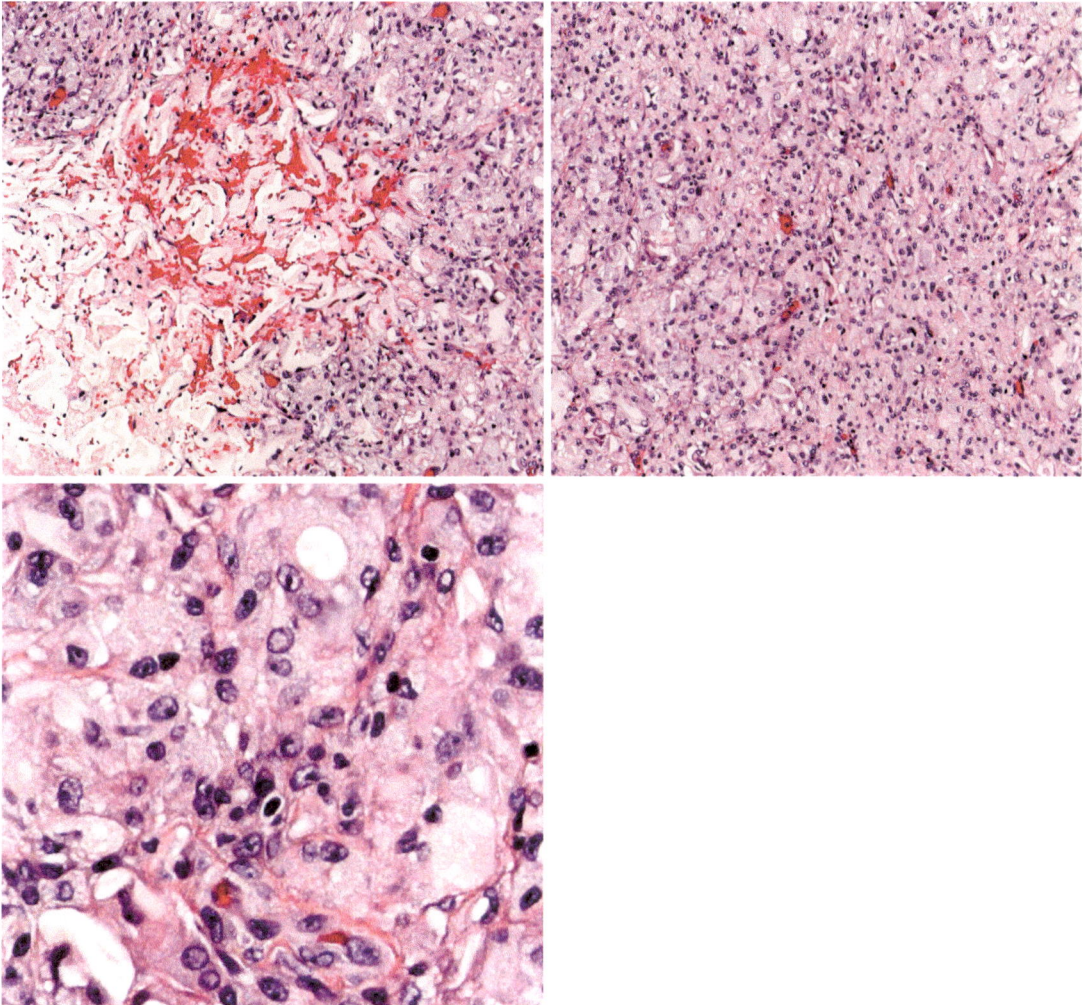

Fig. 2.18 Myospherulosis – here is an example of a different iatrogenic tissue reaction: Gelfoam in the sinonasal tract (*left side upper panel*) provokes an intense histiocytic reaction (*bottom*)

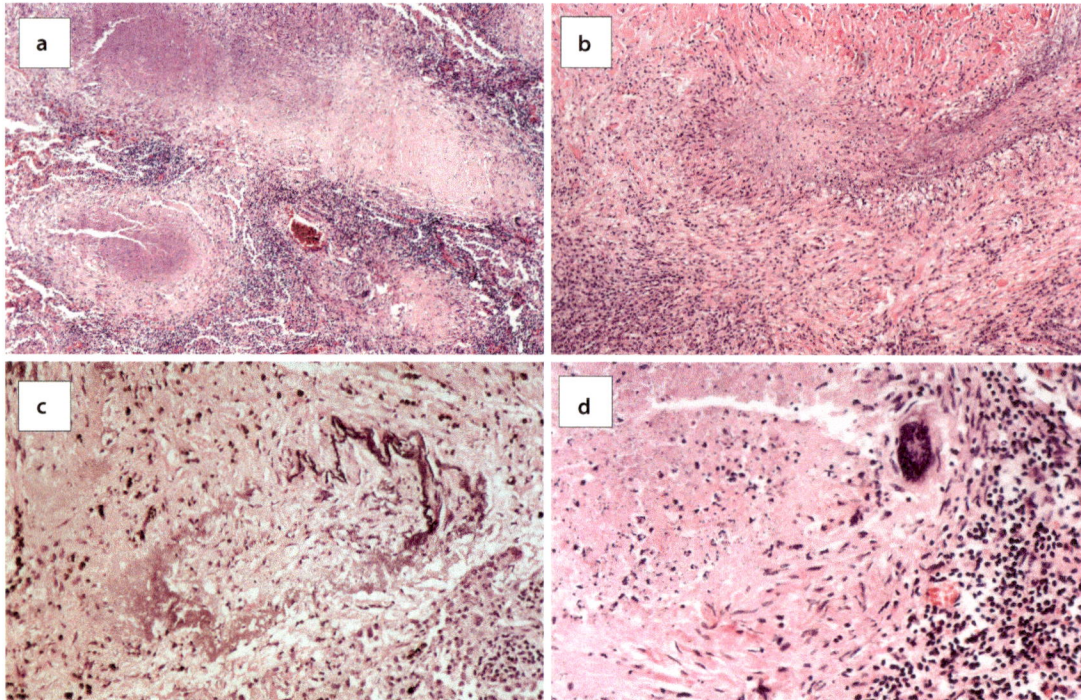

◘ **Fig. 2.19**   Granulomatosis with polyangiitis (Wegener's granulomatosis) – (**a**, **b**) vasculitis leads to geographic zones of necrosis. (**c**) Elastic stain confirms the presence of a disrupted medium sized artery within this necrotic inflammatory process. (**d**) Foreign body type granuloma

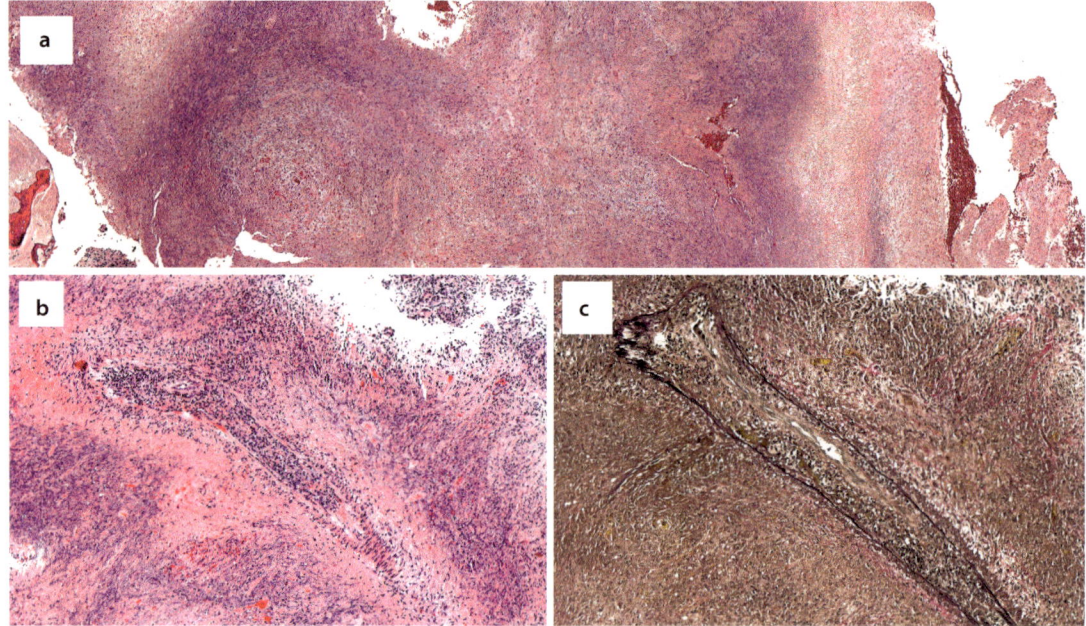

◘ **Fig. 2.20**   This patient has an established diagnosis of granulomatosis with polyangiitis. (**a**) Intranasal biopsy reveals large regions of perivascular necrosis with zones of purulent exudate. (**b**) Vasculitis of varying age can be seen. (**c**) EVG stain confirms prior vasculitis with recannulization

Self Study

1. Which statement is true?
   (a) Rhinophyma is caused by von Frisch bacilli.
   (b) Myospherulosis is caused by mycoplasma.
   (c) Chronic invasive fungal sinusitis is the only condition in which fungal sexual reproduction occurs.
   (d) Invasive fungal hyphae are observable on hematoxylin and eosin stained slides.
2. Which statement/statements is/are true?
   (a) Allergic mucin is composed of degranulated eosinophils, Charcot Leydin crystals, and fungal hyphal fragments.
   (b) Antrochoanal polyps arise at the posterior choanae, and prolapse anteriorly through the nares, and are histologically characterized by a "strange emptiness" and bizarre fibroblasts.
   (c) Iron-like signaling is characteristic of a fungal ball.
   (d) a, b, c
   (e) a and c

Answers

1. Which statement is true?
   (a) Rhinophyma is characterized by pronounced sebaceous hyperplasia, cystically dilated ducts filled with keratin and sebum, vasodilatation in the upper and middle dermis, and perivascular/perifollicular inflammation (Fig. 2.21 **self study**).
   (b) Myospherulosis is a non-infectious inflammatory reaction to agents such as exogenous lipids (e.g., petroleum, lanolin), vitamin E, or traumatized adipose tissue, resulting in the histological hallmark of pseudofungal "spherules".
   (c) Sexual reproduction can be seen in a fungus ball, in the form of fruiting heads.
   (d) Invasive fungal hyphae are observable on hematoxylin and eosin stained slides – **CORRECT**. After systemic therapy, silver stains are necessary to observe hyphae.

2. Which statement/statements is/are true?
   (a) Fungal hyphal fragments are not necessarily present in allergic mucin.
   (b) Antrochoanal polyps arise in the maxilla and can protrude through the posterior choanae.
   (c) Iron-like signaling is characteristic of a fungal ball. **CORRECT**. Iron-like radiographic signaling reflects the iron, manganese, and calcium content of fungal hyphae.

◼ **Fig. 2.21**   Self study

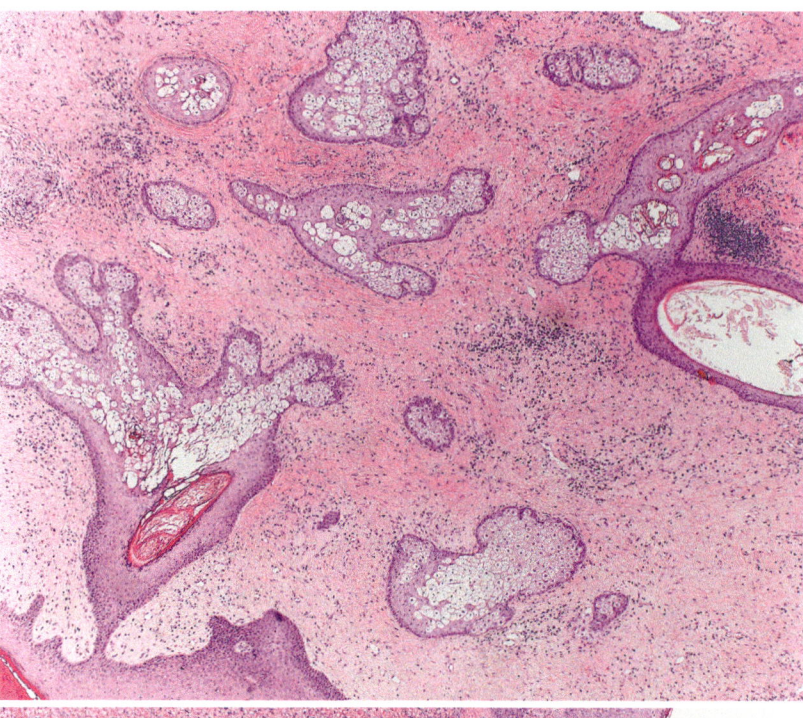

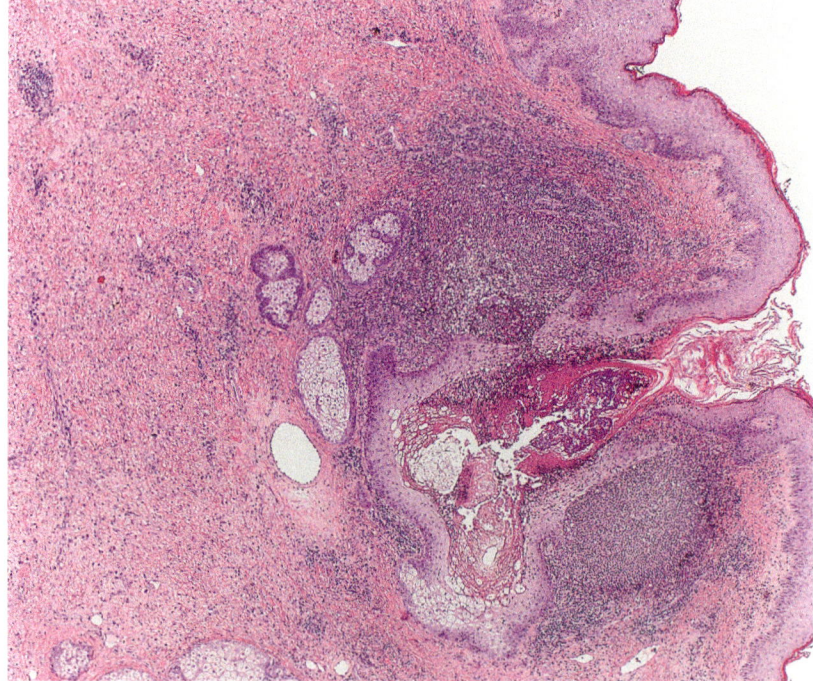

References

1. Ardehali MM, Amali A, Bakhshaee M, Madani Z, Amiri M. The comparison of histopathological characteristics of polyps in asthmatic and nonasthmatic patients. Otolaryngol Head Neck Surg. 2009;140:748–51.
2. Samter M, Beers Jr RF. Intolerance to aspirin. Clinical studies and consideration of its pathogenesis. Ann Intern Med. 1968;68:975–83.
3. Samter M, Beers Jr RF. Concerning the nature of intolerance to aspirin. J Allergy. 1967;40:281–93.
4. Chang JE, White A, Simon RA, Stevenson DD. Aspirin-exacerbated respiratory disease: burden of disease. Allergy Asthma Proc. 2012;33:117–21.
5. Casale M, Pappacena M, Potena M, Vesperini E, Ciglia G, Mladina R, Dianzani C, Degener AM, Salvinelli F. Nasal polyposis: from pathogenesis to treatment, an update. Inflamm Allergy Drug Targets. 2011;10:158–63.

6. Yee KK, Pribitkin EA, Cowart BJ, Vainius AA, Klock CT, Rosen D, Hahn CG, Rawson NE. Smoking-associated squamous metaplasia in olfactory mucosa of patients with chronic rhinosinusitis. Toxicol Pathol. 2009;37: 594–8.

7. Durgam A, Batra PS. Paranasal sinus cholesterol granuloma: systematic review of diagnostic and management aspects. Int Forum Allergy Rhinol. 2013;3:242–7.

8. Mercan H, Edizer DT, Kilic E, Esen T, Ramazanoglu R, Cansiz H. Osseous metaplasia in a nasal polyp: report of a rare case and review of the literature. Ear Nose Throat J. 2012;91:E4–6.

9. Ramachandran K, Thomas MA, Denholm RB. Osseous metaplasia of a nasal polyp. J Otolaryngol. 2005;34:72–3.

10. Srouji S, Kizhner T, Ben David D, Riminucci M, Bianco P, Livne E. The Schneiderian membrane contains osteoprogenitor cells: in vivo and in vitro study. Calcif Tissue Int. 2009;84:138–45.

11. Lou H, Meng Y, Piao Y, Wang C, Zhang L, Bachert C. Predictive significance of tissue eosinophilia for nasal polyp recurrence in the Chinese population. Am J Rhinol Allergy. 2015;29:350–6.

12. Yaman H, Alkan N, Yilmaz S, Koc S, Belada A. Is routine histopathological analysis of nasal polyposis specimens necessary? Eur Arch Otorhinolaryngol. 2011;268:1013–5.

13. Schraven SP, Wehrmann M, Wagner W, Blumenstock G, Koitschev A. Prevalence and histopathology of chronic polypoid sinusitis in pediatric patients with cystic fibrosis. J Cyst Fibros. 2011;10:181–6.

14. Wu X, Amorn MM, Aujla PK, Rice S, Mimms R, Watson AM, Peters-Hall JR, Rose MC, Peña MT. Histologic characteristics and mucin immunohistochemistry of cystic fibrosis sinus mucosa. Arch Otolaryngol Head Neck Surg. 2011;137:383–9.

15. Mostafa HS, Fawzy TO, Jabri WR, Ayad E. Lymphatic obstruction: a novel etiologic factor in the formation of antrochoanal polyps. Ann Otol Rhinol Laryngol. 2014;123:381–6.

16. Taxy JB. Paranasal fungal sinusitis: contributions of histopathology to diagnosis: a report of 60 cases and literature review. Am J Surg Pathol. 2006;30:713–20.

17. Das A, Bal A, Chakrabarti A, Panda N, Joshi K. Spectrum of fungal rhinosinusitis; histopathologist's perspective. Histopathology. 2009;54:854–9.

18. Hedayati MT, Pasqualotto AC, Warn PA, Bowyer P, Denning DW. Aspergillus flavus: human pathogen, allergen and mycotoxin producer. Microbiology. 2007;153: 1677–92.

19. Sandison AT, Gentles JC, Davidson CM. Aspergilloma of paranasal sinuses and orbit in Northern Sudanese. Sabouraudia. 1967;6:57.

20. Miloshev B. Aspergilloma of paranasal sinuses and orbit in Northern Sudanese. Lancet. 1966;1(7440):746.

21. Borish L, Rosenwasser L, Steinke JW. Fungi in chronic hyperplastic eosinophilic sinusitis: reasonable doubt. Clin Rev Allergy Immunol. 2006;30:195–204.

22. Chakrabarti A, Denning DW, Ferguson BJ, Ponikau J, Buzina W, Kita H, Marple B, Panda N, Vlaminck S, Kauffmann-Lacroix C, Das A, Singh P, Taj-Aldeen SJ, Kantarcioglu AS, Handa KK, Gupta A, Thungabathra M, Shivaprakash MR, Bal A, Fothergill A, Radotra BD. Fungal rhinosinusitis: a categorization and definitional schema addressing current controversies. Laryngoscope. 2009;119:1809–18.

23. Ferguson BJ. Eosinophilic mucin rhinosinusitis: a distinct clinicopathological entity. Laryngoscope. 2000; 110:799–813.

24. Guo C, Ghadersohi S, Kephart GM, Laine RA, Sherris DA, Kita H, Ponikau JU. Improving the detection of fungi in eosinophilic mucin: seeing what we could not see before. Otolaryngol Head Neck Surg. 2012;147:943–9.

25. Uri N, Ronen O, Marshak T, Parpara O, Nashashibi M, Gruber M. Allergic fungal sinusitis and eosinophilic mucin rhinosinusitis: diagnostic criteria. J Laryngol Otol. 2013;127:867–71.

26. Nicolai P, Lombardi D, Tomenzoli D, Villaret AB, Piccioni M, Mensi M, Maroldi R. Fungus ball of the paranasal sinuses: experience in 160 patients treated with endoscopic surgery. Laryngoscope. 2009;119:2275–9.

27. Stammberger H, Jakse R, Beaufort F. Aspergillosis of the paranasal sinuses X-ray diagnosis, histopathology, and clinical aspects. Ann Otol Rhinol Laryngol. 1984;93:251–6.

28. Odell E, Pertl C. Zinc as a growth factor for Aspergillus sp. and the antifungal effect of root canal sealants. Oral Surg Oral Med Oral Pathol Oral Radiol Endod. 1995;79:82–7.

29. Senocak D, Kaur A. What's in a fungus ball? Report of a case with submucosal invasion and tissue eosinophilia. Ear Nose Throat J. 2004;83:696–8.

30. Rhodes JC, Bode RB, McCuan-Kirsch CM. Elastase production in clinical isolates of Aspergillus. Diagn Microbiol Infect Dis. 1988;10:165–70.

31. Ibrahim AS, Spellberg B, Walsh TJ, Kontoyiannis DP. Pathogenesis of mucormycosis. Clin Infect Dis. 2012;54:S16–22.

32. Simão I, Gaspar I, Faustino R, Brito MJ. Rhinoscleroma in a 5-year-old Portuguese child. Pediatr Infect Dis J. 2014;33:774–5.

33. Botelho-Nevers E, Gouriet F, Lepidi H, Couvret A, Amphoux B, Dessi P, Raoult D. Chronic nasal infection caused by Klebsiella rhinoscleromatis or Klebsiella ozaenae: two forgotten infectious diseases. Int J Infect Dis. 2007;11:423–9.

34. Chan TV, Spiegel JH. Klebsiella rhinoscleromatis of the membranous nasal septum. J Laryngol Otol. 2007;121: 998–1002.

35. Maguiña C, Cortez-Escalante J, Osores-Plenge F, Centeno J, Guerra H, Montoya M, Cok J, Castro C. Rhinoscleroma: eight Peruvian cases. Rev Inst Med Trop Sao Paulo. 2006;48:295–9.

36. de Pontual L, Ovetchkine P, Rodriguez D, Grant A, Puel A, Bustamante J, Plancoulaine S, Yona L, Lienhart PY, Dehesdin D, Huerre M, Tournebize R, Sansonetti P, Abel L, Casanova JL. Rhinoscleroma: a French national retrospective study of epidemiological and clinical features. Clin Infect Dis. 2008;47:1396–402.

37. Wright J. A nasal sporozoon. (Rhinosporididium kinealyi). NY Med J. 1907;86:1149–53.

38. Justice JM, Solyar AY, Davis KM, Lanza DC. Progressive left nasal obstruction and intermittent epistaxis. JAMA Otolaryngol Head Neck Surg. 2013;139:955–6.

39. Mukherjee B, Mohan A, Sumathi V, Biswas J. Infestation of the lacrimal sac by Rhinosporidium seeberi: a clinicopathological case report. Indian J Ophthalmol. 2013;61:588–90.

40. Choudhury M. Rhinosporidium seeberi in nasal smears. Diagn Cytopathol. 2011;39:593–4.

41. Gichuhi S, Onyuma T, Macharia E, Kabiru J, Zindamoyen AM, Sagoo MS, Burton MJ. Ocular rhinosporidiosis

mimicking conjunctival squamous papilloma in Kenya – a case report. BMC Ophthalmol. 2014;14:45.

42. Mithal C, Agarwal P, Mithal N. Ocular and adnexal rhinosporidiosis: the clinical profile and treatment outcomes in a tertiary eye care centre. Nepal J Ophthalmol. 2012;4:45–8.

43. Norman WG. Rhinosporidiosis in Texas. Arch Otolaryngol. 1960;72:361–2.

44. Lasser A, Smith HW. Rhinosporidiosis. Arch Otolaryngol. 1976;102:308–10.

45. Jimenez JF, Young DE, Hough AJ. Rhinosporidiosis. A report of two cases from Arkansas. Am J Clin Pathol. 1984;82:611–25.

46. Naik RS, Siddiqui RS, Naik V. Urethronasal rhinosporidiosis. J Indian Med Assoc. 1979;72:238–9.

47. Herr RA, Ajello L, Taylor JW, Arseculeratne SN, Mendoza L. Phylogenetic analysis of *rhinosporidium seeberi's* 18S small-subunit ribosomal DNA groups this pathogen among members of the protoctistan mesomycetozoa clade. J Clin Microbiol. 1999;37:2750–4.

48. Vilela R, Mendoza L. The taxonomy and phylogenetics of the human and animal pathogen Rhinosporidium seeberi: a critical review. Rev Iberoam Micol. 2012;29: 185–99.

49. Mc Clatchie S, Warambo MW, Bremner AD. Myospherulosis: a previously unreported disease? Am J Clin Pathol. 1969;51:699–704.

50. Kyriakos M. Myospherulosis of the paranasal sinuses, nose and middle ear. A possible iatrogenic disease. Am J Clin Pathol. 1977;67:118–30.

51. Rosai J. The nature of myospherulosis of the upper respiratory tract. Am J Clin Pathol. 1978;69:475–81.

52. Sindwani R, Cohen JT, Pilch BZ, Metson RB. Myospherulosis following sinus surgery: pathological curiosity or important clinical entity? Laryngoscope. 2003;113:1123–7.

53. Kaul R, Chander B, Dogra SS. Myospherulosis in the nose: a report of an unusual lesion. Indian J Pathol Microbiol. 2014;57:338–9.

54. Coulier B, Desgain O, Gielen I. Sinonasal myospherulosis and paraffin retention cysts suggested by CT: report of a case. Head Neck Pathol. 2012;6:270–4.

55. Syed SP, Wat BY, Wang J. Pathologic quiz case: a 55-year-old man with chronic maxillary sinusitis. Synchronous occurrence of Aspergillosis and myospherulosis. Arch Pathol Lab Med. 2005;129:e84–6.

56. Phillip V, Becker K, Bajbouj M, Schmid RM. Myospherulosis. Ann Diagn Pathol. 2013;17:383–9.

57. Lin HW, Handzel O, Faquin WC, Gopen Q. Myospherulosis from antibiotic ointment in the postoperative mastoid space. Am J Otolaryngol. 2010;31:205–88.

58. Godman GC, Churg J. Wegener's granulomatosis: pathology and review of the literature. AMA Arch Pathol. 1954;58:533–53.

59. Klinger H. Grenzformen der Periarteriitis Nodosa. Frankf Z Pathol. 1931;42:455–80.

60. Wegener F. Ueber generalisierte septische Gefäßerkrankungen. Verh Deut Ges Pathol. 1936;29:202–10.

61. Wegener F. Ueber eine eigenartige rhinogene Granulomatose mit besonderer Beteiligung des Arteriensystems und der Nieren. Beitr Pathol Anat. 1939;102: 30–68.

62. Woywodt A, Haubitz M, Haller H, Matteson EL. Wegener's granulomatosis. Lancet. 2006;367:1362–6.

63. Feder BJ. A Nazi past casts a pall on name of a disease. The New York Times. 2008. http://www.nytimes.com/2008/01/22/health/22dise.html?_r=1&oref=slogin. Accessed 19 Nov 2014.

64. Falk RJ, Gross WL, Guillevin L, Hoffman GS, Jayne DR, Jennette JC, Kallenberg CG, Luqmani R, Mahr AD, Matteson EL, Merkel PA, Specks U, Watts RA, American College of Rheumatology; American Society of Nephrology; European League Against Rheumatism. Granulomatosis with polyangiitis (Wegener's): an alternative name for Wegener's granulomatosis. Arthritis Rheum. 2011;63:863–4.

65. Muller K, Lin JH. Orbital granulomatosis with polyangiitis (Wegener granulomatosis): clinical and pathologic findings. Arch Pathol Lab Med. 2014;138:1110–4.

66. Taylor SC, Clayburgh DR, Rosenbaum JT, Schindler JS. Progression and management of Wegener's granulomatosis in the head and neck. Laryngoscope. 2012;122:1695–700.

67. Gajic-Veljic M, Nikolic M, Peco-Antic A, Bogdanovic R, Andrejevic S, Bonaci-Nikolic B. Granulomatosis with polyangiitis (Wegener's granulomatosis) in children: report of three cases with cutaneous manifestations and literature review. Pediatr Dermatol. 2013;30:e37–42.

68. Olsen KD, Neel 3rd HB, Deremee RA, Weiland LH. Nasal manifestations of allergic granulomatosis and angiitis (Churg-Strauss syndrome). Otolaryngol Head Neck Surg. 1980;88:85–9.

69. Devaney KO, Travis WD, Hoffman G, Leavitt R, Lebovics R, Fauci AS. Interpretation of head and neck biopsies in Wegener's granulomatosis. A pathologic study of 126 biopsies in 70 patients. Am J Surg Pathol. 1990;14:555–64.

70. Del Buono EA, Flint A. Diagnostic usefulness of nasal biopsy in Wegener's granulomatosis. Hum Pathol. 1991;22:107–10.

71. Colby TV, Tazelaar HD, Specks U, DeRemee RA. Nasal biopsy in Wegener's granulomatosis. Hum Pathol. 1991;22:101–4.

72. Bajema IM, Bruijn JA. What stuff is this! A historical perspective on fibrinoid necrosis. J Pathol. 2000;191:235–8.

73. Jennette JC. Nomenclature and classification of vasculitis: lessons learned from granulomatosis with polyangiitis (Wegener's granulomatosis). Clin Exp Immunol. 2011;164 Suppl 1:7–10.

74. Chang SY, Keogh KA, Lewis JE, Ryu JH, Cornell LD, Garrity JA, Yi ES. IgG4-positive plasma cells in granulomatosis with polyangiitis (Wegener's): a clinicopathologic and immunohistochemical study on 43 granulomatosis with polyangiitis and 20 control cases. Hum Pathol. 2013;44:2432–7.

Sinonasal Tract – Benign

© Springer International Publishing Switzerland 2016
M.S. Brandwein, *Textbook of Head and Neck Pathology*,
DOI 10.1007/978-3-319-33323-6_3

Abstract

This chapter covers some common, benign sinonasal entities (Schneiderian papillomas) and uncommon, emerging entities (respiratory epithelial adenomatoid hamartoma and sinonasal serous hamartoma). The latter likely represent benign adenosis-like tumor processes rather than hamartomas. Benign peripheral nerve sheath tumors and ectopic central nervous system entities are also discussed.

Keywords

Respiratory epithelial adenomatoid hamartoma · Seromucinous hamartoma · Schneiderian papillomas · Iinverted papillomas · Nasal glial heterotopia · Glioma · Ectopic meningioma

Glossary

REAH Respiratory epithelial adenomatoid "hamartoma" which represents a true, benign sinonasal neoplasm

COREAH Chondro-osseous component in addition to REAH

SSH Sinonasal seromucinous hamartoma, a benign adenosis type lesion interrelated to REAH.

Schneiderian papillomas Nosology inclusive of the three types of sinonasal papillomas

Nasal glial heterotopia Malformation of displaced glial tissue discontinuous with the intracranial meninges

Encephalocele Herniation of brain tissue and leptomeninges through skull defect which maintains intracranial continuity

Key Points

- Three histologic components of REAH and SSH are proliferating seromucinous tubules, invaginated respiratory epithelium, and stromal changes.
- SSH is characterized by S100+ serous glands lacking a myoepithelial lining (p63 negative).
- REAH is characterized by ductal adenosis surrounded by p63+ basal cells.
- Sinonasal exophytic papillomas invariably arise from the nasal septum.

- Inverted papillomas arise from the lateral nasal wall and antrum.
- If mixed exophytic and inverting patterns present, this likely represents an inverted papilloma from the lateral nasal wall.
- Well-differentiated squamous carcinoma arising from inverted papilloma may be diagnostically challenging; the diagnosis can be based solely on architectural changes.
- Keratinization within an inverted papilloma should raise suspicions for malignant transformation

3.1 Respiratory Epithelial Adenomatoid Hamartoma (REAH)

REAH is a rare and benign sinonasal neoplasm. A male predisposition is noted. REAH usually presents with a single dominant mass ranging from 1 to 4 cm; 70 % arise from the superior nasal cavity and 30 % arise from the nasopharynx or paranasal sinuses [1–7]. There is a propensity for superior nasal cavity REAH to arise from the posterior nasal septum (vomer) and the olfactory cleft. [2, 4] Macroscopically, REAH are firm, polypoid with a distinct pedicle, yellow, gray, or white, with an uneven surface. Interestingly, subclinical REAH may be relatively common and under-recognized. Microscopic subclinical REAH were identified in 35 % of 150 nasal polyposis specimens when surgeons deliberately and separately submitted any polypoid lesions of the olfactory cleft. By comparison, microscopic REAH was retrospectively identified in only 3.9 % of 160 consecutive nasal polyposis specimens routinely processed, supporting the conclusion that REAH is under recognized in the context of nasal polyposis [2].

Recent studies confirm the need for updating REAH nomenclature. "Hamartoma" refers to an oncologically benign malformation of tissues indigenous to an anatomic subsite. Loss of heterozygosity (LOH) studies support the idea that REAH is a benign neoplasm rather than a true hamartoma; 20 % of lesions demonstrated LOH at multiple loci for 9p21 and 9p22 [8]. No clinical recurrences of REAH have been reported. However, microscopic REAH were present adjacent to six of 18 (33 %) low-grade sinonasal adenocarcinoma (SNAC); no microscopic REAH was found adjacent to high-grade SNAC or any intestinal type adenocarcinoma [9]. Taken together, REAH appears to be a benign adenosis-type neoplasm with limited growth potential, probably requiring additional mutational hits to progress to a low-grade malignancy.

Histopathology

The three components of REAH are proliferating seromucinous tubules, invaginated respiratory epithelium, and stromal changes (◘ Fig. 3.1). The proliferating adenosis involves medium to large seromucinous tubules which are lined by ciliated respiratory epithelium. Cystically dilated ducts can be appreciated at low-power. The ductal proliferation produces a crowded, back-to-back appearance. The larger ducts demonstrate parabasal hyperplasia and periductal hyalinization. Occasionally, florid mucinous metaplasia is seen.

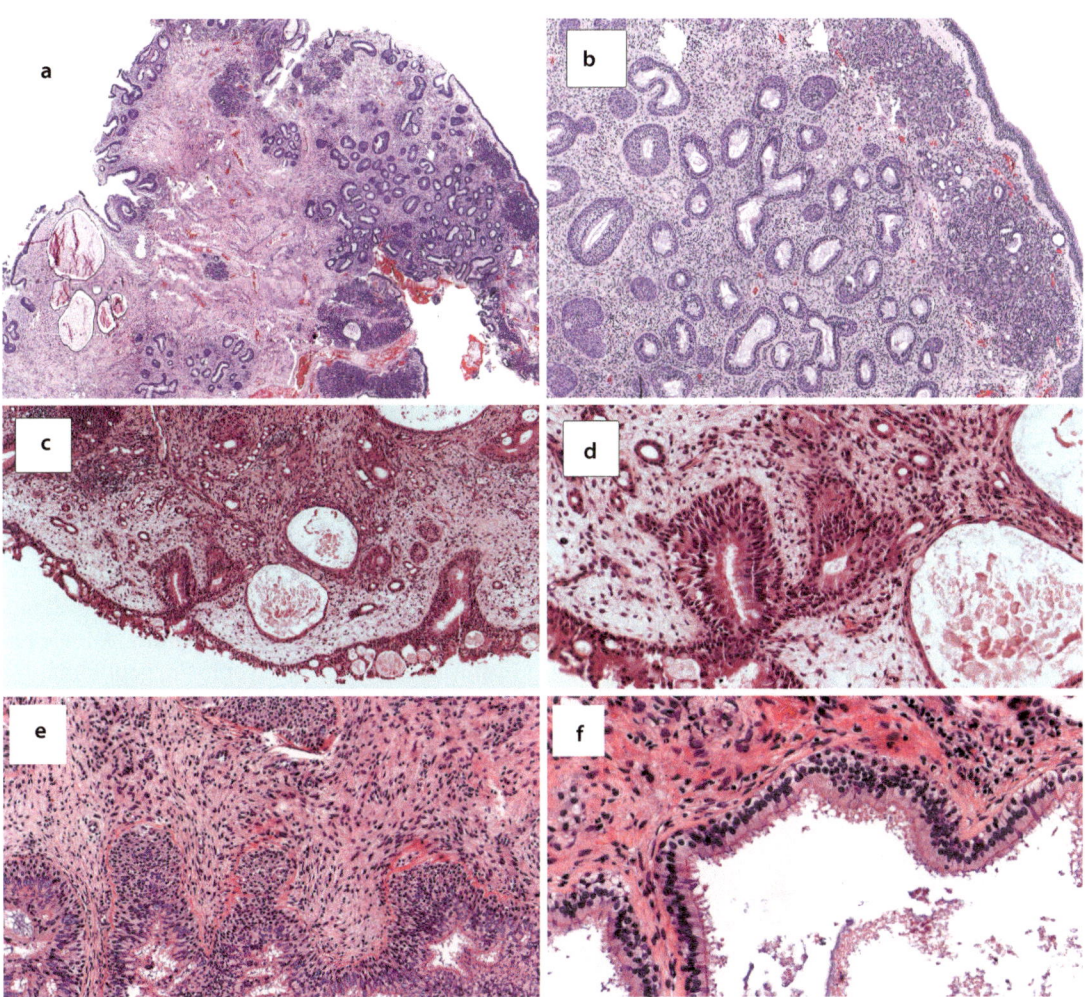

◘ **Fig. 3.1** Respiratory epithelial adenomatoid hamartoma (*REAH*) – (**a**) This case resembles severe chronic sinusitis at first glance, but for the ductal adenosis better observed in **b**. (**b**) Note the proliferation of large ducts with parabasal hyperplasia and adenosis of small ducts immediately below the basement membrane. (**c**) This REAH reveals cystically dilated large ducts and a haphazard pattern of small ductal adenosis. (**d**) This haphazard adenosis could mimic invasive low-grade sinonasal adenocarcinoma (*SNAC*). (**e**) Stromal hypercellularity is another characteristic feature. (**f**) Ciliated epithelium in cystically dilated ducts. This finding is not specific to REAH, but distinguishes REAH from low-grade SNAC

Invagination of ciliated surface respiratory epithelium is another component of REAH. This ciliated epithelium are not specific for REAH, but aids in distinction from low-grade malignancy. The epithelial elements express **CK7+** and are surrounded by **p63**+ basal cells; they are negative for CK20 and CDX2. The stromal changes include inflammation, edema, or hyalinization, and a prominent spindle cell infiltrate.

COREAH includes a chondro-osseous component in addition to REAH [10–12].

- If you see diffuse squamous metaplasia, hyperplasia, goblet cells, and ciliated cells, then consider an inverted papilloma.
- If glandular crowding and no basement membrane, or if pleomorphism is present, then consider intestinal type adenocarcinoma (CK20+, CDX2+).

3.2   Sinonasal Seromucinous Hamartoma

Sinonasal seromucinous hamartoma (SSH, **or** serous hamartoma) is another rare polypoid tumor that arises from the posterior nasal septum (vomer) or the nasopharynx [13–17]. SSH and REAH are interrelated as (1) SSH commonly contains areas of REAH, and (2) budding of serous glands from REAH glands has been observed. The features that distinguish SSH from REAH are (1) **S100+ serous glands in SSH**, and (2) **p63+ basal cells in REAH**. SSH is also a benign adenosis-type neoplasm rather than a hamartoma [14]. Excision is usually curative; only one patient has been reported to have developed a recurrence [13].

■ **Histopathology**
As with REAH, the three histological components of SSH are proliferating seromucinous tubules, invaginated respiratory epithelium, and stromal changes (◘ Figs. 3.1 and 3.2). The proliferating adenosis involves small ductules and serous acini, producing a haphazard lobular pattern. The distinction of SSH from REAH lies with the proliferating serous glands. These small glands are single-layered with little or no myoepithelial lining. They are composed of bland, mitotically inactive cuboidal cells with round to oval nuclei, and cytoplasm that is either clear or eosinophilic, dense, with cytoplasmic granules (modified zymogen granules). Periglandular and periductal hyalinization is present. The proliferating seromucinous tubules are usually **S100+** and **p63 negative**, another point of distinction between SSH and REAH. Additionally, the seromucinous tubules are **CK7+, CK19+**, and negative for CK14 and CK20. As with REAH, the invaginated respiratory epithelium is ciliated. p63 IHC highlights only basal cells around invaginated respiratory epithelium, but not ductules. The lesional stroma contains numerous myofibroblastic spindle cells (calponin +, smooth muscle actin+).

- If glandular crowding present, and no basement membrane or cytologic pleomorphism seen, consider low-grade intestinal type adenocarcinoma.

3.3   Exophytic Papillomas

Three types of histologically distinct papillomas occur in the sinonasal tract: (1) exophytic or fungiform papillomas, (2) inverted papillomas, and (3) oncocytic Schneiderian papillomas [18, 19]. The majority of sinonasal exophytic papillomas arise from the anterior nasal septum. A male predisposition is noted. Exophytic papillomas are grey, white, or pink with a warty or pebbled appearance. They are etiologically associated with low-risk Human Papillomavirus (HPV), especially HPV6/11 [20, 21]. Excision is usually curative.

■ **Histopathology**
The architecture of an exophytic papilloma is characterized by papillary fronds with relatively thin fibrovascular cores covered by mature squamous epithelium (◘ Fig. 3.3). While the squamous epithelium is mature, keratinization should be scant. Respiratory mucosa with goblet cells may be retained. Cytological pleomorphism and mitotic activity should be absent. If there is mixed

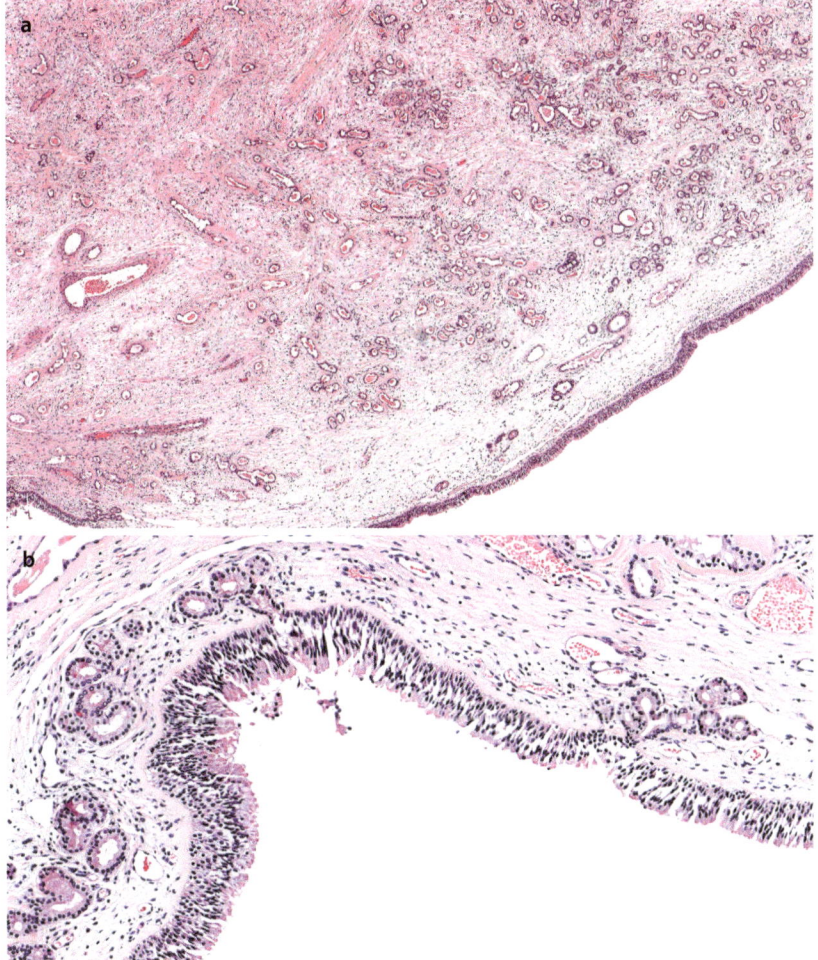

Fig. 3.2 Sinonasal serous hamartoma is distinguished from REAH by the presence of serous glands. (**a**) Proliferation of small, bland serous glands, ducts and tubules with lobular or haphazard patterns. (**b**) The surface respiratory epithelium invaginates into the polyp. These glands may lack myoepithelial lining (Case courtesy of Drs. Bayardo Perez-Ordonez and Ilan Weinreb)

exophytic and inverting patterns, the lesion likely originates from the lateral nasal wall and represents an inverted papilloma.

- If dense keratosis present and lesion confined to the nasal vault, the consider verruca vulgaris (■ Fig. 3.4).
- If a biopsy yields "too much" material, and/or reveals complex papillae and/or pleomorphism, then clinicoradiographic correlation is necessary. Consider squamous cell carcinoma, papillary variant (■ Fig. 3.5).

3.4   Inverted Papillomas

Inverted papillomas tend to occur from the 4rth decade onward, with a peak incidence in the 6th decade and a strong male predominance (approximately 3:1) [18]. Inverted papillomas are distinctly uncommon in children [22]. They usually arise from the lateral nasal wall around the middle turbinate or the ethmoid recess and can expand to fill the maxilla. Inverted papillomas of the ethmoids can erode lamina papyracea to involve the orbit and displace the globe. Bulky inverted papillomas may extend through the posterior choanae and fill the nasopharynx. Isolated frontal and sphenoid sinus inverted papillomas are extremely

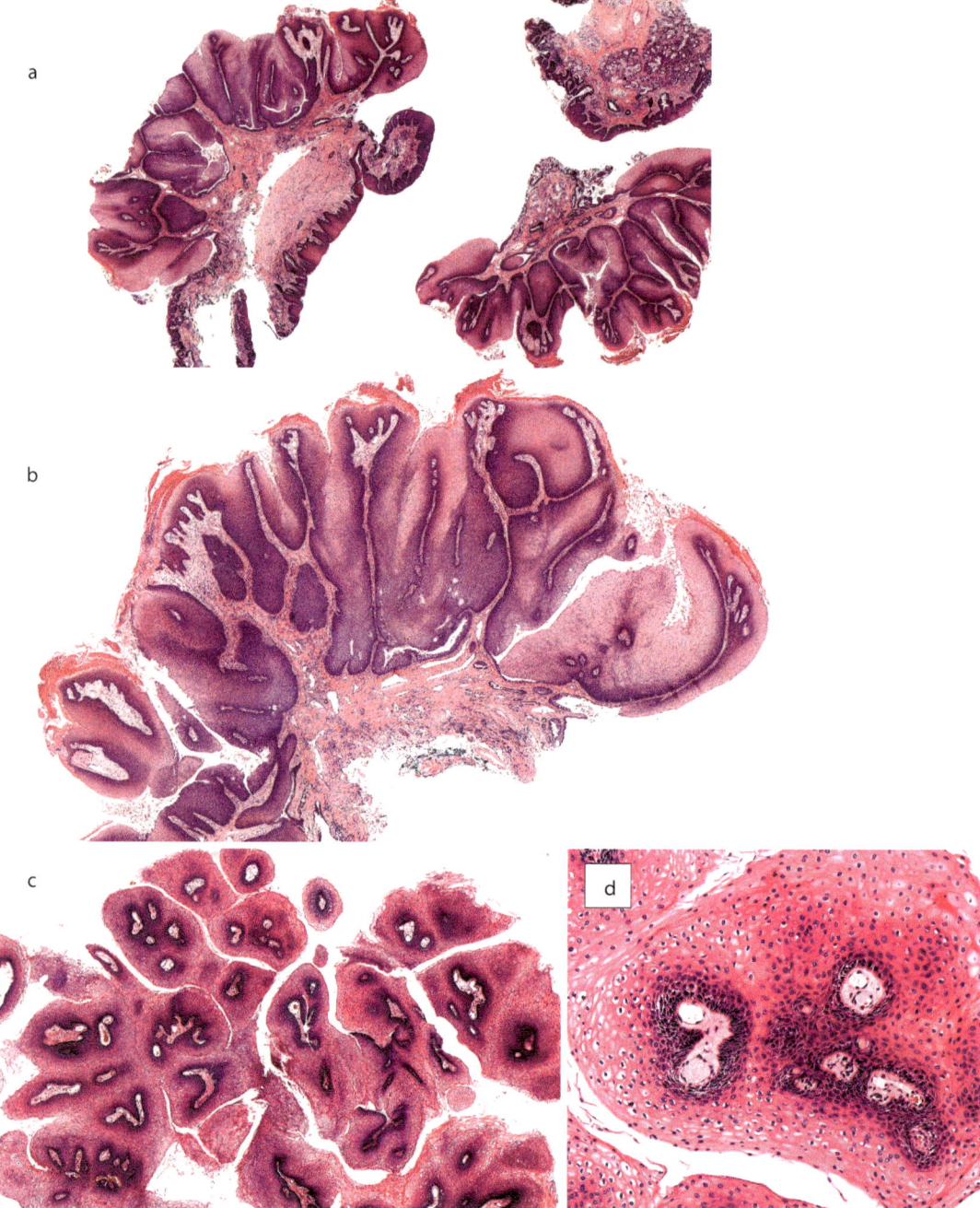

◻ Fig. 3.3 Exophytic papillomas – (**a, b**) sinonasal exophytic papillomas usually arise from the anterior nasal septum and are more sessile than their typical laryngeal or oral counterparts. (**c**) Fibrovascular cores in cross section. (**d**) Mature, keratinizing squamous epithelium

rare. Isolated antral inverted papillomas, without nasal cavity involvement, are uncommon (5 %). *Bona fide* nasal septal inverted papillomas are also distinctly uncommon. [23] Likely, this is due to the tethered septal submucosa which promotes exophytic rather than endophytic growth. Rarely, inverted papillomas can originate from sites such as middle ear or lacrimal apparatus [24, 25]. Bilateral presentation occurs 8 % of cases and may be associated with malignant transformation.

Conservative complete surgical resection via open lateral rhinotomy, or endoscopic approach,

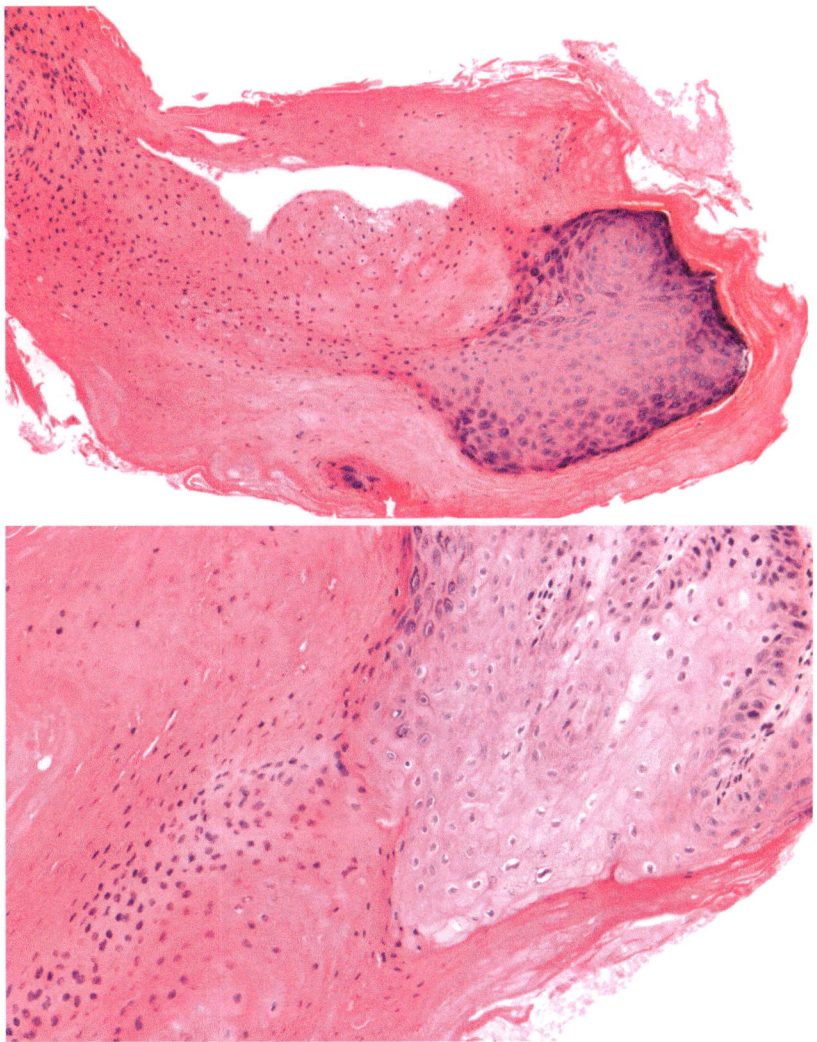

Fig. 3.4 Verruca vulgaris of nasal vault is characterized by a spikey fronds covered by dense hyperkeratosis keratosis with parakeratotic spires (*top*). *Bottom*: Higher power view of parakeratotic spires

will often cure most patients. However long term recurrence rates may be as high as 20 %. Additionally, HPV detection in inverted papillomas is significantly associated with increased likelihood of recurrence, and has been noted to increase with dyplasia [21].

■ **Histopathology**

On gross examination, inverted papillomas are polypoid, white, gray, with "prune-like" pitted surfaces (■ Fig. 3.6). Histologically, they are composed of ribbons and islands of immature "glycogenated" stratified squamous mucosa which "invert" into the loose lamina propria (■ Fig. 3.6). Ciliated columnar epithelium and goblet cells can

be retained. If mixed patterns are seen (e.g., exophytic and inverting, or oncocytic and inverting) then the lesions should be classified as inverted papilloma.

Squamous metaplasia and hyperplasia are commonly observed adjacent to inverted papilloma. However, isolated squamous metaplasia is not specific or predictive for adjacent inverted papilloma. As mentioned, inverted papilloma epithelium has an immature glycogenated appearance. Hyperkeratosis and parakeratosis are uncommon and worrisome, as these findings may portend malignant transformation. Dysplasia is seen in approximately 10 % of inverted papillomas.

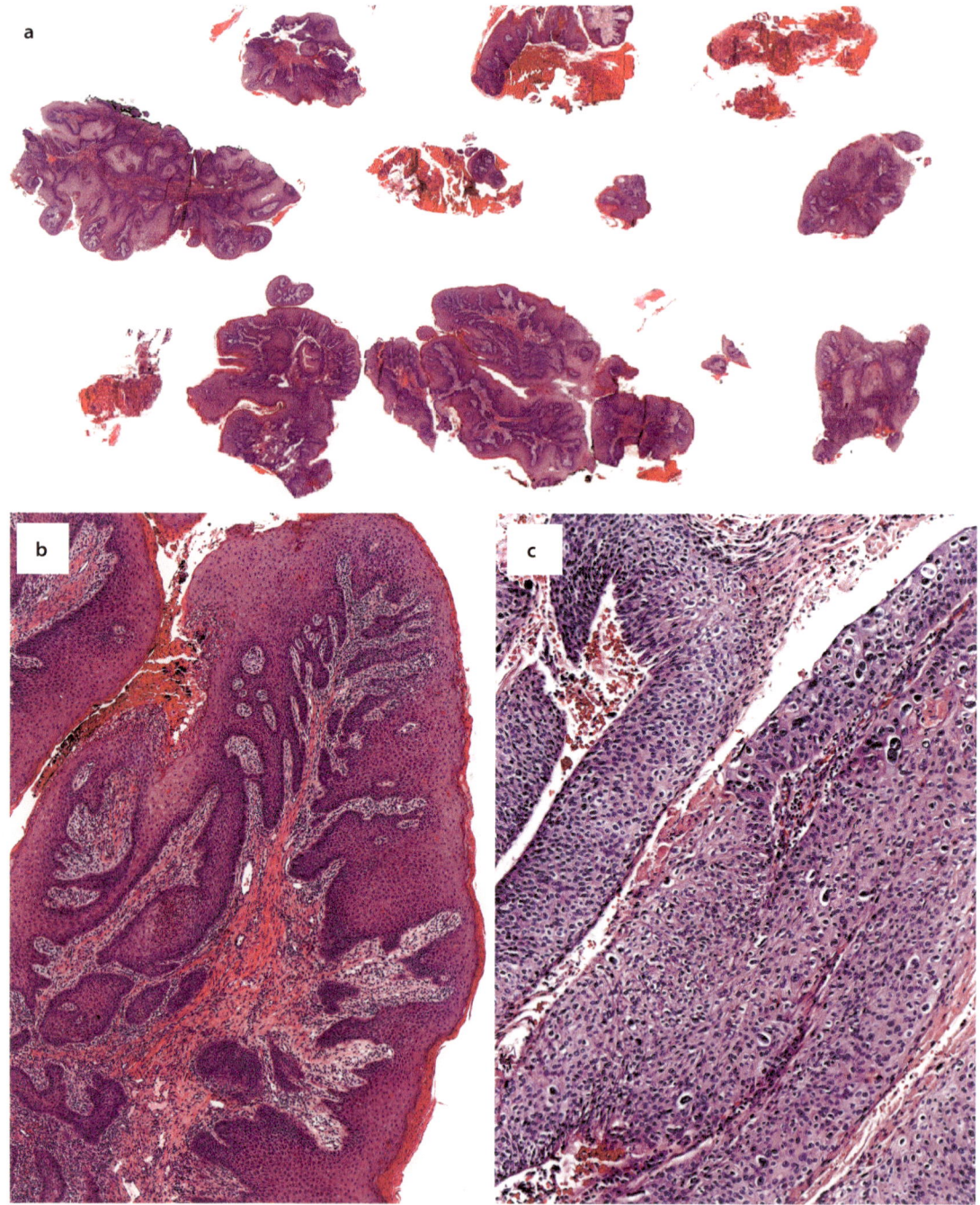

■ **Fig. 3.5** (**a**) Experience will teach you when to suspect more than a papilloma. Biopsy of squamous carcinoma, papillary variant. (**b**) These papillae are not slender or simple as with exophytic papillomas. No pleomorphism is present in this case. (**c**) Recognizing a papillary variant of squamous cell carcinoma is easier when there's pleomorphism

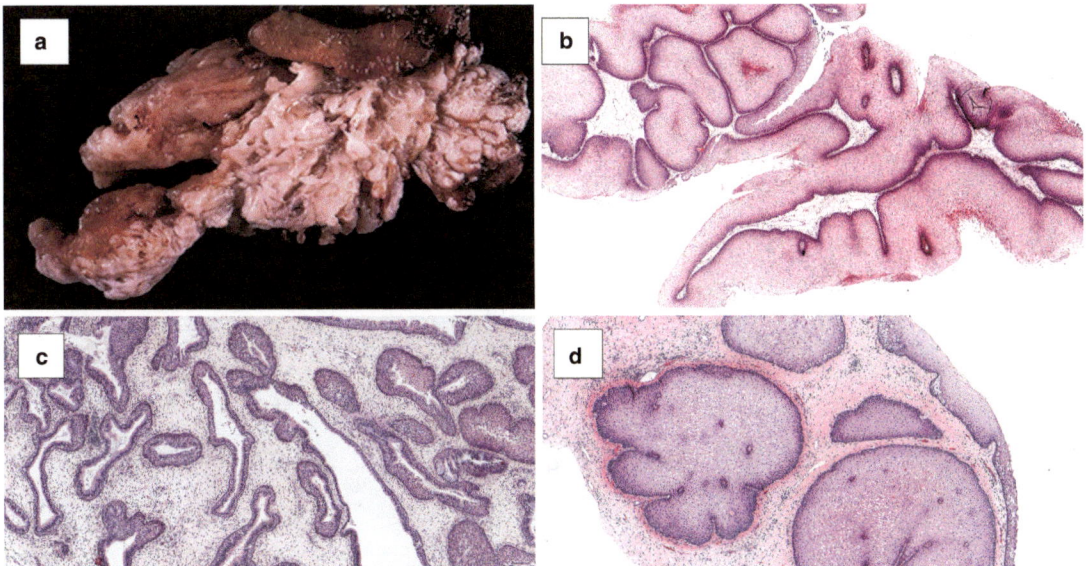

◙ Fig. 3.6 Inverted papilloma – (**a**) *whitish grey* polypoid lesion arising from the lateral nasal wall. The "prune-like" invaginations represent inverting components. (**b–d**) Typical smooth contours of ribbons and islands of nonkeratinizing, "glycogenated" squamous epithelium

---

- Papillae can also be seen in hypertrophic papillary sinusitis, and papillary intestinal type adenocarcinoma; these papillae lack the stratified layers of squamous mucosa of inverted papillomas.

3.5 Oncocytic Schneiderian Papilloma

Oncocytic Schneiderian papillomas (OSP) (previously known as cylindrical cell papillomas), represent the rarest (3–5%) form of Schneiderian papilloma [18, 19, 26, 27]. The male/female predisposition (1.6:1) is less pronounced than with inverted papillomas (3:1). Patients with OSP usually present after the 4rth decade. These lesions may arise from the lateral nasal wall, but they are more likely to affect only the antrum. OSP are soft, ragged, reddish tumors, grossly mimicking malignancy. Curiously, OSP have never been

associated with HPV [21]. The local recurrence and malignant transformation rates for OSP are similar to inverted papillomas: 25–35%, and 9–17%, respectively [18, 21, 28, 29].

■ Histopathology

The brightly eosinophilic epithelium pierced with mucous microcysts, characteristic of OSP, can be appreciated at low-power observation (◙ Fig. 3.7). At higher power, stratified layers of tall oncocytes are observed forming a delicate lace-like pattern. The inverting oncocytic islands can form "star-like" glandular structures. OSP can typically be admixed with inverted papillomas.

- *If cytologic pleomorphism and mitotic activity seen, then consider malignant transformation.*
- *If papillae are lined by a single layer of columnar cells, then consider low-grade papillary intestinal type adenocarcinoma.*

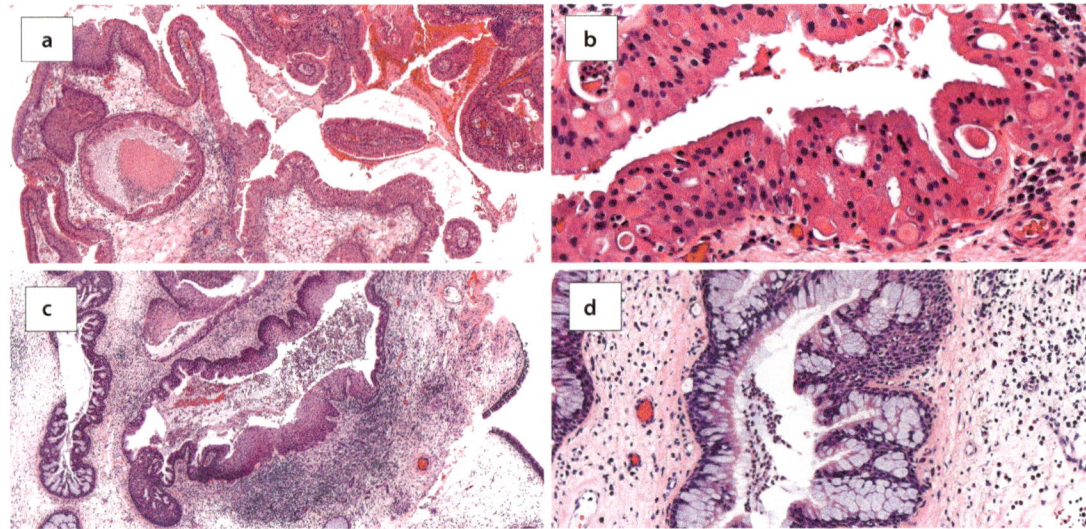

Fig. 3.7 Oncocytic Schneiderian Papilloma (*OSP*) – (**a**) intense cytoplasmic eosinophilia seen at low-power. (**b**) The epithelium is composed of stratified tall oncocytes pierced with glandular spaces. (**c**) OSP can be commonly admixed with typical inverted papilloma. (**d**) This OSP is unusual due to goblet cell hyperplasia

3.6   Carcinoma-ex-inverted Papilloma

Approximately 10 % of inverted papillomas undergo malignant transformation. This is significantly associated with the detection of high-risk HPV [18, 19, 21, 30]. Clinically, carcinoma-ex-inverted papilloma may manifest as a *de-novo* presentation, or be associated with recurrent inverted papillomas.

■ Histopathology

Most commonly, malignant transformation gives rise to squamous cell carcinoma (SCC) but other carcinomas (e.g., mucoepidermoid carcinoma, undifferentiated carcinoma) may also develop [30]. Malignant transformation can be recognized at low-power as an alteration in the silhouette of the inverting islands. Rather than the smooth contours of inverted papilloma, the epithelial islands are larger and more confluent, with complex shapes (■ Fig. 3.8). Nuclear pleomorphism, increased mitotic figures, apoptosis, and necrosis are seen. Keratinization in an inverted papilloma should raise the suspicion for malignant transformation. A rarer phenotype of malignant transition demonstrates crowded, confluent inverted islands, keratinization (paradoxical maturation), smooth contours, and limited pleomorphism. This well-differentiated SCC-ex-IP can be difficult to recognize; the diagnosis is based solely on architectural changes (■ Figs. 3.9 and 3.10). The differential diagnosis of SCC-ex-IP includes the transitional variant of SCC (■ Fig. 3.11).

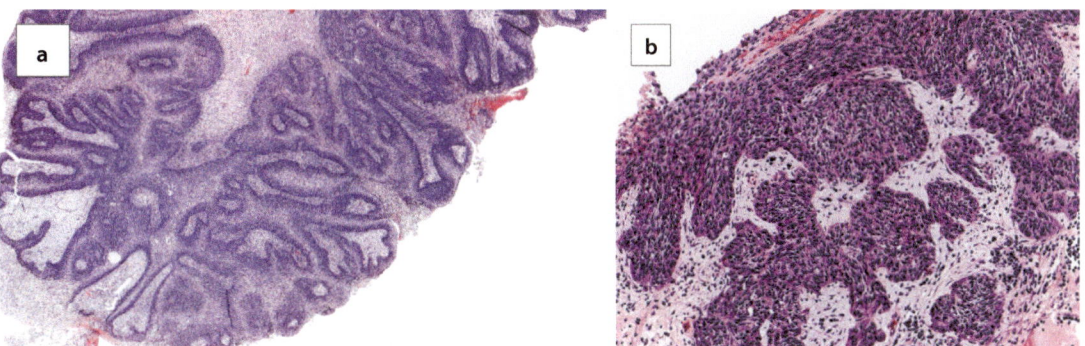

🔲 **Fig. 3.8** Carcinoma-ex-inverted papilloma – (**a**) the transitional pattern suggests an origin from inverted papilloma. (**b**) Frankly pleomorphic infiltrating squamous carcinoma

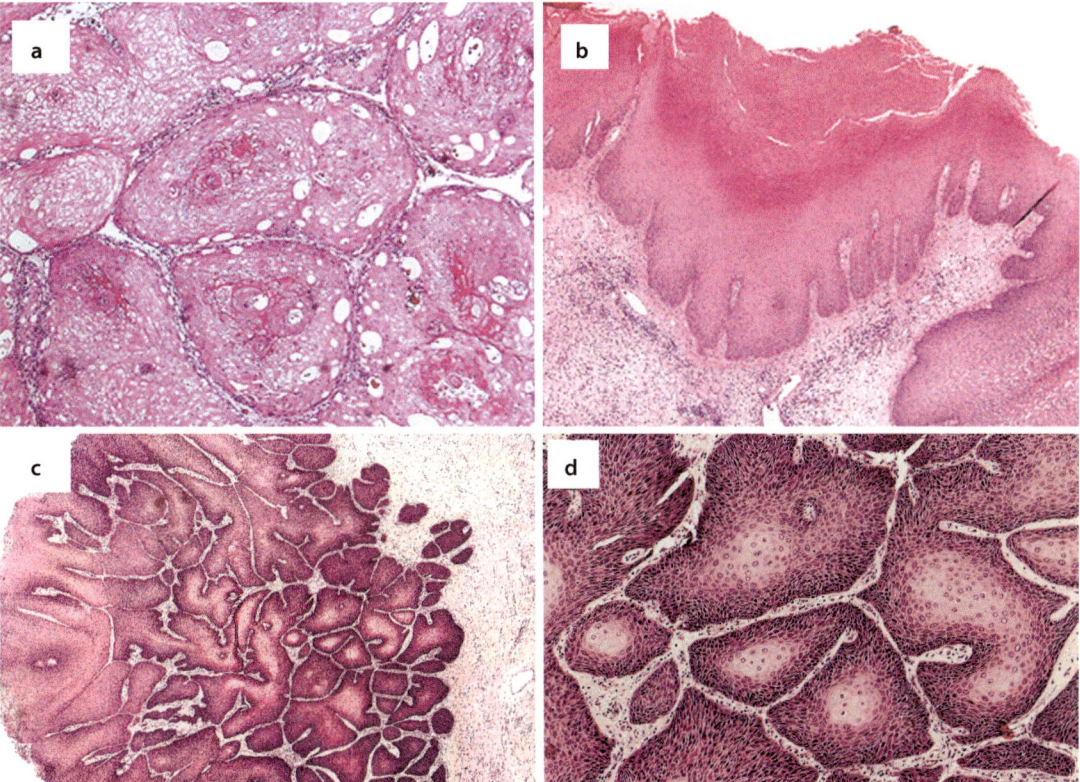

🔲 **Fig. 3.9** (**a–d**) SCC-ex-inverted papilloma – sometimes, the diagnosis of well differentiated squamous carcinoma must be is based *only* on tumor architecture, not cytologic pleomorphism. Crowding of islands and keratinization speak for malignant transformation

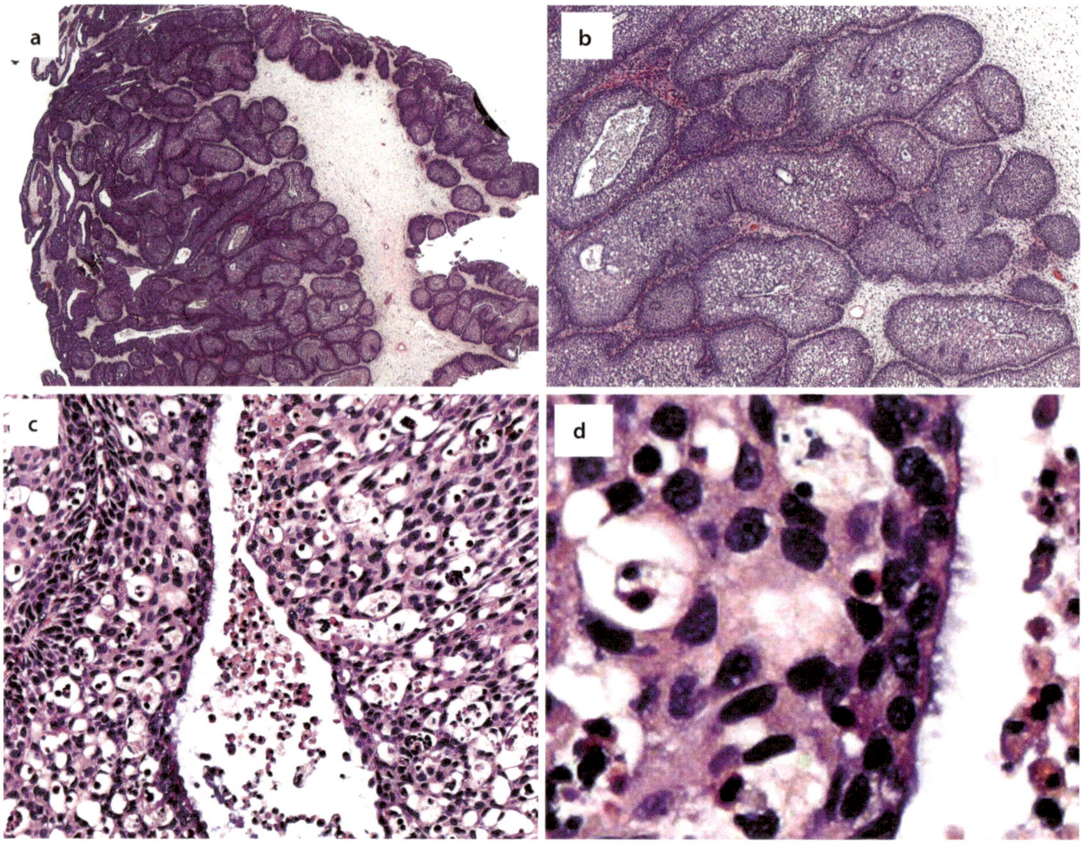

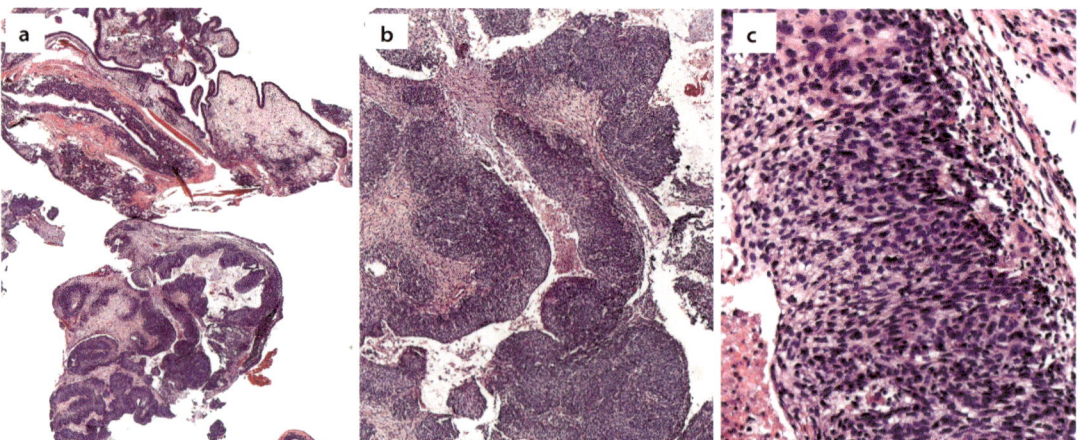

◘ **Fig. 3.10** (**a**, **b**) The smooth contours are those of inverted papilloma, but the crowded appearance, and limited intervening stroma tells you something more is happening. (**c**, **d**) The architectural crowding and pleomorphism warrant a diagnosis of SCC-ex-inverted papilloma. Do not be deterred by the lack of frank invasion. Clinicoradiographic correlation will determine the extent of surgery, and the degree of invasion in the resection specimen will determine the prognosis

◘ **Fig. 3.11** (**a**, **b**) Low- and intermediate-power views of transitional variant of SCC enters the differential diagnosis of SCC-ex-inverted papilloma. Notice the smooth ribbon contours and maturation. (**c**) Recognizing directional maturation in a neoplasm allows you to conclude that this is a carcinoma, rather than adenocarcinoma. (*D*=down: these tumor cells recapitulate basal reserve cells. *U*=up: these are maturing flattened tumor cells.) A common question is, "How far can I go here?" The diagnostic criteria for the head and neck differ from other sites, for instance, urinary tract. You need not see any irregular shaped islands invading stroma. On a biopsy, this histology warrants the diagnosis of transitional variant of SCC. If this represents the worst pattern of invasion on a resection specimen, then you would conclude that this represents a "non aggressive pattern of invasion". Lastly, notice the ciliated epithelium in (**d**). This would not be seen in transitional variant of SCC

3.7   Neurofibromas

Neurofibroma is a benign peripheral nerve sheath tumor that arises from a nerve trunk. Most neurofibromas occur sporadically and not associated with von Recklinghausen's disease (neurofibromatosis type 1, NF-1). Sinonasal neurofibromas are extremely rare, usually sporadic, and most commonly originate in the nasal vestibule [31]. Excision is curative.

▪ Histopathology

At low-power, neurofibromas are characterized by relatively uniform cellularity. Interlacing fascicles and bundles of bland spindle cells are embedded in a fibrous or loose myxoid stroma. Coarse collagen bundles are present within the stroma with a characteristic "shredded carrot" appearance. The spindled tumor cells have irregular, wavy, bland nuclei. "Comma-shaped" spindle cells are a helpful finding. Residual nerve axons are seen within and at the periphery of neurofibroma.

The plexiform neurofibroma contains tortuous, hyperplastic, hypercellular nerves within a background of diffuse neurofibroma (◘ Fig. 3.12). Focal cytologic atypia or rare mitoses can be seen. Nuclear palisading and perivascular hyalinization are absent. Infiltrating mast cells are another characteristic finding. Neurofibromas are S100+ and SOX10+. CD34 highlights fibroblasts and calretinin stains rare cells.

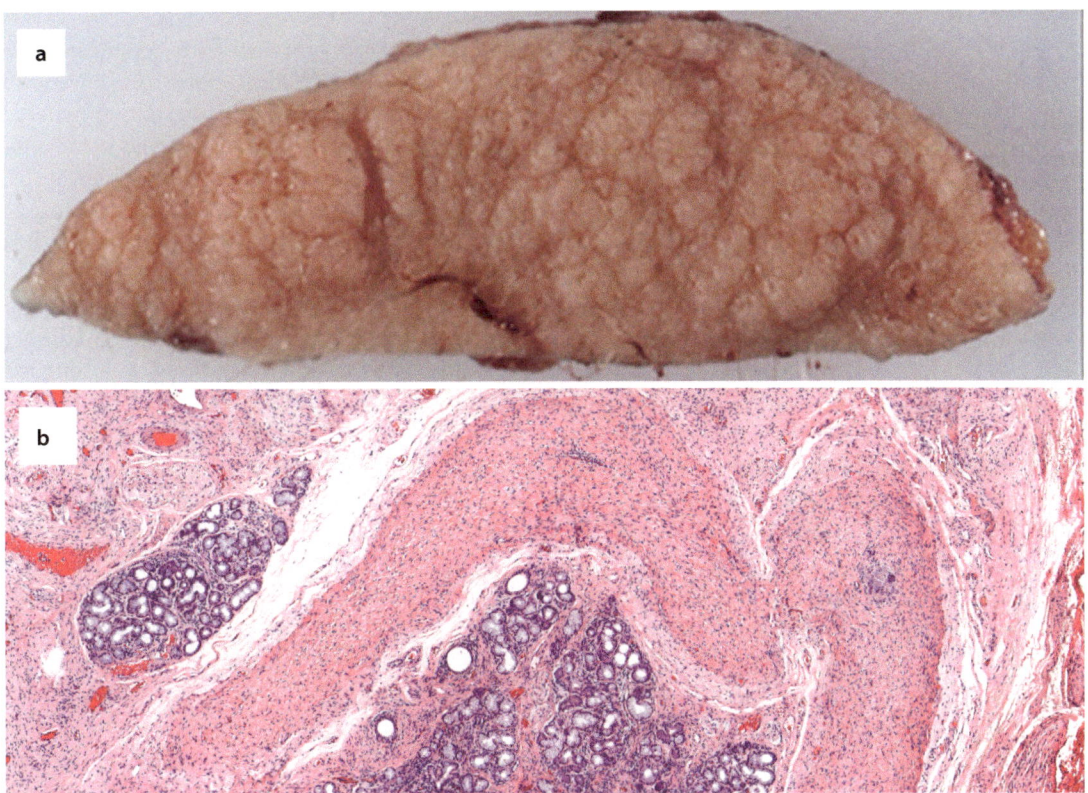

◘ **Fig. 3.12**   (**a**) Plexiform neurofibroma is usually associated with neurofibromatosis type 1. The overlying skin is hyperplastic and hyperpigmented. Multiple subcutaneous nodules are mobile and stringy; the sensation of palpating them has been likened to a "bag of worms". (**b, c**) Plexiform neurofibromas are composed of hypercellular nerves embedded in a loose tumor stroma of wavy spindle cells. (**d**) Stromal infiltrate of bland spindle cells which can be extremely long and wavy. *Inset*: "Comma"-shaped cells are seen

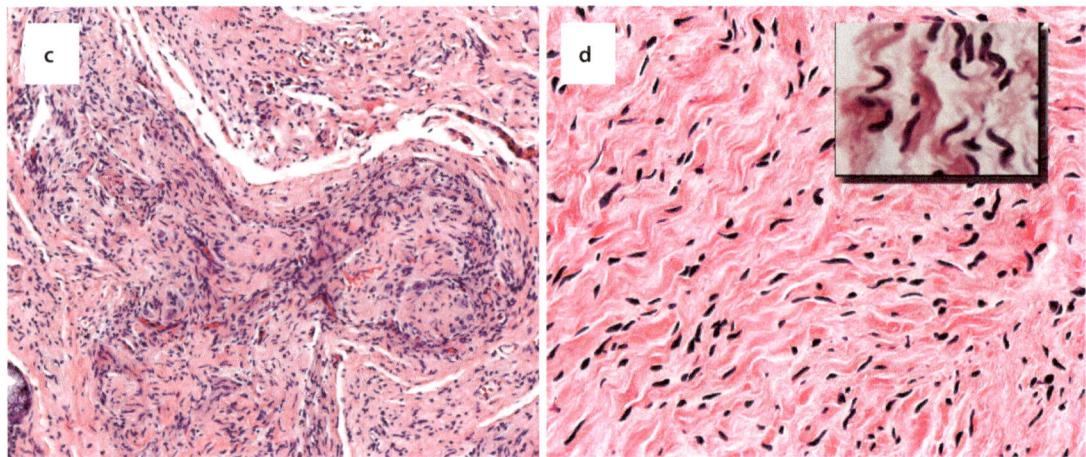

▫ Fig. 3.12 (continued)

3.8   Schwannomas

A schwannoma is a benign peripheral nerve sheath tumor arising from myelinated nerves. It forms a discrete expansile mass that forms eccentrically from the nerve trunk. Most head and neck Schwannomas are solitary and originate from soft tissue peripheral nerves, or cervical, spinal, or cranial nerves (e.g., "acoustic neuromas" of cranial nerve VIII). Sinonasal Schwannomas are extremely uncommon and represent only 4% of all head and neck Schwannomas. They originate from the 1rst and 2nd branches of the trigeminal nerve and autonomic plexi. The nasal cavity and ethmoid sinuses are most common sinonasal sites [32–36]. Sinonasal Schwannomas can also extend superiorly into the anterior cranial fossa. The olfactory nerves lack myelinated Schwann cells; not surprisingly, Schwannomas are not seen here.

▪ Histopathology

Sinonasal Schwannomas are unencapsulated and may infiltrate local bone. At low-power, Schwannomas demonstrate alternating hypercellular and hypocellular zones, referred to as Antoni A and Antoni B areas (▫ Fig. 3.13). The Antoni A areas have greater cellularity and are composed of fusiform tumor cells with wavy nuclei that form whorls and pallisading fascicles. The stroma is relatively hyalinized. Verocay bodies represent a distinctive arrangement of groups of spindle cells that line up with each other along their long axis. Antoni B areas are less cellular. The fusiform tumor cells are present within a loose matrix which may form microcysts. Perivascular hyalinization is a common and helpful diagnostic feature. Ancient Schwannomas are characterized by calcification, cystic necrosis, nuclear degeneration, and loss of Antoni A areas. Schwannomas are S100+ and calretinin+. CD34 highlights hypocellular Antoni B areas

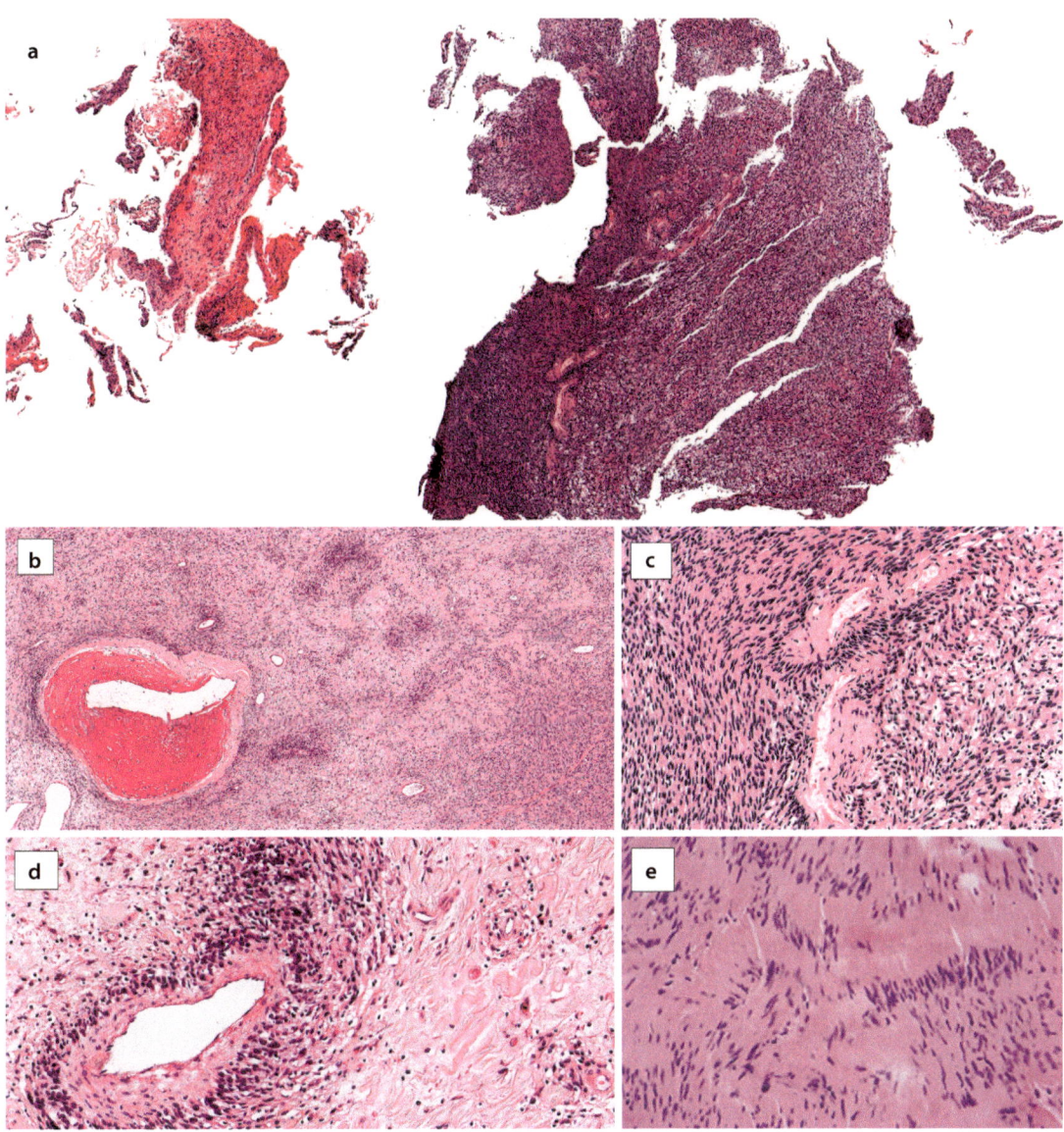

◘ **Fig. 3.13** Sinonasal schwannoma (**a**) Perivascular hyalinization is a very helpful hint. You can already see this at low-power. (**b**) Perivascular hyalinization (**c**) Characteristic areas of dense cellularity (Antoni A) and collagen deposition (**d**) Paucicellular areas (Antoni B) (**e**) Palisading tumor cells line up to form Verrucay bodies

3.9   Meningiomas

Meningiomas are benign tumors arising from meningeal arachnoid cells with a predisposition to affect middle-aged females. Extracranial meningiomas can arise by the following mechanisms:

Type 1: Direct extension of an intracranial tumor after bony resorption. 20 % of intracranial meningiomas extend to skull, scalp, orbit, sinonasal tract, temporal bone, skull base, etc.

Type 2: Extracranial metastasis from an intracranial tumor.

Type 3: Arachnoid cells sequestered around suture lines, cranial nerves, or vessels exiting foramina.

Type 4: Ectopic arachnoid cells with no demonstrable intracranial component or association with cranial nerves or foramina.

A recent publication on extracranial meningiomas demonstrates that temporal bone meningiomas have a significant predisposition for females, and scalp meningiomas have a significant predisposition for males [37]. Sinonasal meningiomas are extremely rare; most commonly they involve the nasal cavity alone or the nasal cavity plus paranasal sinuses. Meningiomas are generally indolent tumors. Patient outcome for sinonasal meningiomas is influenced by resectability and potential for local morbidity due to tumor size [38]. An excellent outcome can be expected for completely resected WHO 1 sinonasal meningiomas. The 5 year disease-specific survivals are 92.4 %, 88.9 and 50 %, for WHO 1, WHO 2, and WHO 3 extracranial meningiomas, respectively [37].

Meningioma: WHO Grade 1 (Lack anaplasia)
Meningotheliomatous Mixed (Transitional)
Psammomatous
Fibroblastic
Angiomatous
Microcystic
Secretory
Metaplastic
Lymphoplasmacyte-rich

Meningioma: WHO Grade 2
Atypical meningioma
Chordoid meningioma
Clear cell meningioma

Meningioma WHO Grade 3
Anaplastic meningioma
Papillary meningioma
Rhabdoid meningioma

▪ Histopathology

WHO Grade 1 meningiomas are subclassified as follows:

Meningotheliomatous – This is the most common pattern which is characterized by whorls and lobules of syncytial spindled and epithelioid tumor cells (◨ Fig. 3.14). The bland tumor cells have abundant eosinophilic cytoplasm, indistinct cell membranes, round to oval nuclei, and intranuclear cytoplasmic pseudoinclusions. Psamomma bodies are typical.

Fibrous – have a prominent spindle cell pattern with interlacing collagen.

Mixed (Transitional) – have meningothelial plus spindled components.

Angiomatous – are characterized by prominent vascularity.

Psammomatous – are characterized by abundant concentric and confluent calcifications.

Metaplastic – This variant is extremely rare. Metaplastic meningiomas demonstrate mesenchymal differentiation (e.g., lipid, xanthomatous, smooth muscle, osseous, chondroid, myxoid). EMA expression is retained [39].

Secretory – Tumor cells have round intracytoplasmic inclusions that are PAS+/CK7+/CEA+, and represent "pre-psammoma" bodies.

An infiltrative growth pattern is common in all patterns and grades of meningioma. While EMA+ is typical, it can be focal or weak [38].

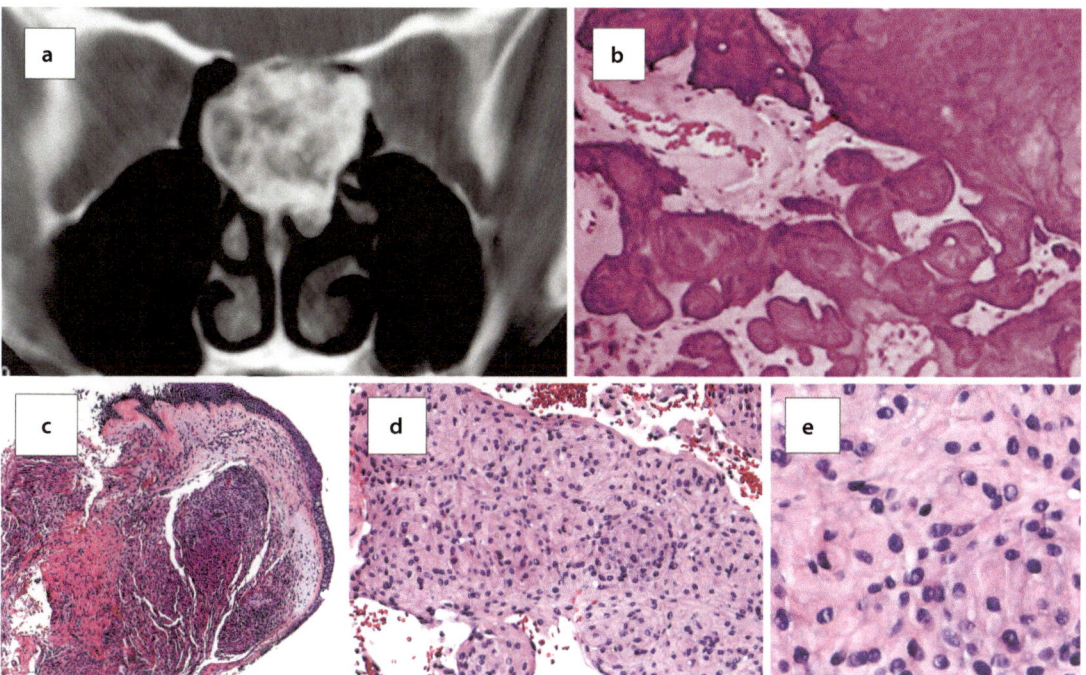

Fig. 3.14 Ectopic sinonasal meningioma – (**a**) heterogenous, expansile, calcified tumor in the superior nasal cavity. The radiographic differential diagnosis includes chondrosarcoma, pleomorphic adenoma, psammomatoid ossifying fibroma, and olfactory neuroblastoma. (**b**) Coalescing calcifications. (**c**) Typical meningothelial whorls (**d**, **e**) Meningotheioma cells can be epithelioid and spindled

> • *Psammoma bodies can also be present in psammomatoid ossifying fibroma and olfactory neuroblastoma – neither express EMA.*

WHO Grade 2 (■ Fig. 3.15)

Fifteen to 35 % of intracranial meningiomas are classified as WHO Grade 2 (atypical meningioma) [40]. Atypical meningiomas are character- ized by increased cellularity, pleomorphism, high nuclear/cytoplasmic ratio (small cell changes), and prominent nucleoli. The tumor grows in a sheet-like pattern, rather than a lobular growth pattern. Atypical meningiomas infiltrate brain tissue. Zones of necrosis are present. The mitotic rate is 4–19/10 HPF.

WHO Grade 3

These meningioma variants are frankly malig- nant, cytologically, with a mitotic rate of >20 mitoses/10 HPF. Rhabdoid or papillary features can be present.

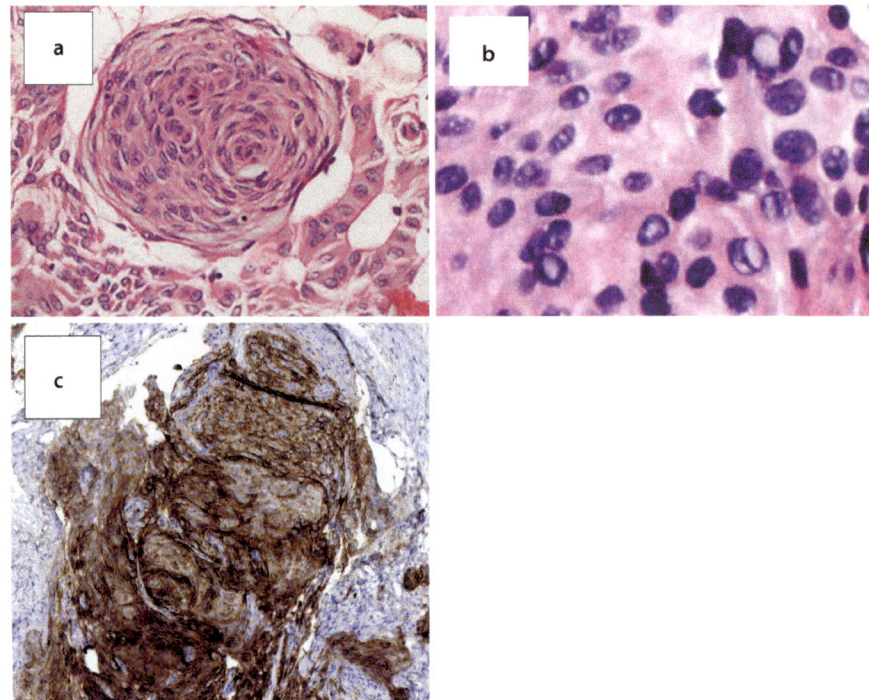

■ **Fig. 3.15**   Ectopic sinonasal meningioma (**a**) typical meningothelial whorls (**b**) Note intranuclear holes. (**c**) EMA expression, while characteristic, is *not* expressed in every meningioma

3.10   Nasal Glial Heterotopia (NGH)

NGH represents a congenital malformation of displaced glial tissue which is discontinuous with the intracranial meninges. Although NGH has been incorrectly referred to as a "glioma" it is not a neoplasm. Encephalocele represents herniation of brain tissue and leptomeninges through a skull defect; intracranial continuity is maintained. Encephaloceles can be due to congenital malformation or trauma or surgery. NGH and congenital encephalocele are usually brought to attention during infancy. As babies are obligate nasal breathers, any neonatal nasal obstruction will manifest as respiratory distress soon after birth.

Approximately 60 % of NGH are exclusively extranasal, presenting as subcutaneous nodules around the nasal bridge [41]. Approximately 10 % of NGH have both subcutaneous and intranasal components, whereas approximately 30 % of NGH are entirely intranasal, presenting as polyp-oid lesions of the superior nasal cavity or nasopharynx [42–44]. Infants with congenital encephaloceles may have episodes of meningitis. Patients with acquired encephaloceles can present with cerebrospinal fluid rhinorrhea.

■ **Histopathology**

Nasal glial heterotopia demonstrate fibrillary neuroglia with a prominent network of glial fibers (■ Fig. 3.16). Astrocytes can show gemistocytic change (Greek: fill up) and appear enlarged and star-shaped. These large astrocytic cells may mimic histiocytes. Actual neuronal cells are rarely identified. The presence of choroid plexus, ependymal cells, and pigmented retinal cells have also been reported. Encephaloceles are histologically identical to normal brain, but include degeneratives changes such as hemorrhage and fibrosis. Nasal glial heterotopia and encephaloceles express glial fibrillary acid protein (GFAP). The distinction between nasal glial heterotopia and encephalocele is made on clinicoradiographic correlation.

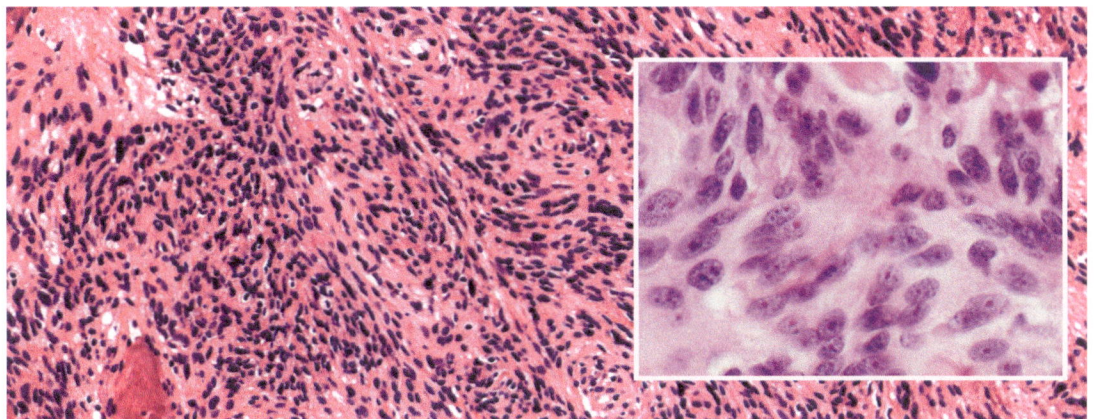

Fig. 3.16 Recurrent atypical meningioma with intranasal component. Intracranial extension, necrosis, and elevated Ki-67 (20 %) were documented in the index neoplasm, warranting classification as WHO II atypical meningioma. Here we see hypercellularity, nuclear pleomorphism and prominanet nucleoli (*Inset*)

3.11 Osteomas

Head and neck osteomas are indolent boney growths that are either peripheral (arising from periosteum, attached to the cortical plate), central (arising from endosteum, expanding into medullary space), or intracavitary (originating in the paranasal sinuses). The most common head and neck osteoma is the peripheral type [45–49]. The frontal sinus is most common site for an intracavitary osteoma, followed by the ethmoid and maxillary sinuses. A male predominance is seen. Osteomas may be symptomatic depending on location and size, but most are found incidentally on radiographs.

Most head and neck osteomas are single and sporadic; a significant proportion of sporadic patients have > one osteoma [48]. Gardener's syndrome (familial adenomatous polyposis) represents an autosomal dominant syndrome associated with multiple intestinal adenomatous polyps developing in the first or second decade of life; progression to colonic adenocarcinoma is inevitable without prophylactic colectomy. Multiple bilateral pigmented retinal lesions on ophthalmic fundoscopic examination (congenital hypertrophy of the retinal pigment epithelium) are characteristic and diagnostic for familial adenomatous polyposis. Syndromic patients also develop multiple soft tissue tumors (epidermoid inclusion cysts, fibromas, and desmoids). Twenty five to 50 % of syndromic patients have multiple bony lesions such as peripheral mandibular or cranial osteomas and sinonasal osteomas [50, 51].

■ **Histopathology**

Osteomas can be classified as either compact (ivory), cancellous (mature, or mixed type). Compact osteomas are composed of dense cortical lamellar bone (■ Figs. 3.17 and 3.18). Cancellous osteomas contain mature trabecular bone with intervening fibroconnective tissue. Osteomas can also appear "osteoblastoma-like", these are composed of trabeculae of woven bone rimmed by active osteoblasts and osteoclasts, localized to the base of the lesion, with peripheral bone maturation [47, 49]. Osteoma bone can appear Paget-like with irregular cement-lines.

> • *If the differential diagnosis is osteoma versus*
>   *osteoblastoma, then radiographically:*
>   *Osteoma with osteoblastoma-like areas*
>   *= densely ossified intracavitary lesion*
>   *Osteoblastoma = expansile calcified mass*

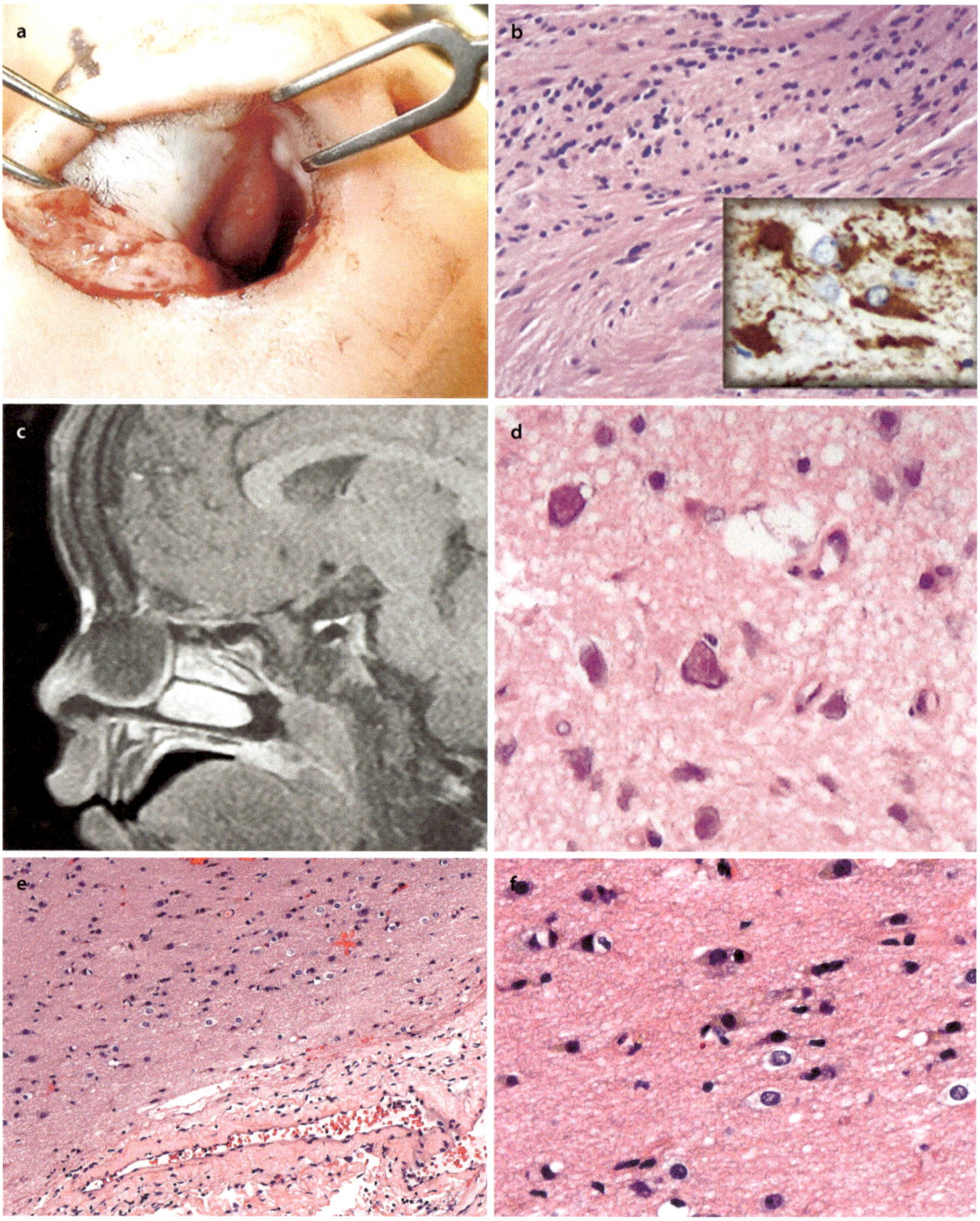

Fig. 3.17 Nasal glial heterotopia – (**a**) typical presentation as an intranasal polyp in a child. (**b**) Neuropil and glial cells. *Inset*: glial fibrillary acidic protein. (**c**) Sagital T1-weighted, fat suppressed MR image of an anterior nasal fossa mass that extends to the anterior skull base, without an intracranial component. There is *no* caudal distortion of the undersurface of the frontal lobe, as one would see in an encephalocele. (**d**) Glial cells and laminated calcifications. (**e, f**) Adult encephalocele, neutropil and glial cells

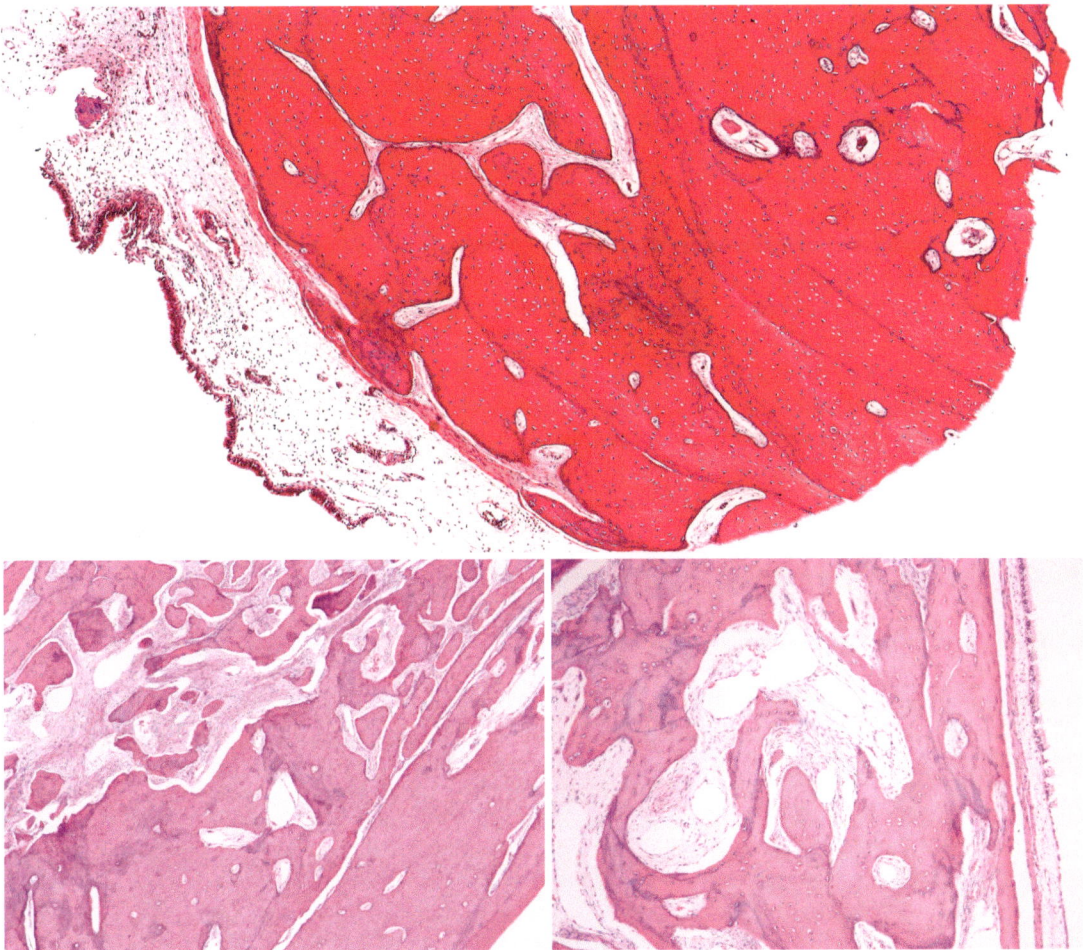

◘ Fig. 3.18 Paranasal sinus osteoma – *Upper panel*: compact osteoma: discreet mass within the Schneiderian mucosa composed of dense cortical bone. Note the parallel blue cement lines of mature bone. *Bottom panels*: a cancellous-type osteoma composed of trabecular bone. Here, the blue cement lines are irregular, representing immature trabecular bone

Self Study

1. Which statement is true regarding ◘ Fig. 3.19?
   (a) This represents a benign hamartomatous process.
   (b) This is worrisome for carcinoma – ex-inverted papilloma.
   (c) These lesions appear red and ragged on gross examination.
   (d) This lesion must arise from the nasal septum.

2. Which statement is true regarding ◘ Fig. 3.20?
   (a) The mature, keratinized squamous epithelium is typical for exophytic papilloma.
   (b) This lesion must arise from the nasal septum.

   (c) The epithelium of this inverted papilloma is bland and benign.
   (d) The architectural changes are worrisome for carcinoma-ex-inverted papilloma.

3. Which statement/statements is/are true regarding ◘ Fig. 3.21?
   (a) This represents a benign hamartomatous process.
   (b) The proliferating ductules are single-layered with little or no basal cell lining.
   (c) There is a propensity for the olfactory cleft.
   (d) a + b.
   (e) a, b, c.

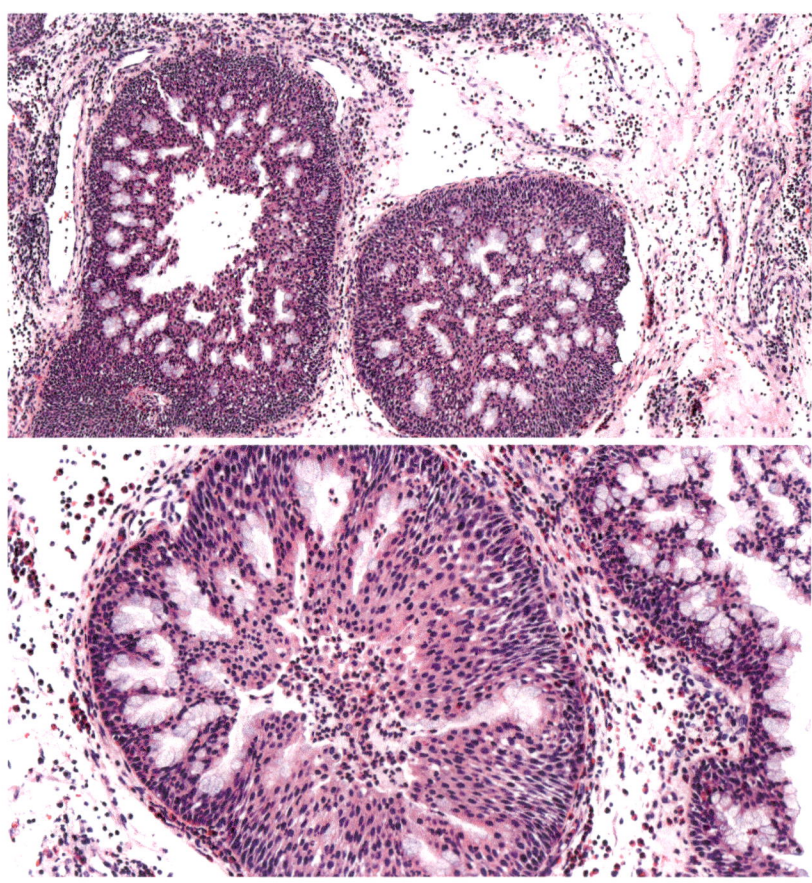

◘ **Fig. 3.19**   Self study

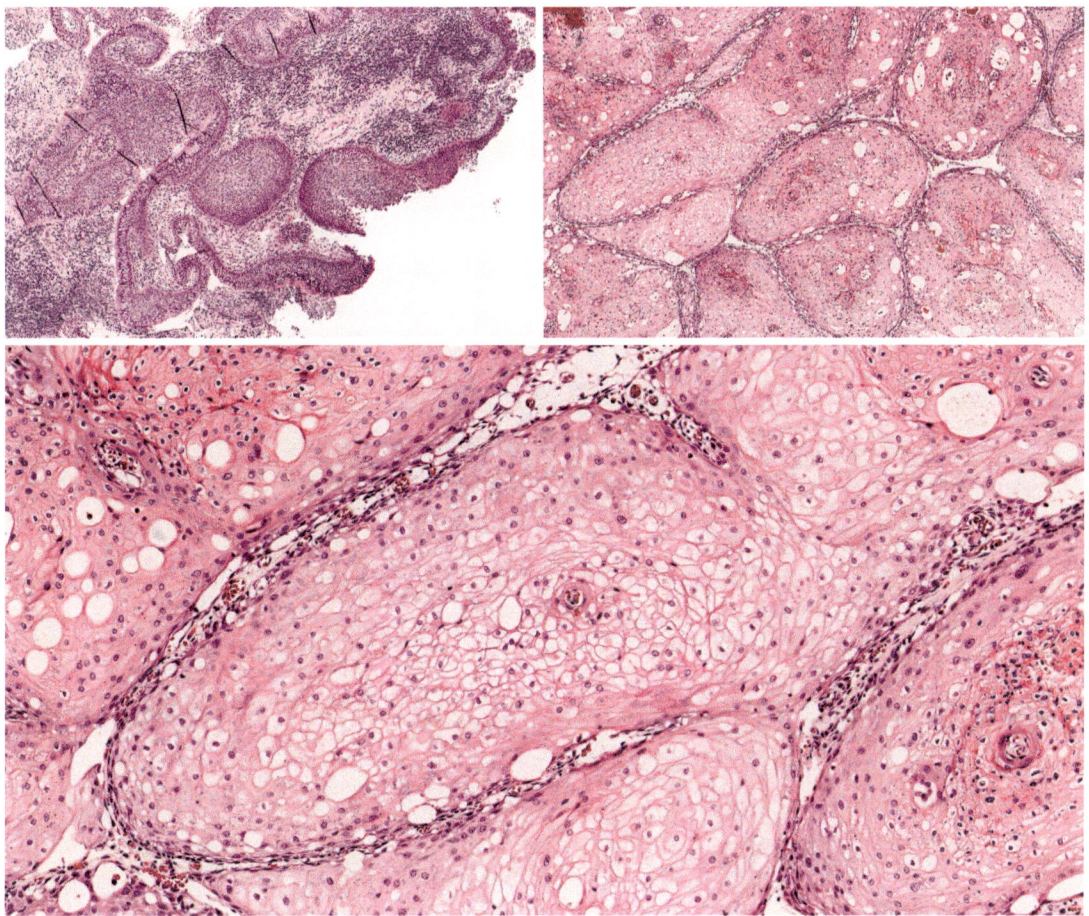

■ **Fig. 3.20** Self study

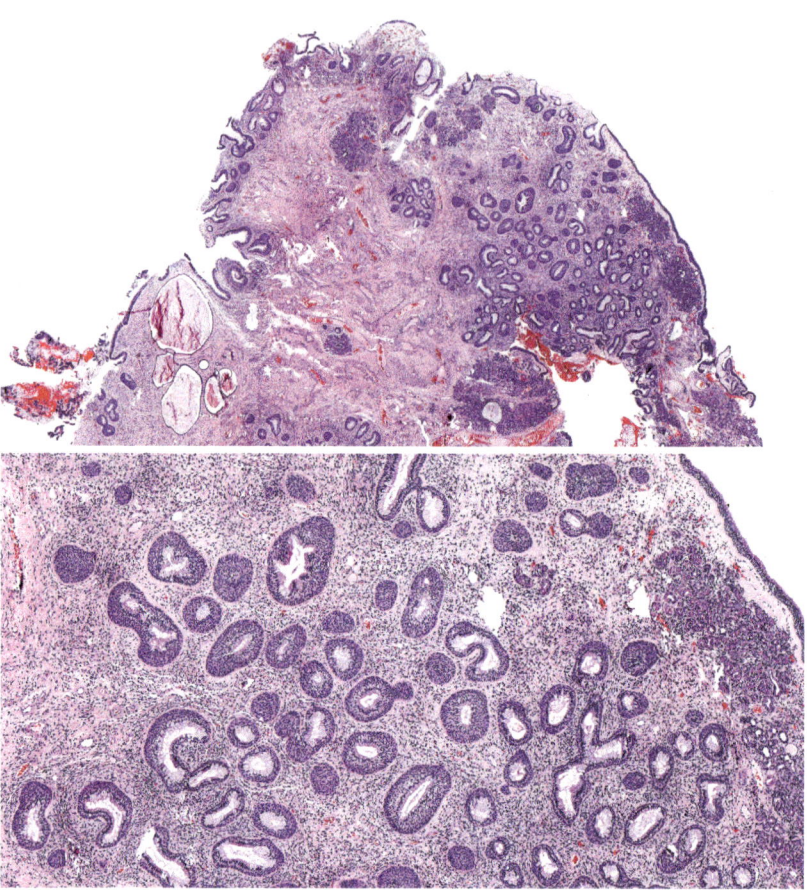

◘ Fig. 3.21   Self study

Answers

1. Which statement is true regarding ◘ Fig. 3.19?

    This is an oncocytic Schneiderian papilloma. Stratified columnar oncocytes are appreciated in the bottom panel. The goblet cell hyperplasia here is somewhat unusual.

    (a)   This represents a benign hamartomatous process. *No.*

    (b)   This is worrisome for carcinoma – ex-inverted papilloma. *No.*

    (c)   These lesions appear red and ragged on gross examination **CORRECT.**

    (d)   This lesion must arise from the nasal septum. *These typically arise from the antrum or lateral nasal wall.*

2. Which statement is true regarding ◘ Fig. 3.20?

    (a)   The mature, keratinized squamous epithelium is typical for exophytic papilloma. *No papillary structures are seen.*

    (b)   This lesion must arise from the nasal septum. *The upper left panel demonstrates the typical mucosa of antrum/lateral nasal wall.*

    (c)   The epithelium of this inverted papilloma is bland and benign. Bland yes, but see below.

    (d)   The architectural changes are worrisome for carcinoma-ex-inverted papilloma. **CORRECT This represents a well-differentiated keratinizing squamous carcinoma-ex-inverted papilloma. As with other well-differentiated keratinizing squamous carcinomas, the lack of pleomorphism can cause some diagnostic confusion. More commonly, carcinoma-ex-inverted papilloma is cytologically pleomorphic.**

3. Which statement/statements is/are true regarding ◘ Fig. 3.21?

    (a)   This represents a benign hamartomatous process. *No. This is an example of respiratory epithelial adenomatoid "hamartoma"*

(REAH) which represents a clonal proliferation rather than a hamartoma.

(b) The proliferating ductules are single-layered with little or no basal cell lining. *No. The ductal elements here are surrounded by **p63**+ basal cells.*

(c) There is a propensity for the olfactory cleft. **CORRECT.** *There is a propensity for superior nasal cavity REAH to arise from the posterior nasal septum (vomer) and the olfactory cleft.*

References

1. Wenig BM, Heffner DK. Respiratory epithelial adenomatoid hamartomas of the sinonasal tract and nasopharynx: a clinicopathologic study of 31 cases. Ann Otol Rhinol Laryngol. 1995;104:639–45.
2. Gauchotte G, Marie B, Gallet P, Nguyen DT, Grandhaye M, Jankowski R, Vignaud JM. Respiratory epithelial adenomatoid hamartoma: a poorly recognized entity with mast cell recruitment and frequently associated with nasal polyposis. Am J Surg Pathol. 2013;37:1678–85.
3. Metselaar RM, Stel HV, van der Baan S. Respiratory epithelial adenomatoid hamartoma in the nasopharynx. J Laryngol Otol. 2005;119:476–8.
4. Cao Z, Gu Z, Yang J, Jin M. Respiratory epithelial adenomatoid hamartoma of bilateral olfactory clefts associated with nasal polyposis: three cases report and literature review. Auris Nasus Larynx. 2010;37:352–6.
5. Vira D, Bhuta S, Wang MB. Respiratory epithelial adenomatoid hamartomas. Laryngoscope. 2011;121:2706–9.
6. Eloy JA, Friedel ME, Eloy JD, Mirani NM, Liu JK. Bilateral olfactory fossa respiratory epithelial adenomatoid hamartomas. Arch Otolaryngol Head Neck Surg. 2011;137:820–2.
7. Fitzhugh VA, Mirani N. Respiratory epithelial adenomatoid hamartoma: a review. Head Neck Pathol. 2008;2:203–8.
8. Ozolek JA, Hunt JL. Tumor suppressor gene alterations in respiratory epithelial adenomatoid hamartoma (REAH): comparison to sinonasal adenocarcinoma and inflamed sinonasal mucosa. Am J Surg Pathol. 2006;30:1576–80.
9. Jo VY, Mills SE, Cathro HP, Carlson DL, Stelow EB. Low-grade sinonasal adenocarcinomas: the association with and distinction from respiratory epithelial adenomatoid hamartomas and other glandular lesions. Am J Surg Pathol. 2009;33:401–8.
10. Flavin R, Russell J, Phelan E, McDermott MB. Chondro-osseous respiratory epithelial adenomatoid hamartoma of the nasal cavity: a case report. Int J Pediatr Otorhinolaryngol. 2005;69:87–91.
11. Choi E, Catalano PJ, Chang KG. Chondro-osseous respiratory epithelial hamartoma of the sinonasal tract. Otolaryngol Head Neck Surg. 2006;134:168–9.
12. Nomura K, Oshima T, Maki A, Suzuki T, Higashi K, Watanabe M, Kobayashi T. Recurrent chondro-osseous respiratory epithelial adenomatoid hamartoma of the nasal cavity in a child. Ear Nose Throat J. 2014;93:E29–31.
13. Weinreb I, Gnepp DR, Laver NM, Hoschar AP, Hunt JL, Seethala RR, Barnes EL, Chetty R, Perez-Ordoñez B. Seromucinous hamartomas: a clinicopathological study of a sinonasal glandular lesion lacking myoepithelial cells. Histopathology. 2009;54:205–13.
14. Ambrosini-Spaltro A, Morandi L, Spagnolo DV, Cavazza A, Brisigotti M, Damiani S, Jain S, Eusebi V. Nasal seromucinous hamartoma (microglandular adenosis of the nose): a morphological and molecular study of five cases. Virchows Arch. 2010;457:727–34.
15. Fleming KE, Perez-Ordoñez B, Nasser JG, Psooy B, Bullock MJ. Sinonasal seromucinous hamartoma: a review of the literature and a case report with focal myoepithelial cells. Head Neck Pathol. 2012;6:395–9.
16. Weinreb I. Low grade glandular lesions of the sinonasal tract: a focused review. Head Neck Pathol. 2010;4:77–83.
17. Khan RA, Chernock RD, Lewis Jr JS. Seromucinous hamartoma of the nasal cavity: a report of two cases and review of the literature. Head Neck Pathol. 2011;5:241–7.
18. Barnes L. Schneiderian papillomas and nonsalivary glandular neoplasms of the head and neck. Mod Pathol. 2002;15:279–97.
19. Hyams VJ. Papillomas of the nasal cavity and paranasal sinuses. A clinicopathological study of 315 cases. Ann Otol Rhinol Laryngol. 1971;80:192–206.
20. Syrjänen K, Syrjänen S. Detection of human papillomavirus in sinonasal papillomas: systematic review and meta-analysis. Laryngoscope. 2013;123:181–92.
21. Lawson W, Schlecht NF, Brandwein-Gensler M. The role of the human papillomavirus in the pathogenesis of Schneiderian inverted papillomas: an analytic overview of the evidence. Head Neck Pathol. 2008;2:49–59.
22. Eavey RD. Inverted papilloma of the nose and paranasal sinuses in childhood and adolescence. Laryngoscope. 1985;95:17–22.
23. Kelley JH, Joseph M, Carroll E, Goodman ML, Pilch BZ, Levinson RM, Strome M. Inverted papilloma of the nasal septum. Arch Otolaryngol. 1980;106:767–71.
24. Wenig BM. Schneiderian-type mucosal papillomas of the middle ear and mastoid. Ann Otol Rhinol Laryngol. 1996;105:226–33.
25. Fechner RE, Sessions RE. Inverted papilloma of the lacrimal sac, the paranasal sinuses and the cervical region. Cancer. 1977;40:2303–8.
26. Barnes L, Bedetti C. Oncocytic Schneiderian papilloma: a reappraisal of cylindrical cell papilloma of the sinonasal tract. Hum Pathol. 1984;15:344–51.
27. Vorasubin N, Vira D, Suh JD, Bhuta S, Wang MB. Schneiderian papillomas: comparative review of exophytic, oncocytic, and inverted types. Am J Rhinol Allergy. 2013;27:287–92.
28. Kaufman MR, Brandwein MS, Lawson W. Sinonasal papillomas: clinicopathologic review of 40 patients with inverted and oncocytic schneiderian papillomas. Laryngoscope. 2002;112:1372–7.
29. Karligkiotis A, Bignami M, Terranova P, Gallo S, Meloni F, Padoan G, Lombardi D, Nicolai P, Castelnuovo P. Oncocytic Schneiderian papillomas: clinical behavior and outcomes of the endoscopic endonasal approach in 33 cases. Head Neck. 2014;36:624–30.

30. Nudell J, Chiosea S, Thompson LD. Carcinoma ex-Schneiderian papilloma (malignant transformation): a clinicopathologic and immunophenotypic study of 20 cases combined with a comprehensive review of the literature. Head Neck Pathol. 2014;8:269–86.

31. Azani AB, Bishop JA, Thompson LD. Sinonasal tract neurofibroma: A clinicopathologic series of 12 cases with a review of the literature. Head Neck Pathol. 2015;9:323–33.

32. Mey KH, Buchwald C, Daugaard S, Prause JU. Sinonasal schwannoma—a clinicopathological analysis of five rare cases. Rhinology. 2006;44:46–52.

33. Buob D, Wacrenier A, Chevalier D, Aubert S, Quinchon JF, Gosselin B, Leroy X. Schwannoma of the sinonasal tract: a clinicopathologic and immunohistochemical study of 5 cases. Arch Pathol Lab Med. 2003;127:1196–9.

34. Blake DM, Husain Q, Kanumuri VV, Svider PF, Eloy JA, Liu JK. Endoscopic endonasal resection of sinonasal and anterior skull base schwannomas. J Clin Neurosci. 2014;21:1419–23.

35. Ohashi R, Wakayama N, Kawamoto M, Tsuchiya S, Okubo K. Solitary nasal schwannoma: usefulness of CD34 and calretinin staining for distinction from histological mimics. J Nippon Med Sch. 2013;80:300–6.

36. Suh JD, Ramakrishnan VR, Zhang PJ, Wu AW, Wang MB, Palmer JN, Chiu AG. Diagnosis and endoscopic management of sinonasal schwannomas. ORL J Otorhinolaryngol Relat Spec. 2011;73:308–12.

37. Rushing EJ, Bouffard JP, McCall S, Olsen C, Mena H, Sandberg GD, Thompson LD. Primary extracranial meningiomas: an analysis of 146 cases. Head Neck Pathol. 2009;3:116–30.

38. Thompson LD, Gyure KA. Extracranial sinonasal tract meningiomas: a clinicopathologic study of 30 cases with a review of the literature. Am J Surg Pathol. 2000;24:640–50.

39. Tang H, Sun H, Chen H, Gong Y, Mao Y, Xie Q, Xie L, Zheng M, Wang D, Zhu H, Che X, Zhong P, Zheng K, Li S, Bao W, Zhu J, Wang X, Feng X, Chen X, Zhou L. Clinicopathological analysis of metaplastic meningioma: report of 15 cases in Huashan hospital. Chin J Cancer Res. 2013;25:112–8.

40. Backer-Grøndahl T, Moen BH, Torp SH. The histopathological spectrum of human meningiomas. Int J Clin Exp Pathol. 2012;5:231–42.

41. Pereyra-Rodríguez JJ, Bernabeu-Wittel J, Fajardo M, Torre C, Sánchez-Gallego F. Nasal glial heterotopia (nasal glioma). J Pediatr. 2010;156:688.

42. Park YH, Kim SW, Cho SH, Choi YW. Nasopharyngeal glioma causing respiratory distress in a neonate: transoral endoscopic excision. Ear Nose Throat J. 2010; 89:E11–3.

43. Ohta N, Ito T, Sasaki A, Aoyagi M. Endoscopic treatment of intranasal glioma in an infant presenting with dyspnea. Auris Nasus Larynx. 2010;37:373–6.

44. Hu J, Ta J, Deisch J, Lee S, Wareham R. Image-guided transoral resection of recurrent parapharyngeal space glial heterotopia. Int J Pediatr Otorhinolaryngol. 2014; 78:366–9.

45. Pons Y, Blancal JP, Vérillaud B, Sauvaget E, Ukkola-Pons E, Kania R, Herman P. Ethmoid sinus osteoma: diagnosis and management. Head Neck. 2013;35:201–4.

46. Boffano P, Roccia F, Campisi P, Gallesio C. Review of 43 osteomas of the craniomaxillofacial region. J Oral Maxillofac Surg. 2012;70:1093–5.

47. McHugh JB, Mukherji SK, Lucas DR. Sino-orbital osteoma: a clinicopathologic study of 45 surgically treated cases with emphasis on tumors with osteoblastoma-like features. Arch Pathol Lab Med. 2009;133:1587–93.

48. Larrea-Oyarbide N, Valmaseda-Castellón E, Berini-Aytés L, Gay-Escoda C. Osteomas of the craniofacial region. Review of 106 cases. J Oral Pathol Med. 2008;37:38–42.

49. Lehmer LM, Kissel P, Ragsdale BD. Frontal sinus osteoma with osteoblastoma-like histology and associated intracranial pneumatocele. Head Neck Pathol. 2012;6:384–8.

50. Harned RK, Buck JL, Olmsted WW, Moser RP, Ros PR. Extracolonic manifestations of the familial adenomatous polyposis syndromes. AJR Am J Roentgenol. 1991;156:481–5.

51. Smud D, Augustin G, Kekez T, Kinda E, Majerovic M, Jelincic Z. Gardner's syndrome: genetic testing and colonoscopy are indicated in adolescents and young adults with cranial osteomas: a case report. World J Gastroenterol. 2007;13:3900–3.

Sinonasal Malignancies

© Springer International Publishing Switzerland 2016
M.S. Brandwein, *Textbook of Head and Neck Pathology*,
DOI 10.1007/978-3-319-33323-6_4

Abstract

One way to tame the diagnostic diversity of sinonasal malignancies is a problem solving approach that categorizes tumors into basic histological patterns (e.g. small blue round cell, basaloid, epithelioid, rhabdoid, etc). For example, rhabdomyosarcoma shares space next to INI-deficient carcinoma as both have rhabdoid elements. Melanoma shares space next to the dendritic cell sarcomas, as both enter the differential diagnosis of epithelioid tumors. But this approach has its limitations; tumor heterogeneity is just one of many limitations. Flipping pages, "matching pictures", seeking quick Google answers, are all for rookies. There is no substitute for patiently studying and "listening" to slides. Some tumors refused to be tamed. BRD4-NUT Translocation Midline Carcinoma, a newly described entity with important treatment considerations shares space here with "basaloid" carcinomas. But tumor morphology is really quite variable. This particular diagnosis transcends histology, requiring confirmation of the NUT-BRD translocation (either by FISH or immunohistochemistry). Happily, nut midline carcinoma seems to be the only member of the list below which transcends histology to such a degree. In retrospect, re-examining many "foolers" (for instance, adamantinoma-like EFT) will reveal some histological "off-ness" with respect to the initial diagnosis. The vast majority of sinonasal malignancies still can be diagnosed correctly (on resection, if not biopsy), using a solid histopathologic foundation and a rational immunohistochemical approach.

Keywords

Sinonasal undifferentiated carcinoma · BRD4-NUT Translocation Midline Carcinoma · INI-deficient Sinonasal Carcinoma · Ewing's Family Tumor · Dendritic cell sarcoma · Sinonasal extranodal NK/T-cell lymphomas · Sinonasal Teratocarcinosarcoma

Glossary

BRD4-NUT Translocation Midline Carcinoma defined by specific balanced translocation of chromosomes 15 (*NUT* (**nu**clear protein in **t**estis) gene) and 19 *BRD* (**bro**mo**d**omain-containing protein)

Follicular dendritic cell sarcoma The most common dendritic cell sarcoma: CD21+, CD23+, and CD35+

Interdigitating cell sarcoma CD123+, negative for CD21, CD23, CD35

Sinonasal extranodal NK/T-cell lymphomas endemic to Asia, Central America, and South America, with natural killer (NK), NK *precursor* or T-cell phenotype, EBV+

PAX3-FOX01, PAX7-FOX01 balanced translocations detected in 60%, and 20% of alveolar rhabdomyosarcomas, respectively

Homer-Wright pseudorosettes tumor cells aligned around neurofibrillary processes

Flexner-Wintersteiner rosettes glandular structures formed by columnar/cuboidal cells, evidence of true olfactory differentiation.

Glomangiopericytoma synonym for sinonasal hemangiopericytoma, which is not hemangiopericytoma-*like*, but is the real deal.

Biphenotypic sinonasal sarcoma an emerging entity associated with following translocations: PAX3-MAML3, PAX3-NCOA1, or PAX3-FOXO1. May represent low-grade sinonasal fibrosarcoma that varies with additional mesenchymal differentiation and the degree of reactive changes of Schneiderian mucosa.

Key Points

- The importance of recognizing BRD4-NUT Translocation Midline Carcinoma is in its unresponsiveness to usual chemotherapy protocols. Patients should be referred for clinical trials using bromodomain inhibitors (BETi) and histone deacetylase inhibitors (HDACi).
- Consider the dendritic cell sarcomas when dealing with a keratin negative epithelioid neoplasm. Nuclear grooves, deep invaginations, and multinucleated/syncitial tumor cells are characteristic histologic findings.
- 20% of Ewing's family tumor (EFT) are histologic variants (atypical EFT); confirmation of *EWS-FLI1* fusion can be useful for this group.

4.1   Small Blue Round Cell ± Basaloid

4.1.1   Sinonasal Undifferentiated Carcinoma (SNUC)

SNUC is an unfortunate, high-grade malignancy lacking any specific differentiation [1–6]. Most patients with SNUC present with large tumors extending beyond the sinonasal tract into orbit and brain. Not uncommonly, some sort of occupational exposure history can be elicited. SNUC has been reported in a 12 year-old child [7], in a 19 year-old with Gorlin's Syndrome [8], and in conjunction with multifocal heterotopic neuroglia [9]. An aggressive clinical course is common and patients may develop distant metastases to lungs and bone. An overall disease-specific mortality rate of 52.7% was established by systematic literature review of 167 patients [10]. Aggressive multimodality treatment approach is recommended [11–14].

■ Histopathology

SNUC is one of the most pleomorphic sinonasal malignancies encountered. It can form solid, discohesive sheets of tumor cells mimicking lymphoid neoplasia, or discrete carcinomatous islands mimicking squamous carcinoma, or trabeculae and ribbons in a loose stroma mimicking a neuroendocrine carcinoma (☐ Fig. 4.1). SNUC is an exclusionary diagnosis; the key to recognizing SNUC is excluding tumors demonstrating keratinization or gland

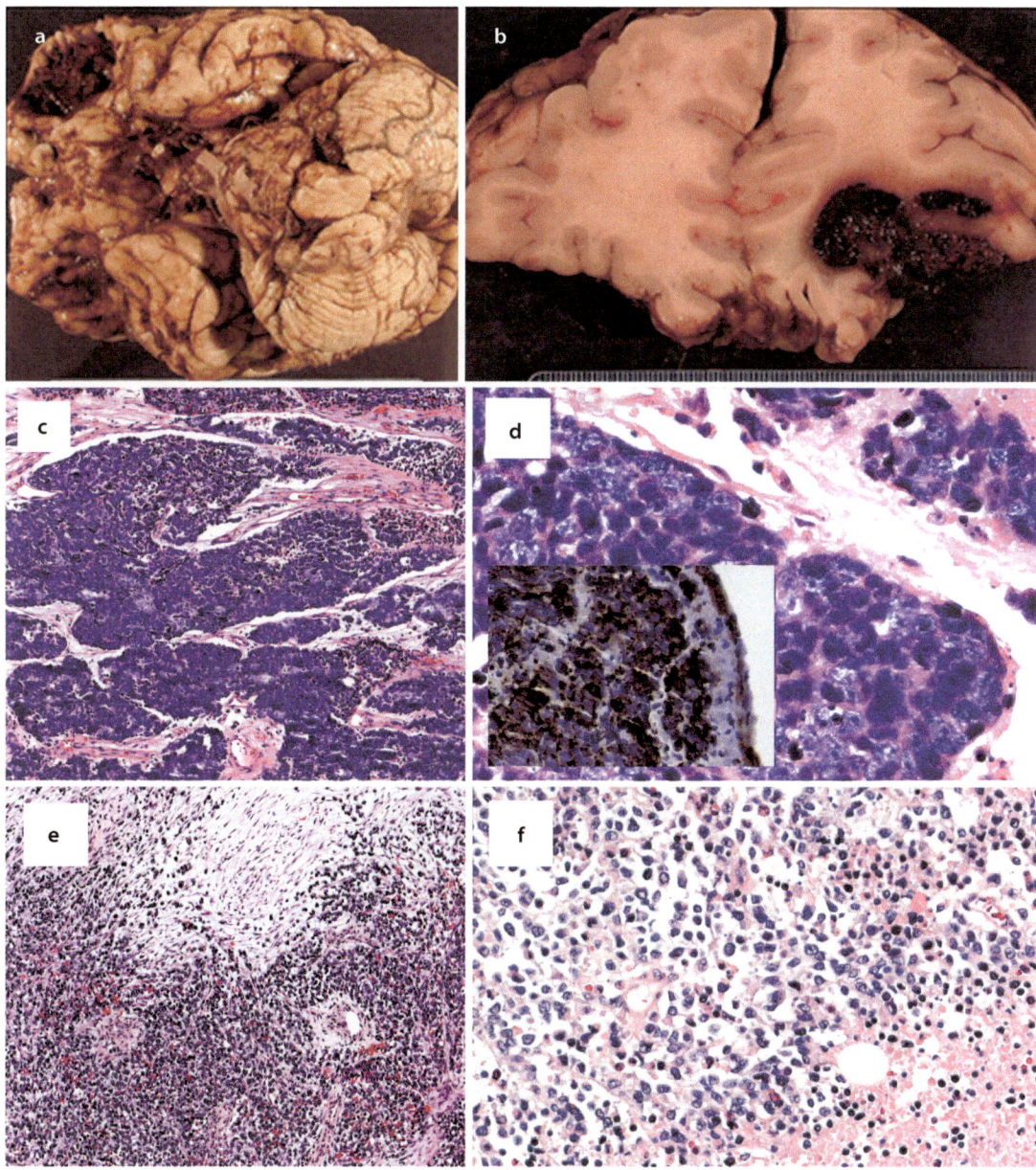

☐ **Fig. 4.1** Sinonasal undifferentiated carcinoma (SNUC) – (**a**, **b**) Intracranial extension of SNUC. (**c**) Poorly-differentiated carcinoma with cohesive islands. (**d**) Highly pleomorphic tumor cells. No cytoplasmic keratinization should be seen by light microscopy. *Inset*: Immunohistochemistry for keratin. (**e**, **f**) Another example of SNUC, which is more discohesive

formation (■ Fig. 4.2). Tumor cells are highly pleomorphic with high nuclear/cytoplasmic ratio. The carcinoma cells can be small or large, round or spindled. Nuclear chromatin is coarse and nucleoli are prominent. Mitotic activity is very brisk. Necrosis and tumor vascular emboli are common features. Although evidence of squamous differentiation excludes the diagnosis of SNUC, mucosal *in-situ* carcinoma can be seen. Osteoclast-like giant cells are a rare feature of SNUC. Immunohistochemically, SNUC will express cytokeratins and EMA; expression of S100, NSE and p63 is rare (■ Table 4.1).

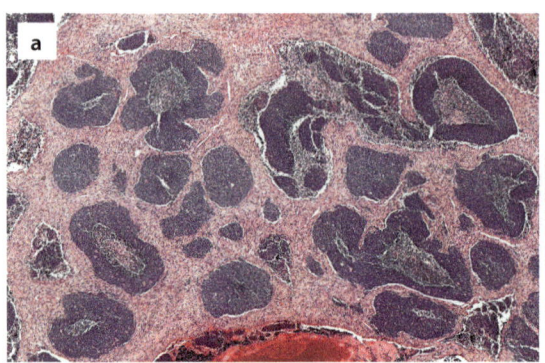
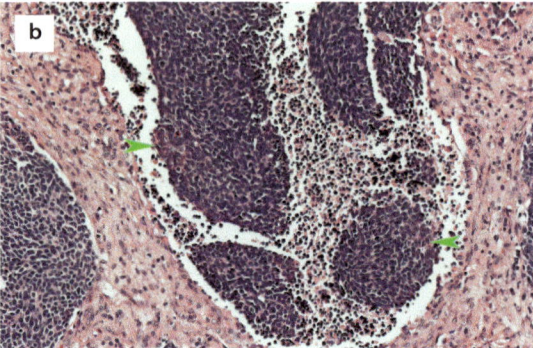

■ Fig. 4.2 (**a**) Poorly differentiated squamous cell carcinoma. (**b**) Finding focal keratinization (*arrows*) excludes the diagnosis of SNUC

■ Table 4.1   Sinonasal malignancies: selected differential diagnoses

Tumor	General features
Sinonasal Undifferentiated Carcinoma (**SNUC**)	No keratinization or intercellular bridges should be seen in SNUC Invariably high-grade and usually high-stage tumor (■ Fig. 4.1) CK8+ 100%, CK19+ 50%, CK7+ 50%, NSE+ 18%, EMA+ 18%[immunoquery 2/19/15] P63 negative or focal [11] Diffuse p16+ unrelated to HPV [12]
Squamous cell carcinoma (**SCC**)	Basaloid or poorly differentiated SCC – Look for keratinization or intercellular bridges (■ Fig. 4.2)
BRD4-NUT Translocation Midline Carcinoma (**NMC**)	Monotonous basaloid tumor cells, rounded nuclei, abrupt keratinization in 33% of NMC (■ Fig. 4.3). Presence of EBV should be excluded. Diagnosis can be established FISH with probes for 15q14 NUT breakpoint, or diffuse nuclear expression of NUT protein by IHC
Sinonasal HPV-related Adenoid-Cystic-like Carcinoma	Intermediate- to high-grade adenoid cystic carcinoma with evidence of myoepithelial differentiation. Limited ductal differentiation. Associated with high-risk HPV
Nasopharyngeal Carcinoma	Thenasopharynx and nasal cavity are anatomically contiguous, but pathologically worlds apart. Beware of potential anatomic confusion on pathology requisition forms Nasopharyngeal carcinoma is frequently EBER+, p63+
Melanoma	Primary sinonasal melanoma is more common than metastatic disease. Pleomorphic epithelioid, sarcomatoid, or plasmacytoid tumor cells, abundant mitoses S100+ 96%, Mart-1 88%, HMB45 45%, MITF+ 76% [immunoquery 2/19/15]
Sinonasal Neuroendocrine Carcinoma (**SNEC**)	Greater pleomorphism than ONB, with mixed carcinomatous and neuroendocrine features

◘ **Table 4.1** (continued)

Tumor	General features
Olfactory Neuroblastoma (**ONB**)	Origin: superior nasal cavity. Relatively bland with finely dispersed chromatin. Even Hyams Grade III/IV ONB is less pleomorphic than SNEC. Homer-Wright pseudorosettes and psammomatoid calcifications can be seen. **Synaptophysin** +, **chromogranin** +, **calretinin + Cam5.2 + 31** %[immunoquery 2/19/15]
INI-deficient Sinonasal Carcinoma	Sinonasal carcinoma lacking overt squamous or glandular differentiation, with subtle rhabdoid tumor cell component and complete loss of SMARCB1 (INI) expression by IHC
Ewings Family Tumor (EFT)	EFT: Current nomenclature for Primitive Neurectodermal Tumor/ Ewing's Sarcoma. Monotonous neoplasm with a number of variants, characterized by *EWS-FLI1* fusion (>90%), followed by *EWS-ERG*. Rarer *EWS* fusion partners: *ETV1, E1AF*, and *FEV*. **Diffuse CD99 + FLI1 +**
Rhabdomyosarcoma	Should be considered in the differential diagnosis for adult, as well as pediatric sinononasal tumors. See discussion for the wide range of histology Desmin+, MyoD1+, degree of nuclear myogenin expression can correlate with histologic variants. INI expression preserved FISH with FOX01 break-apart probe for diagnosis of alveolar rhabdomyosarcoma

4.1.2 BRD4-NUT Translocation Midline Carcinoma (Nut Midline Carcinoma, NMC)

NMC represents a rare, recently described aggressive variant of squamous carcinoma defined by a specific balanced translocation of chromosomes 15 and 19. Although NMC may develop in childhood, it occurs over a wide patient age range. More than one third of NMC arise in the head and neck; other sites include mediastinum and lung. A recent report including outcome data on 54 NMC patients revealed a 2-year progression-free survival rate of only 9%, a 2-year overall survival rate of 19%, and a median overall survival was 6.7 months [15]. Importantly, NMC are not responsive to standard chemotherapeutic agents.

As a variant of squamous carcinoma, NMC is uniquely characterized by a simple genetic karyotype. The *NUT* (**nu**clear protein in **t**estis) gene on chromosome 15 is translocated to chromosome 19, partnering with *BRD4* (**br**omodomain-containing protein **4**) in the majority of NMC. An alternative rearrangement partner is *BRD3-NUT* for a subset of NMC (Nut-variant carcinomas) [16–20]. NUT protein is expressed solely in testicular or ovarian post-meiotic germ cells. BRD protein is a member of the BET family of chromatin readers (**b**romodomain and **e**xtra **t**erminal). BRD binds acetylated chromatin-binding bromodomains which are important to the recruitment of positive transcriptional elongation factors. It is hypothesized that the BRD-NUT fusion protein promotes proliferation and blocks differentiation through a cascade of p300 activation, BRD4-NUT accumulation, and further p300 sequestration. The fusion protein leads to overall decreased chromatin acetylation and decreased transcription of differentiation genes through downstream activation of *MYC*. The impact of the fusion protein is reversed by blocking either *BRD-NUT* or *MYC* activation [20]. Blocking *BRD-NUT* results is irreversible squamous differentiation and tumor growth arrest. There is ongoing development of molecular targeted therapies for NMC patients using bromodomain inhibitors (BETi) and histone deacetylase inhibitors (HDACi).

■ **Histopathology**

NMC is composed of islands of monotonous basaloid tumor cells, with round nuclei and an undifferentiated appearance. "Abrupt kerati-

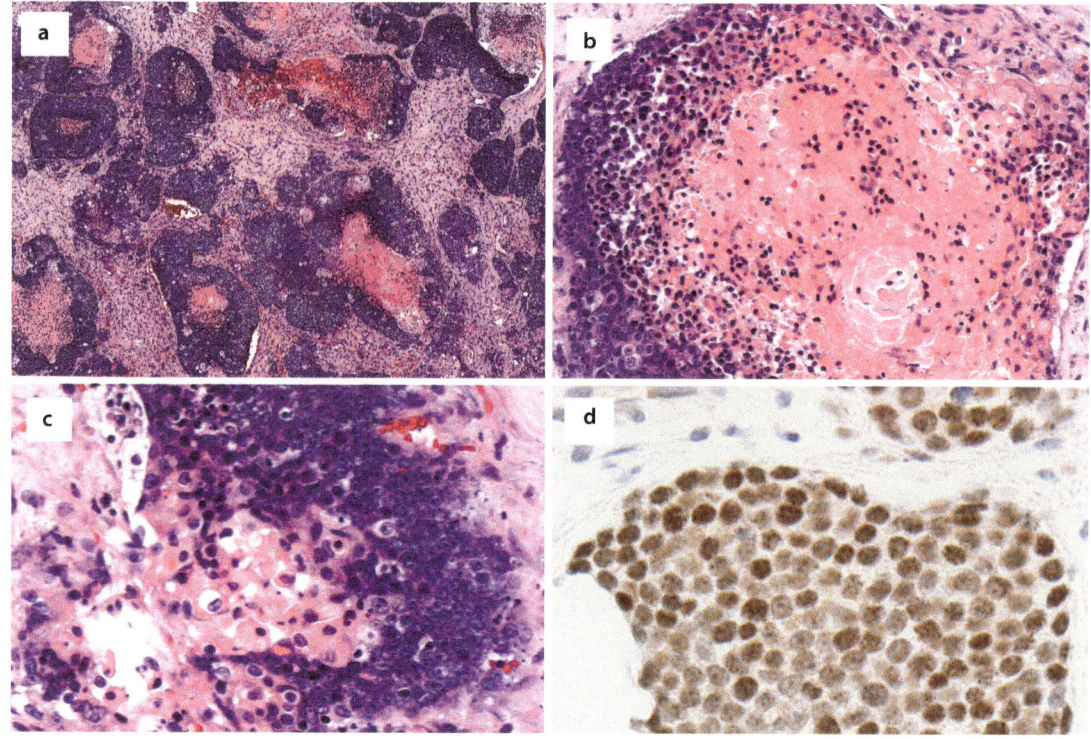

☐ **Fig. 4.3**   BRD4-NUT Translocation Midline Carcinoma – (**a**, **b**) Islands of "small blue round cell neoplasm" with central eosinophilia. (**c**) "Abrupt keratinization" adjacent to undifferentiated malignant cells. (**d**) Nuclear expression of BRD4-NUT fusion protein (Courtesy of Dr. Christopher French, MD)

nization" is seen in 33 % of cases (21/63); seeing this should bring the possibility of NMC to mind (☐ Fig. 4.3). The "abruptness" refers to the sharp delineation between the areas of squamous differentiation and undifferentiated malignant component. However, the majority of NMC lack abrupt keratinization. Other histologies associated with NMC include anaplastic carcinoma, poorly-differentiated carcinoma, round cell tumor, and trabecular and cord-like patterns [21]. Mesenchymal chondroid differentiation has been described [22].

The diagnosis of NMC can be established by immunohistochemistry. The NUT protein is diffusely expressed with a speckled nuclear pattern (Cell Signaling, Danver, MA). IHC for NUT protein has been recommended in the work-up of all poorly-differentiation midline carcinomas in children and adolescents. The IHC profile of NMC includes variable expression of Cam 5.2, CK7, CK20, and p63. IHC markers for muscle and neuroendocrine differentiation, CD99, Fli-1, and EBER, are all negative. NMC has also been associated with p16 over expression, unrelated to HPV [23].

4.1.3   Sinonasal Human Papillomavirus-Related Adenoid-Cystic-Like Carcinoma

Sinonasal Human Papillomavirus-related Adenoid-Cystic-like Carcinomais recently proposed nosology for a group of sinonasal malignancies that are similar, if not identical, to intermediate- or high-grade adenoid cystic carcinomas [24–27]. Sinonasal Human Papillomavirus-related Adenoid-Cystic-like Carcinoma is composed of basaloid tumor cells forming cribriform, microcystic, or solid patterns with well-delineated fibrous tumor stroma. Peripheral pallisading of tumor cells may be seen. Myoepithelial differentiation is confirmed (calponin, s100, p63, actin). These tumors can be associated with squamous carcinoma-*in-situ*, although this does not exclude, *a priori*, the diagnosis of adenoid cystic carcinoma. Ductal differentiation is minimal and perineural invasion is uncommon; the lack of these features is atypical for adenoid cystic carcinomas. The "adenoid cystic-*like*" terminology was based on the absence of *MYB-NF1B* rearrangement by FISH in six studied cases. The *MYB-NF1B* rearrangement can be detected by FISH in archival samples in 44, and 49 % of adenoid cystic carcinomas [28, 29]. Human papillomavirus (HPV) status was accessed first by ISH; a large group of adenoid cystic carcinomas were screened using high-risk HPV probes and then HPV type-specific probes. ISH positive cases were validated by quantitative polymerase chain reaction (qPCR) with GP5/6 consensus primers. It would have been more appropriate to use qPCR for initial screening, as this technique is much more sensitive than ISH. HPV 31/33, followed by HPV16 were the most common HPV types. Earlier, Boland and colleagues demonstrated HPV by ISH in 2 of 27 adenoid cystic carcinomas; interestingly both tumors were sinonasal and high-grade. *MYB-NF1B* rearrangement was not assessed in this study [30]. No associations between HPV, sinonasal origin, or high-grade, were found in 50 adenoid cystic carcinomas studied by our group [31]. More studies will be necessary to establish if these HPV+ sinonasal carcinomas are truly distinct from conventional adenoid cystic carcinoma.

4.2 Small Blue Round Cell ± Epithelioid

4.2.1 Transitional Variant Squamous Carcinoma

The transitional variant of squamous carcinoma is included here as it's common in the sinonasal tract, and frequently enters into the differential diagnosis of sinonasal small blue round cell tumors.

▪ Histopathology
The transitional variant of squamous carcinoma is composed of smooth ribbons and rounded islands of nonkeratinizing carcinoma resembling urothelial carcinoma, hence the appellation "transitional" (◘ Fig. 4.4). The criteria for diagnosing invasive bladder carcinoma (small irregular shaped islands, desmoplastic reaction) does not apply in the present context. The transitional variant of squamous carcinoma is characterized by a pushing, nonaggressive, pattern of invasion. It is the abundance of these smoothly contoured ribbons of carcinoma that mitigates against the possibility of an "in-situ" carcinoma. The transitional variant demonstrates

◘ **Fig. 4.4** Squamous carcinoma, transitional variant – Histologic variants of squamous carcinoma will be covered in "Volume 2, Chapter 8: Oral Cavity: Malignant and Precursor Lesions". However, the transitional variant is common in the sinonasal tract and may enter the differential diagnosis of "small blue round cell tumors". (**a**) A question often heard regarding this morphology is, "How far would you go?" The implication is that there *should* be some hesitancy in diagnosing invasion. (**b**) On the contrary, the transitional pattern is an example of "nonaggressive pattern of invasion". The smooth ribbon-like contours should not dissuade one from recognizing invasion, albeit non-aggressive. What is true in one context (e.g. urinary bladder) is not necessarily true in a different context. Look for the "Down/Up" orientation – reflecting the polarity of tumor maturation. One side of the ribbon recapitulates the basal reserve layer (*white and blue arrowheads*). The opposite side recapitulates mucosal maturation, with flattening of tumor cells (*white and red arrowheads*)

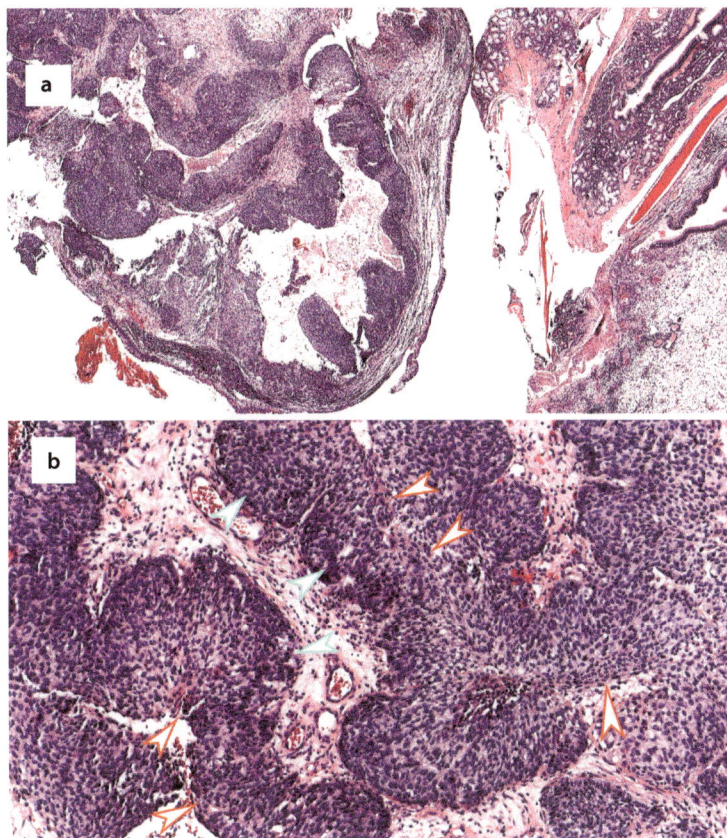

the polarity of maturation. One side of the ribbon recapitulates the basal reserve layer and is composed of basaloid tumor cells with limited cytoplasm. The opposite side of the ribbon recapitulates mucosal maturation, with flattening of the tumor cells. Identifying this polarity on a biopsy excludes the possibility of an adenocarcinoma.

4.2.2 Sinonasal Melanoma (SNM)

Mucosal melanomas represent 1.3 % of all melanomas, the most common site is the sinonasal tract. However, sinonasal melanomas (**SNM**) are extremely rare, with an incidence of 0.05 cases/100,000 population as per the SEER (Surveillance, Epidemiology, and End Results) tumor registry [32]. Nasal cavity, especially nasal septum, is most commonly affected [33–37]. Antral involvement is usually secondary to nasal cavity origin. It is extraordinarily rare for primary SNM to arise in the ethmoids, frontal, or sphenoid sinuses [36]. Patient age range is 50–70 years. An initial diagnosis of SNM need not prompt cutaneous work-up. When skin melanomas metastasize to the head and neck, it is usually in the context of disseminated

disease, and involves larynx or pharynx. The overall patient prognosis for SNM is extremely poor. SEER data demonstrates an overall 5-year survival rate of 24 % [33]. Most patients with SNM who develop local recurrence ultimately die of disease. Occasional patients with SNM remain disease-free for long periods, only to develop explosive, fatal recurrence.

The 6th AJCC edition (American Joint Cancer Committee) staged SNM along with all other sinonasal malignancies. A distinct SNM staging scheme debuted in the 7th AJCC edition, notable for the omission of the T1/T2 categories [38, 39]. ▣ Tables 4.2 and 4.3 present the new 8th AJCC staging criteria for all sinonasal malignancies, and specifically for mucosal melanomas which includes SNM, respectively [40]. Note the addition of extranodal extension (ENE); this upstages N status. ENE_g (gross extranodal extension) is defined as tumor extension either grossly apparent to the naked eye at the time of dissection, or microscopic extension > 2 mm beyond lymph node capsule.

Primary surgery is the therapeutic mainstay; published data support the idea that postoperative adjuvant radiotherapy improves locoregional control, although overall survival is not impacted [41, 42].

▣ **Table 4.2**   American Joint Cancer Committee staging criteria (8th edition) sinonasal malignancies

Maxillary sinus		
	TX	Primary tumor cannot be assessed
	To	No evidence of primary tumor
	Tis	*Carcinoma-in-situ (CIS)*
	T1	Tumor limited to sinus mucosa, no bony erosion/destruction
	T2	Tumor with bony erosion/destruction including hard palate and/or middle nasal meatus Excludes extension to posterior maxillary wall/pterygoid plates
	T3	Tumor invades bone of posterior maxillary wall, subcutaneous tissues, orbital floor, medial orbit, pterygoid fossa and/or ethmoids
	T4a	Tumor invades anterior orbit, skin of cheek, pterygoid plates, infratemporal fossa, cribriform plate, sphenoid or frontal sinuses
	T4b	Tumor invades orbital apex, dura, brain, middle cranial fossa, cranial nerves other than maxillary division of trigeminal nerve, nasopharynx, or clivus
Nasal cavity and ethmoid sinuses		
	Tx	Primary tumor cannot be assessed
	To	No evidence of primary tumor
	Tis	*Carcinoma-in-situ*
	T1	Tumor restricted to one subsite with/without bony invasion

◘ **Table 4.2**	(continued)
T2	Tumor invades two contiguous subsites or extends into an adjacent region within the nasoethmoidal complex, with/without bony invasion
T3	Tumor invades medial orbit, orbital floor, maxillary sinus, palate, or cribriform plate
T4a	Tumor invades anterior orbital contents, skin of nose or cheek, minimal anterior cranial fossa extension, pterygoid plates, sphenoid or frontal sinuses
T4b	Tumor invades orbital apex, dura, brain, middle cranial fossa, cranial nerves other than maxillary division of trigeminal nerve, nasopharynx, or clivus

Regional lymph nodes (N)

Nx	Cannot be assessed
No	No regional lymph node metastasis
N1	Metastasis in a single ipsilateral lymph node ≤ 3 cm, no ENE*
N2a	Metastasis in a single ipsilateral or contralateral lymph node ≤ 3 cm with ENE* or single ipsilateral lymph node > 3 cm but ≤ 6 cm, no ENE*
N2b	Metastasis in multiple ipsilateral lymph nodes ≤ 6 cm, no ENE*
N2c	Metastasis in bilateral or contralateral lymph nodes, ≤ 6 cm, no ENE*
N3a	Metastasis in a lymph node > 6 cm, no ENE*
N3b	Metastasis in a single ipsilateral node > 3 cm in greatest dimension with ENE* or multiple ipsilateral, contralateral or bilateral nodes any with ENE*

Distant metastasis (M)

Mx	Cannot be assessed
Mo	No distant metastasis
M1	Distant metastasis

Reproduced with permission from AJCC Cancer Staging Manual 8th edition, 2016

Resected positive lymph nodes require examination for presence and degree of extranodal extension (ENE). ENE_m (microscopic extranodal extension) is defined as ENE ≤ 2 mm. ENE_g (gross ENE) is defined as either tumor extension apparent to the naked eye dissection, or microscopic extension > 2 mm beyond lymph node capsule. Either ENE_g or ENE_m is used to define pathological ENE+ nodal status.

Anatomic stage and prognostic groups			
If T...	and N...	and M...	then stage
CIS	0	0	0
1			1
2			2
3			3
1, 2, 3	1		
4a	0, 1		4A
1, 2, 3, 4a	2		
Any T	3		4B
4b	Any N		
Any T		1	4C

▫ Table 4.3 American Joint Cancer Committee staging criteria (8th Edition) for mucosal melanomas (which includes SNM)

Primary tumor (T)

T3	Polypoid mass involving mucosa and soft tissues, regardless of size
T4a	Melanoma involving cartilage, bone, deep soft tissue, skin
T4b	Advanced melanoma involving brain, dura, lower cranial nerves (CIX, X, XI, XII), masticator space, prevertebral space, carotid artery, mediastinum

Regional lymph nodes (N)

Nx	Cannot be assessed
No	No regional lymph node metastasis
N1	Regional lymph node metastases present

Distant metastasis (M)

Mo	No distant metastasis
M1	Distant metastasis

Reproduced with permission from AJCC Cancer Staging Manual 8th edition, 2016

Anatomic stage and prognostic groups

If T...	and N...	and M...	then stage
3	0	0	**3**
4a			**4A**
3, 4a	1		
4b	Any N		**4B**
Any T		1	

■ Mutations

The mutational profile of SNM differs from cutaneous melanoma; few SNM patients might actually benefit from *BRAF* or *cKIT* targeted therapies. Generally, mutually exclusive *NRAS*, *BRAF*, and *cKIT* mutations are most common in cutaneous melanomas. Activating *NRAS* mutations are frequent in sun-damage melanomas, whereas *BRAF*V600E mutations are more common in non-sun exposed melanomas. *KIT* mutations are least common in cutaneous melanomas, and more common in mucosal melanomas. SNM mutational profiling demonstrates that *NRAS* muta-

tions are most common, and detected in 14–22 % of cases [43–46]. *NRAS*, *cKIT*, and *BRAF* mutations are also mutually exclusive in SNM. *cKIT* mutations are detected in 4–18 % of SNM, and activating mutations are not predicted by immunohistochemistry. The *BRAFV600E* mutation, a treatment target typical of non-ultraviolet related skin melanomas, has not been detected in SNM.

■ Histopathology

Melanoma is characterized by five possible cell phenotypes: epithelioid, spindled, undifferentiated, pleomorphic, and clear cell types. Epithelioid melanoma cells are large, with abundant pink "dirty" cytoplasm and vesicular nuclei with prominent pinkish nucleoli (▫ Fig. 4.5). Spindled melanoma cells mimic sarcoma. Undifferentiated melanoma cells are small to medium, with dark nuclei and high nuclear/cytoplasmic ratio. They may have a plasmacytoid appearance with eccentric nuclei and intranuclear holes. The pleomorphic phenotype is self-descriptive. Clear melanoma cells vary in size from small to large "balloon-cells" (▫ Fig. 4.6). All melanomas are invariably mitotically active.

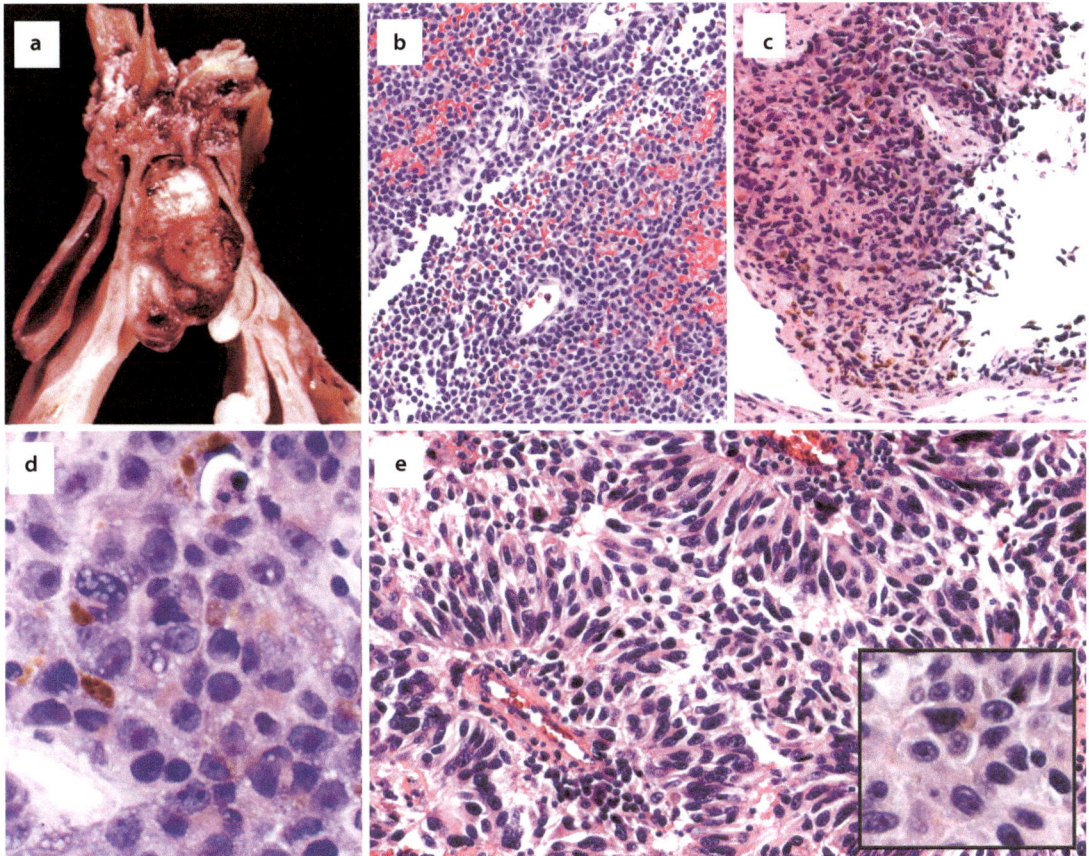

Fig. 4.5 Melanoma – (**a**) Polypoid pigmented tumor in the superior nasal cavity. (**b**) Discohesive undifferentiated plasmacytoid cells. (**c**) Infiltrating pleomorphic cells and melanophages. (**d**) Note intranuclear holes and amphophilic nucleoli. (**e**) Metastatic melanoma from primary oral melanoma, 19 years prior. Note the deceptive neuroendocrine appearance of the spindled melanoma cells as they form perivascular trabeculae (*Inset*: Cytoplasmic melanin)

Melanoma can form a number of possible growth patterns with variable degree of cohesion. The organoid nested pattern is most commonly seen. Melanoma can form syncitial sheets; it can also be discohesive and form alveolar patterns. Trabecular and pseudopapillary growth patterns are possible. Sarcomatoid spindled melanoma produces interlacing fascicles (**◘** Fig. 4.7). The peritheliomatous pattern demonstrates viable melanoma cells closest to vessels, and necrotic tumor away from vessels.

In evaluating resection specimens, the adjacent mucosa should be evaluated for Pagetoid spread of melanoma cells (**◘** Fig. 4.6). The melanoma cells stand out as larger, atypical, epithelioid cells with clearing artifact between the melanoma cells and epithelium.

Immunohistochemical profile: S100+ 96%, Mart-1 88%, HMB45 45%, MITF+ 76% immunoquery 2/19/15

A rare potential immunohistochemical pitfalls is that melanomas can express epithelial markers and desmin [47, 48].

◘ Table 4.4 details histologic findings which are significantly predictive of outcome [37, 49–51]. These variables should be included in the pathology report as it will allow for better data abstraction by tumor registries, which enhances the level of pathology detail in the SEER database.

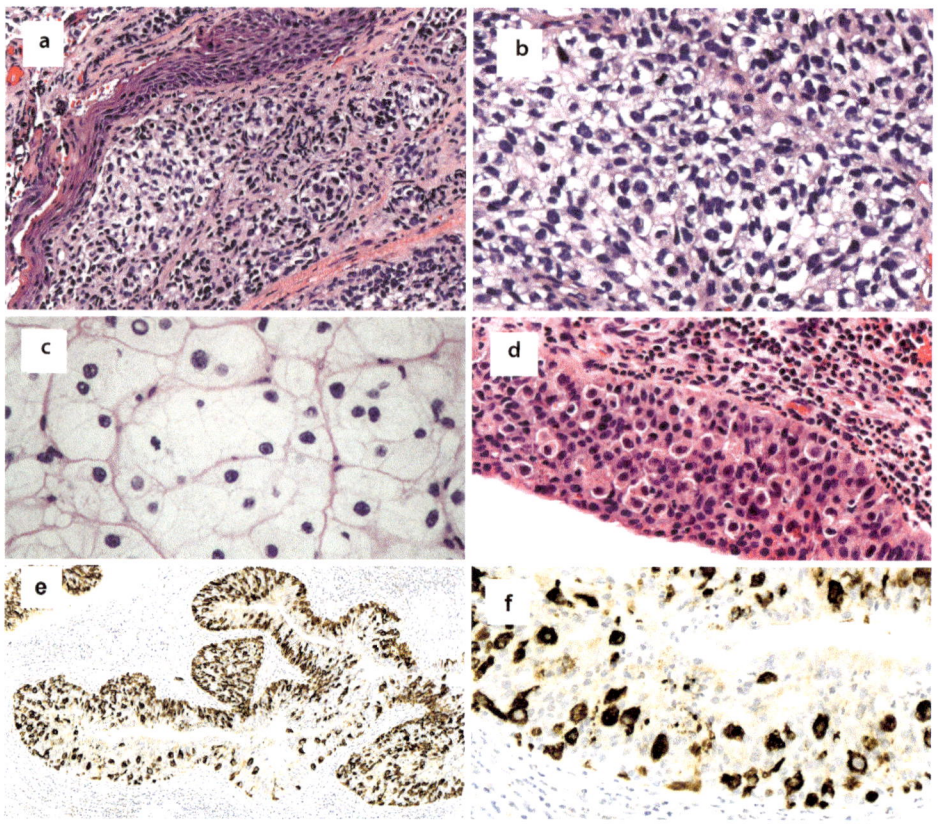

◘ **Fig. 4.6**   Melanoma – (**a**, **b**) Clear cell variant. (**c**) Balloon cell melanoma – notice intranuclear holes. (**d**) Intramucosal Pagetoid spread of melanoma in adjacent respiratory mucosa. The melanoma cells stand out as larger, atypical, epithelioid cells with clearing artifact between the melanoma cells and epithelium. (**e**, **f**) The full extent of Pagetoid spread of melanoma is revealed with IHC for S100

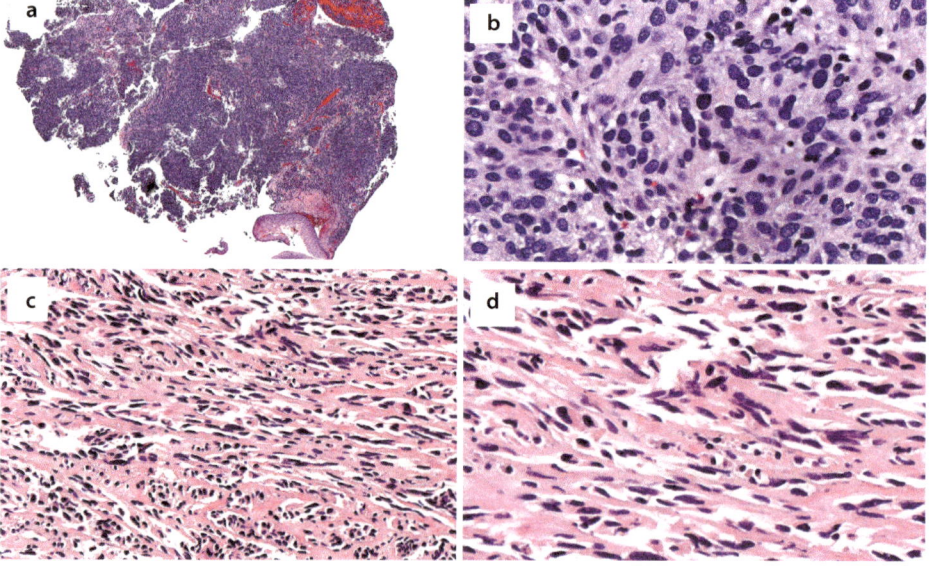

◘ **Fig. 4.7**   (**a**, **b**) Nasal septal melanoma, epithelioid and spindled morphology. The abundant cytoplasm has a "tinge of tan". (**c**, **d**) Metastatic melanoma, spindle cell variant. This tumor strongly expressed S100, but not HMB-45 or MART-1, typical of the spindle cell and desmoplastic variants

□ Table 4.4 Potential histologic prognosticators for sinonasal melanoma

Histologic variable	Report	Anatomic sites	Finding
Mitoses	Mochel 2015	Sinonasal	>2 mitoses/mm² correlated with development of local recurrence and metastasis (p = 0.04 each)
	Shuman 2011	Sinonasal, oral	Fewer mitoses/mm² correlated with improved disease-free survival (HR 1.09, 95 % CI 1.03, 1.16, p = 0.002). No cut-off given.
	Thompson 2003	Sinonasal	>10 mitoses/10 HPF correlated with disease specific mortality (p = 0.026)
Predominant undifferentiated histology	Thompson 2003	Sinonasal	Predominant undifferentiated histology (small to medium cells, high nuclear/cytoplasmic ratio, no specific architecture) correlated with disease specific mortality (p = 0.033)
Necrosis	Mochel 2015	Sinonasal	Any necrosis correlated with decreased overall survival (p = 0.04)
Ulceration	Shuman 2011	Sinonasal, oral	Decreased overall survival (HR 3.71, 95 % CI 1.43, 9.63, p = 0.01)
Pseudopapillary architecture	Moreno 2010	Sinonasal	Higher rate of locoregional failure, p = 0.0144
Degree of pigmentation	Moreno 2010	Sinonasal	5 year overall survival, 47.6 %, no pigmentation versus 0 %, grouped levels of pigmentation, p = 0.0183

4.2.3　Dendritic Cell Sarcoma

Dendritic Cell Sarcoma is a neoplastic grouping of rare and related tumors derived from antigen-presenting immune accessory cells. This group includes **Langerhans cell histiocytosis, disseminated juvenile xanthogranulomas, follicular dendritic cell-, interdigitating dendritic cell-, fibroblastic reticular cell-, blastic plasmacytoid dendritic cell-, and true histiocytic sarcomas** are included within this group [52–62]. Dendritic cell sarcomas tend to affect middle-aged individuals without gender predominance, involving lymph nodes or extranodal sites. Although dendritic cell sarcomas only rarely affect the sinonasal tract [63–66], they are discussed in this chapter as one might need to consider these diagnoses when faced with keratin-negative epithelioid tumors (□ Table 4.4). Misdiagnoses are common; dendritic cell sarcomas are often first diagnosed as carcinoma, meningioma, "inflammatory pseudotumor", or "malignant fibrous histiocytoma".

Follicular dendritic cells produce a structural meshwork of antigen presenting cells within lymphoid germinal centers. These cells arise from mesenchymal stromal precursors, and express markers of follicular dendritic differentiation (CD21, CD23, CD35). Follicular dendritic cell sarcomas (FDCS) represent the most common dendritic cell sarcoma; they typically arise in cervical lymph nodes. Extranodal FDCS will affect head and neck sites (tonsils, pharynx). There are two histological FDCS variants: sarcomatoid FDCS, which is composed of spindle cells forming storiform, fascicular, or whorled patterns, and inflammatory pseudotumor-like FDCS, which has a marked lymphoplascytic infiltrate. The hyaline vascular variant of Castleman's disease may also be associated with FDCS.

Interdigitating dendritic cells arise from hematopoetic precursors (Langerhan's cells, myeloid precursors, lymphoid precursors) and are normally present in T-cell rich areas, such as the paracortical region of lymph node. They express S100, CD68, and CD123, but lack Birbeck

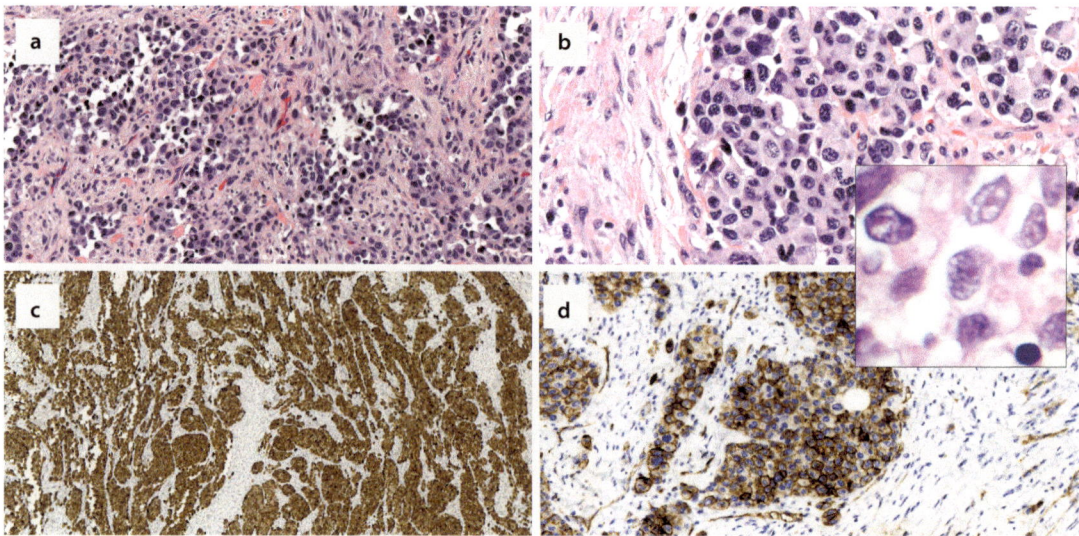

◘ Fig. 4.8   Interdigitating Dendritic Cell Sarcoma: (**a**) Somewhat cohesive epithelioid malignant cells. (**b**) The tumor nuclei are grooved and tapered at one end (*Inset*); they are morphologically distinct from the typical nuclei of squamous carcinoma (**c**) S100. (**d**) CD123

granules, and are CD1a-negative. Interdigitating dendritic cell sarcoma (IDCS) is the second most common dendritic sarcoma. Most commonly, IDCS presents with solitary cervical lymph node involvement; one third of IDCS develop at various extranodal sites. Multifocal systemic IDCS is rare. IDCS have been associated with other hematological or solid malignancies (e.g. B-cell lymphoma, chronic lymphocytic leukemia, mycosis fungiodes).

Dendritic cell sarcomas should be considered at least intermediate-grade sarcomas. They are treated surgically; the decision to include adjuvant radiation and chemotherapy (with lymphoma-type protocols) is made on an individual basis. The prognosis of FDCS is significantly poorer for patients with intraabdominal tumors on multivariate analysis [50]. Patients may develop local recurrence or metastases to other lymph nodes, lung, marrow, or liver.

■ **Histopathology**
Dendritic cell sarcomas are epithelioid, and form a variety of growth patterns. While the first impression they may evoke is that of a carcinoma, in retrospect, there is always something a little "off" in the patterns for carcinoma. The growth pattern

variations are: sheets-like, sarcomatoid fascicles, storiform, circular meningioma-like whorls, follicular-like, trabecular, and pseudovascular (◘ Figs. 4.8, 4.9 and 4.10). As a generalization, carcinomas usually demonstrate architectural homogeneity. Sheet-like, storiform, and fascicular growth patterns speak against the diagnosis of carcinoma. The tumor cells can be spindled, oval, or polygonal, or epithelioid with abundant eosinophilic and fibrillary cytoplasm. Cell membranes are indistinct. The tumor nuclei are oval to round, with vesicular chromatin, thin nuclear membranes, and prominent small to medium nucleoli. Nuclear grooves, deep invaginations and multinucleated/syncitial tumor cells are characteristic findings. Bilobed Reed-Sternberg-like nuclei can be seen. Mitotic activity will be variable. Long interconnected cell processes, an ultrastructural feature, may be discerned on IHC.

It is difficult to distinguish FDCS from IDCS based purely on histology. Both FDCS and IDCS can have intratumoral lymphocytes. Perivascular lymphocytes have been described in FDCS. Plasma cell and eosinophil infiltrate has been observed with IDCS. A sinusoidal lymph node pattern may be observed in IDCS; emperipolesis has also been described in IDCS.

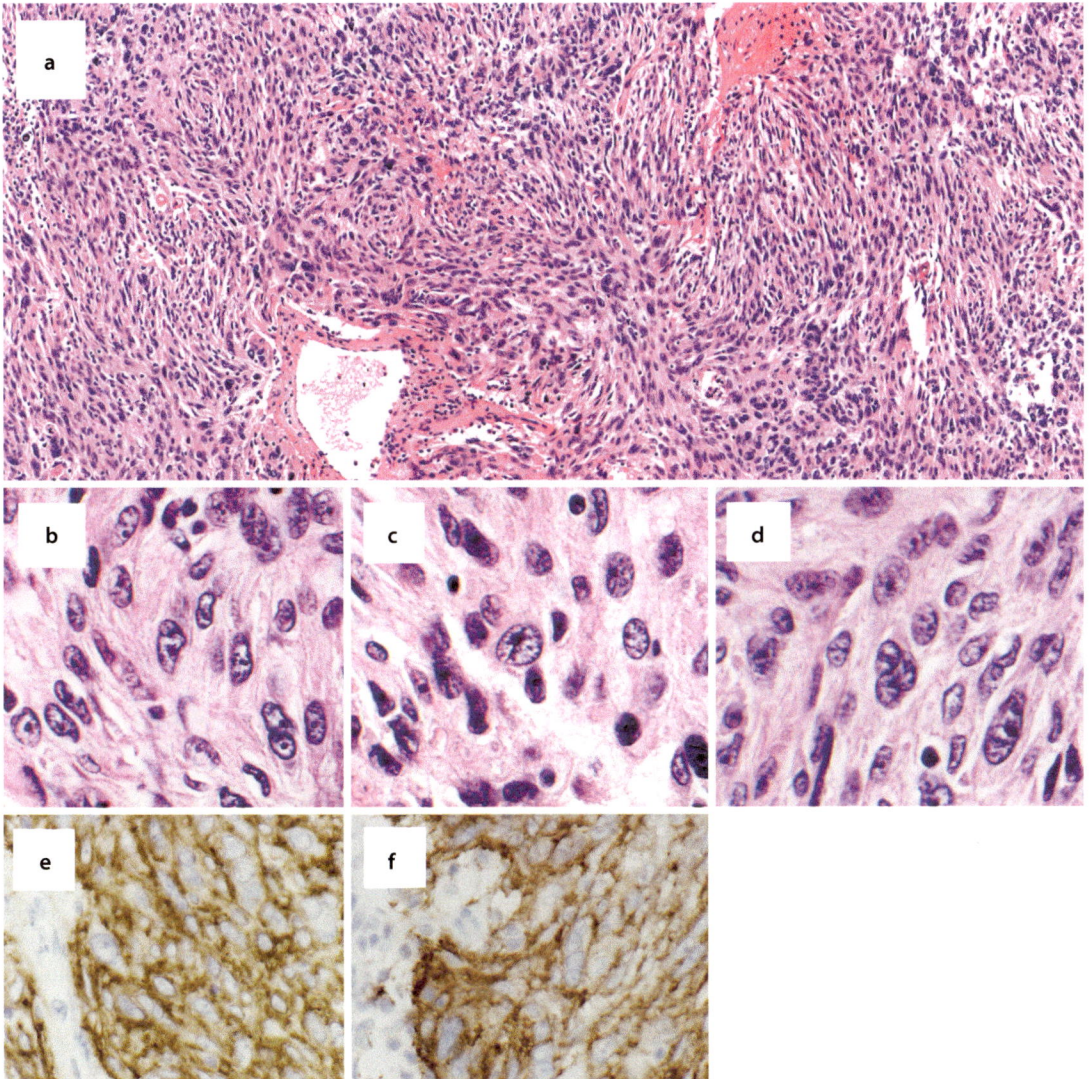

Fig. 4.9 Follicular Dendritic Cell Sarcoma: (**a**) Whorls of spindled tumor cells. (**b**) Nuclei are tapered at one end. (**c**) Cleaved nuclei. (**d**) Multinucleated tumor cells. These findings suggest dendritic cell origin. (**e**) CD21. (**f**) CD35

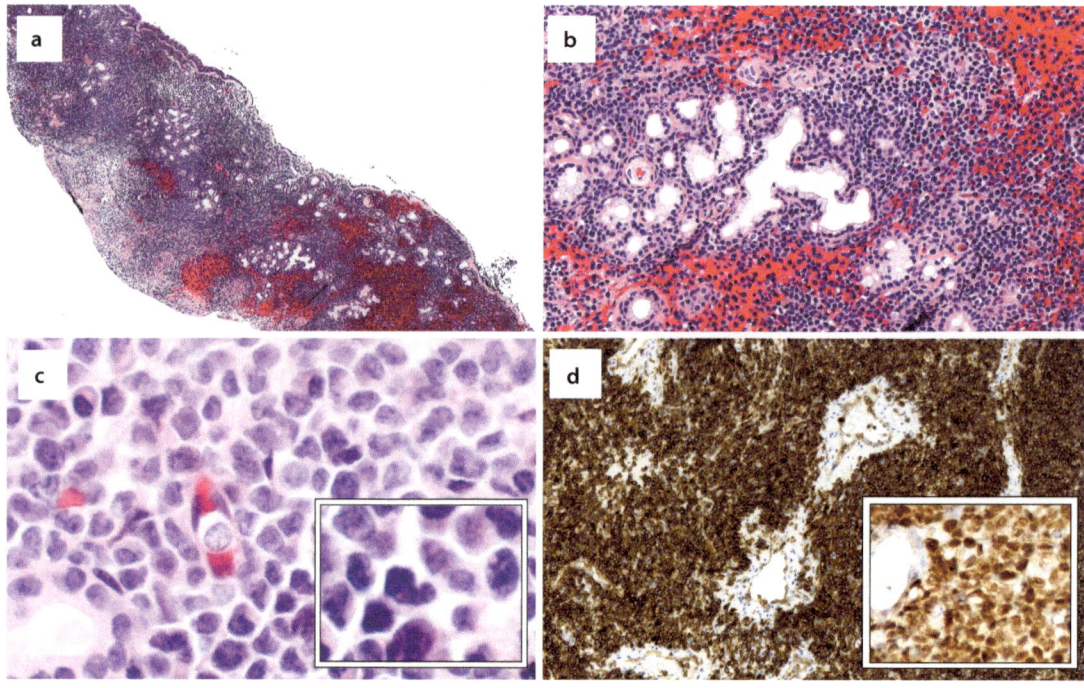

□ **Fig. 4.10**   Blastic plasmacytoid dendritic cell sarcoma: (**a**, **b**) monotonous, discohesive, mononuclear cells. (**c**) *Inset*: Irregular blast-like nuclei with fine chromatin. The neoplasm was CD4dim, CD56hi, CD2dim, CD117dim, HLA-DR hi, nuclear TdT+, and CD45d low/+, by flow cytometry. (**d**) Diffuse CD123 expression. *Inset*: TdT

4.2.4 **Extramedullary Plasmacytoma**

"Plasma cell dyscrasia" describe a disease group characterized by monoclonal proliferation of plasmacytes, orlymphocytoid plasmacytes, producing monoclonal immunoglobulins. **Multiple myeloma (MM)** is the most common disease of this group, which also includes Waldenstrom's macroglobulinemia, heavy chain disease, and primary amyloidosis. Plasmacytic proliferation limited to one bone marrow site is classified as **solitary plasmacytoma (SP)**. The diagnosis of MM is rendered when multiple bone marrow lesions are discovered; MM usually affects patients over 40 years old (median age within sixth and seventh decades) with roughly equal gender distribution. Focal plasmacytic proliferation in **extra-marrow soft tissue** is classified as **extramedullary plasmacytoma (EMP)**. Ten percent of EMP patients have multiple lesions at other soft tissue extramedullary sites. Eighty percent of EMP are diagnosed in the head and neck, most often the sinonasal tract, which is also associated with male predominance [67–73]. Conversely, EMP represents 3–4% of all sinonasal cavity tumors. EMP and MM can overlap; EMP is the initial

manifestation of MM in 5% of patients. EMP may progress to MM in 8–36% of patients. In contrast, SP progresses to MM in 60% of patients.

The diagnosis of a sinonasal EMP should prompt systemic work-up (blood, bone survey, bone marrow study, urine and serum proteins). Small EMP may be treated by primary surgery or radiotherapy, whereas surgery plus adjuvant radiotherapy is indicated for larger EMP. Chemotherapy is reserved for high-grade or large lesions, or refractory/relapsed disease. Local recurrence can develop in approximately 20% of patients with head and neck EMP after a mean of 36 months; the 10-year overall local recurrence–free rate is around 80% [67].

■ **Histopathology**

Tumor histology will follow tumor grade. A diffuse infiltrate of discohesive neoplastic plasma cells is seen. Well-differentiated clonal plasma cells can look completely normal or only mildly atypical. If you see that >5% of plasma cells are bi-nucleated, then be suspicious for a monoclonal plasma cell proliferation. Intranuclear inclusions (Dutcher bodies) can be seen. Mott cells, with grape-like bunches of cytoplasmic globules may also be observed. Moderately-differentiated tumors dem-

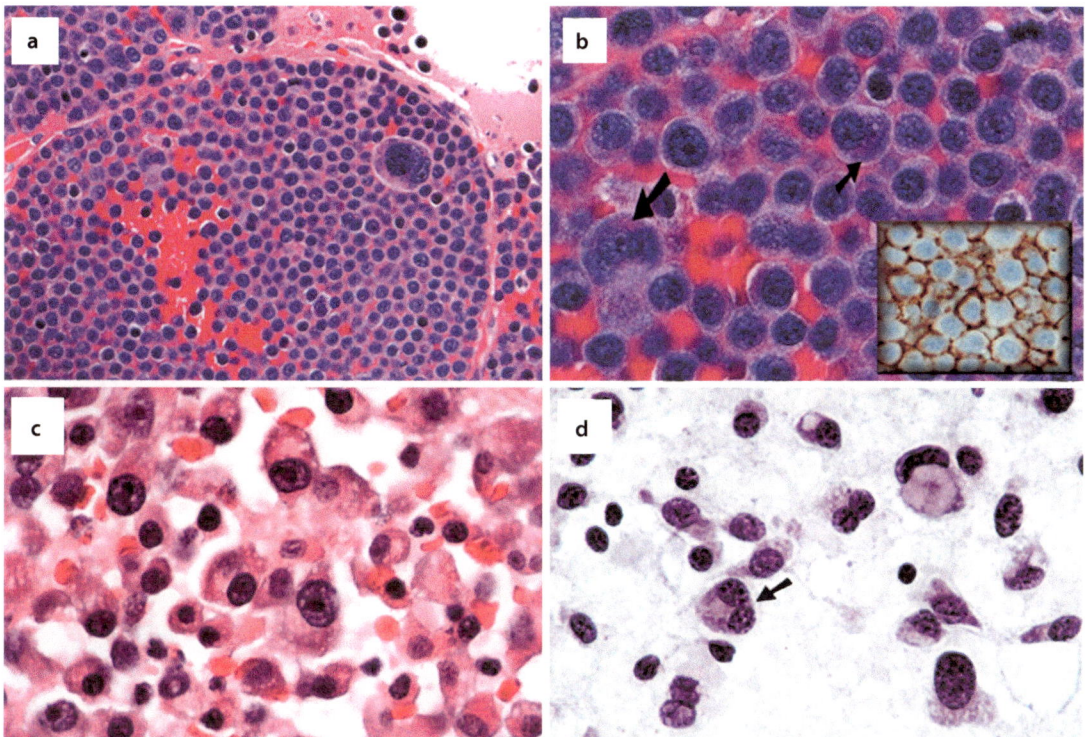

☐ Fig. 4.11 Plasmacytoma: (**a–d**) discohesive atypical plasma cells with characteristic binucleated cells (*arrows*) and perinuclear hofs (*arrows*). *Inset*: Membranous CD138

onstrate moderate atypia and pleomorphism, but are still recognizable as plasmacytic in origin. Chromatin can be recognized as having "clock-face" morphology. A prominent perinuclear hof can be observed; binucleate plasma cells can be seen (☐ Fig. 4.11). Poorly-differentiated plasmacytic tumors are comprised of bizarre malignant cells and multinucleated cells; they are hardly recognizable as plasmacytic. Interspersed among the bizarre cells, some tumor cells with differentiated plasmacytic features (perinuclear hof, clock-face chromatin, binucleate cells) may be observed.

Immunohistochemically, plasmacytes express **CD138**, **EMA**, and lack B-cell markers (**CD20**, **PAX-5**, **and usually CD79a**). With respect to **Kappa/lambda ISH**, the usual light chain clone **is** IgG kappa. Poorly-differentiated extramedullary plasmacytoma may lack light chain production.

4.2.5 Sinonasal T-Cell and B-Cell Lymphomas

Ten percent of head and neck lymphomas are diagnosed at extranodal sites such as Waldeyer's ring, the sinonasal tract, or the thyroid [74]. Sinonasal lymphomas (**SNL**) are more common in Asian populations; they are the second most common extranodal lymphoma after intestinal lymphoma. SNL can be classified as **natural killer (NK)/T-cell** type, **NK** *precursor*/T-cell, and **B-cell**. From a historical perspective, sinonasal extranodal NK/T-cell lymphomas (**SN-ENKTL**) were classified as the nebulous but sinister sounding "lethal midline granulomas". Epstein Barr virus (**EBV**) positive SN-ENKTL are endemic to Asia, Central America, and South America. Western SNL are often diffuse, large, B-cell lymphomas (**SN-DLBCL**), EBV-negative, and affect Caucasians, Asians, or Hispanics. Recent SEER18 database analysis demonstrates that SN-DLBCL are three times more common than SN-ENKTL (1054 versus 328, respectively) [75]. Mean patient age for SN-DLBCL is significantly older than SN-ENKTL (67.8 years versus 51.7, respectively). SN-ENKTL typically localize to the nasal cavity, whereas SN-DLBCL can involve the nasal cavity or maxilla [76–79]. **Angiocentric T-cell lymphomas** characteristically invade around and into vessels, and are associated with necrosis and bone invasion. These lymphomas may be diagnostically challenging as malignant cells are scanty and embedded within dense inflammation.

SN-ENKTL, especially angiocentric variants, may present with, or develop, multiorgan lymphoma affecting skin, liver, larynx, kidney, breast, testis, and prostate. NK/T-cell SNL may also be associated with hemophagocytic syndrome, a fatal complication that may be etiologically associated with EBV reactivation. Sinonasal lymphomas are treated by combination local radiotherapy and chemotherapy, usually with anthracycline-based regimens (CHOP: cyclophosphamide/doxorubicin/vincristine/prednisone). The addition of rituximab has improved outcomes for patients with SN-DLBCL [80]. Patient outcome for SN-ENKTL is significantly poorer compared with SN-DLBCL. The 5- and 10-year disease-specific survival rates for SN-DLBCL, and SN-ENKTL, are 72.8%, and 46.8%, respectively, versus 38.4%, and 13.9%, respectively, in groups matched for age, stage, and treatment [74].

■ **Histopathology**

The most common B-cell SNL is diffuse, large B-cell lymphoma (**SN-DLBCL**). Rarer B-cell SNL subtypes include Burkitt's lymphoma, Burkitt-like lymphoma, and marginal zone B-cell lymphoma types. Large malignant lymphocytes have angulated, irregular nuclear contours, vesicular chromatin, nuclear cleaves, and multiple nucleoli. As a generalization, lymphoma cells are characterized by fine chromatin, as compared with carcinomas, which demonstrate coarse chromatin. Bizarre multilobated nuclei and multinucleated tumor cells are seen. Mitotic activity is brisk. Immunoblastic B-cells have very large, vesicular nuclei, single, prominent, central, pink nucleolus, and plasmacytoid cytoplasm. If >90% of lymphoma cells are immunoblastic, then the tumor should be classified as diffuse large B-cell, *immunoblastic variant*.

SN-ENKTL composed of variable proportion of atypical, small to large T-cells (■ Fig. 4.12). Cytological atypia can vary from slight to pronounced, with large atypical lymphocytes, oval, indented, or convoluted nuclei, and clear cytoplasm. The diagnostic cells can be obscured by necrosis, cellular debris, fibrin, mixed inflammation (■ Fig. 4.13). Look for angioinvasion of atypical lymphocytes which may be limited and subtle (■ Fig. 4.14). The sinonasal seromucinous glands and ducts may also be infiltrated by atypical lymphocytes.

> **SN-DLBCL: CD20+, CD79a+, Pax-5+, CD19+, CD22+,**
> **Plasmacytoid B-cells: CD20−, CD79a+, Pax-5+, CD138+,CD45−**
> **SN-ENKTL: CD4+, no pan-T (CD3−, CD5−)**
> **Most common NK: membranous CD56+/NCAM+**
> **Less common NK: CD16+, CD57+**
> **Less common NK: CD56−, but EBV+, CD4+, cytotoxic markers+(perforin+, TIA+, granzyme B+)**

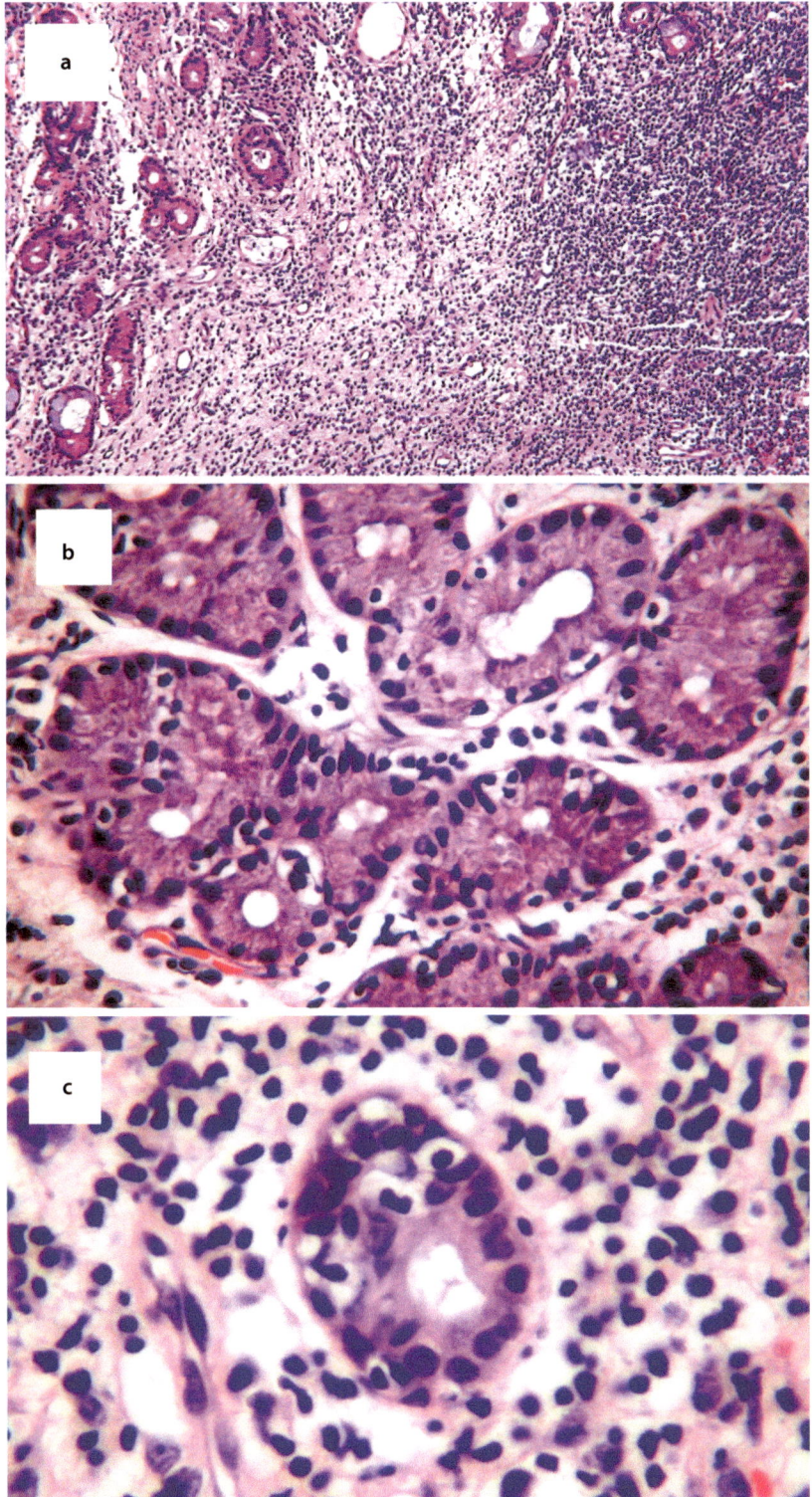

Fig. 4.12 Sinonasal T-cell lymphoma: (**a**) diffuse lymphocytic infiltrate. (**b**, **c**) Atypical angulated lymphocytes (CD3+/CD56−) infiltrate seromucinous ducts. These findings are suspicious for sinonasal T-cell lymphoma. Definitive diagnosis requires T-cell immunoglobulin-like receptor studies

■ **Fig. 4.13** This case illustrates "listening to the slides". A number of technical limitations hampered interpretation of this biopsy. Yet, I noticed how I hyperventilated very time I looked at that slide. The inset demonstrates intraepithelial CD3+ T-cells. Rebiopsy and T-cell receptor studies lead to the diagnosis of **T-cell lymphoma**

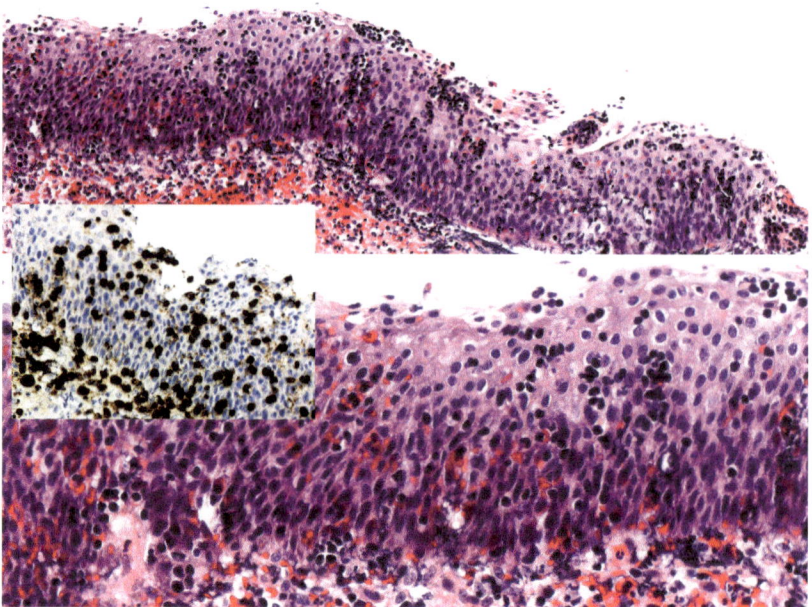

■ **Fig. 4.14** Angiocentric T-cell lymphoma: A necrotic vessel infiltrated by a mixture of atypical T/NK-cells (CD3+, CD56+) and small B cells

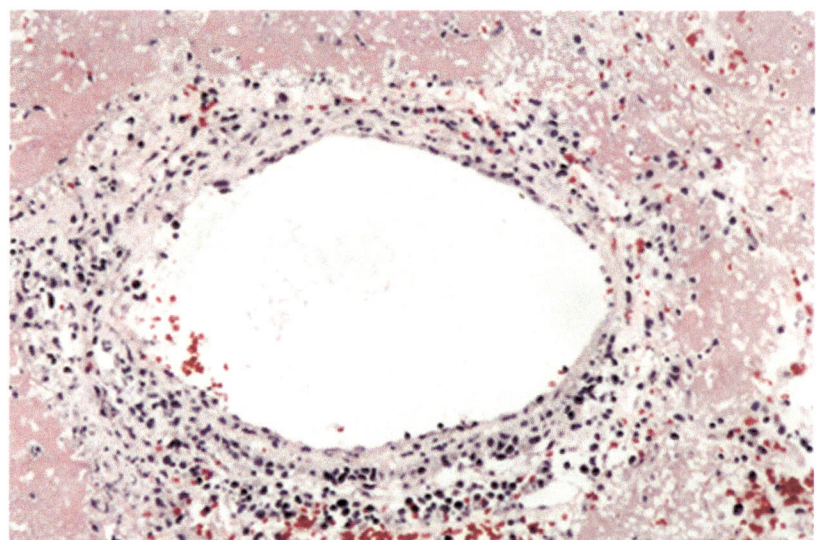

4.3   Small Blue Round Cell ± Rhabdoid ± Myxoid

4.3.1   Rhabdomyosarcoma

Sinonasal rhabdomyosarcoma (SNRMS), which is considered a disease of children and young adults, is an extremely rare malignancy. It should be included in the differential diagnosis of adult sinonasal malignancies as it may be seen at any age. SEER SNRMS data, which commences in 1973, is inherently flawed as diagnoses were not re-reviewed [81, 82]. Reliable institutional studies confirm that the embryonal variant of sinonasal rhabdomyosarcoma is more common in pediatric patients whereas the alveolar variant of sinonasal rhabdomyosarcoma is more common in adults [83–85]. Alveolar rhabdomyosarcoma (**ARMS**) is distinguished from embryonal rhabdomyosarcoma (ERMS) by balanced PAX-FOX01 translocations (also known as PAX-FKHR). PAX3-FOX01 t(2;13)(q35;q14) is detected in 60 % of ARMS; PAX7-FOX01 t(1;13)(p36;q14) is detected in 20 % of ARMS. PAX3 and PAX7 encode transcription factors; FOX01 contains a Forkhead DNA binding domain at its N-terminus and a transcriptional activation domain at its C-terminus. The respective fusion oncoproteins increase transcription of target genes compared to wild-type PAX3 or PAX7. Importantly, 20 % of ARMS are PAX-FOX01 rearrangement-negative, constituting a molecularly heterogenous group that may contain **mixed embryonal and alveolar histologies**; they are associated with a more favorable outcome compared with PAX-FOX01 positive ARMS [86, 87]. Patients with SNRMS are treated by combination surgery, chemotherapy and radiation. ◘ Tables 4.5, 4.6 and 4.7 demonstrate risk stratification based on staging, clinical, and pathological data. Within the subset of patients with SNRMS, age greater than 18 years, and diagnosis of ARMS, are associated with poorer outcomes [83, 84].

■ **Histopathology**

Rhabdomyosarcomas are classified as either **embryonal**-, **alveolar**-, **and pleomorphic-types**, and further subclassified into variants as below. Malignant rhabdomyoblasts have angulated nuclei, prominent nucleoli and a variable amount eosinophilic cytoplasm. The degree of rhabdomyoblastic differentiation varies. Strap cells, tadpole cells, plump rhabdomyoblasts, and wreath cells are evidence of muscle differentiation (◘ Fig. 4.15).

Embryonal rhabdomyosarcoma (ERMS), classic variant: Rhabdomyoblasts embedded in a loose myxoid matrix. Tumor cellular density is variable.

Dense patternvariant ERMS: [88]. The distinction between this variant and ARMS can be challenging. This variant has a solid growth pattern and closely aggregated tumor cells. The rhabdomyoblasts are primitive with scanty cytoplasm, central nuclei, and limited histologic evidence of rhabdomyoblastic differentiation. The degree of nuclear pleomorphism is greater than that seen in ARMS, and there is no alveolar arrangement.

Sclerosingvariant ERMS has been described in children and has an affinity for head and neck. Primitive rhabdomyoblasts are arranged in cords within a dense hyalinized stroma that can may mimic osteoid. Small nests of rhabdomyoblastscan mimic classic ARMS.

Epithelioid ERMS [88] has been described in adults. This variant is composed of large "rhabdoid" cells with round eccentric vesicular nuclei, prominent nucleoli, and abundant eosinophilic to amphophilic cytoplasm. The rhabdomyoblasts form a cohesive sheet-like pattern.

Botryoid ERMS is a grossly polypoid tumor with subepithelial aggregation of rhabdomyoblasts ("cambrium layer").

Spindle variant ERMS is composed of long spindle cells, whorls, intersecting fascicles, resembling smooth muscle neoplasia.

Alveolar rhabdomyosarcoma (ARMS) is characterized by either the PAX3-FOX01 or PAX7-FOX01 rearrangement. The diagnosis is confirmed with the FOX01 break-apart probe and FISH, or RT-PCR for fusion transcripts. Cytologically, ARMS rhabdomyoblasts have scanty eosinophilic cytoplasm and monomorphic round nucleoli, with vesicular chromatin and inconspicuous nucleoli.

▣ **Table 4.5**   Dendritic cell sarcomas: immunohistochemical distinction

	S100	CD68	CD163	CD21[a]	CD23	CD35[a]	CD123	CD1a	KERATINS	CD45
Follicular dendritic cell	±	±	±	+ (may be focal)	+	+ (may be focal)	–	–	–	–
Interdigitating dendritic cell	+	±	±	–	–	–	+	–	–	+
True histiocytic	±	+	+	–	–	–	–	–	–	–
Langerhans histiocytosis	+	±	±	–	–	–	–	+	–	–
Fibroblastic reticular cell tumor[b]	–	–	–	–	–	–	–	–	b	–

[a]CD21/35 cocktail recommended [50]

[b]**Fibroblastic reticular cell tumor** is the rarest dendritic cell sarcoma, which expresses desmin, smooth muscle actin, factor XIIIa, and is further subclassified by keratin expression.

Indeterminate dendritic cell tumors morphologically resemble Langerhans cells and express S100; they are negative for follicular dendritic markers and CD1a

Table 4.6 Rhabdomyosarcoma: AJCC staging

	Primary site	Tumor size	Lymph nodes	Metastases
Stage 1	**Favorable**: Orbit, head & neck (excluding parameningeal), genitourinary (excluding bladder or prostate), bile ducts	Any	Negative/positive	No
Stage 2	**Unfavorable**: Bladder, prostate, extremities, parameningeal (nasopharynx, infratemporal fossa, pterygopalatine fossa, middle ear, and mastoid sinus) or any other non-stage 1 site	≤5 cm	Negative	No
Stage 3	**Unfavorable**	≤5 cm	Positive	No
		>5 cm	Negative/positive	
Stage 4	**Any**			Yes

Reproduced with permission from AJCC Cancer Staging Manual 8th edition, 2016

Table 4.7 Rhabdomyosarcoma – clinical groups

	Lymph nodes	Surgery
Group I	Negative	Complete resection
Group II	Negative	Residual microscopic sarcoma
	Positive	Complete resection
	Positive	Residual microscopic sarcoma
Group III	Negative/positive	Grossly incomplete resection
Group IV	**Distant metastases**	

Classic ARMS is composed of nests of rhabdomyoblasts separated by delicate fibrous septae. There is a discohesiveness in the center and periphery of the nests, which impart the alveolar phenotype (**Fig. 4.16**). **Solid ARMS** is composed of sheets of round rhabdomyoblasts without any intervening fibrous septae. Solid ARMS is the variant most likely to be fusion negative.

Pleomorphic Rhabdomyosarcoma (Adult-type) is composed large, atypical, and bizarre multinucleated polygonal rhabdomyoblasts with a sheet like growth pattern.

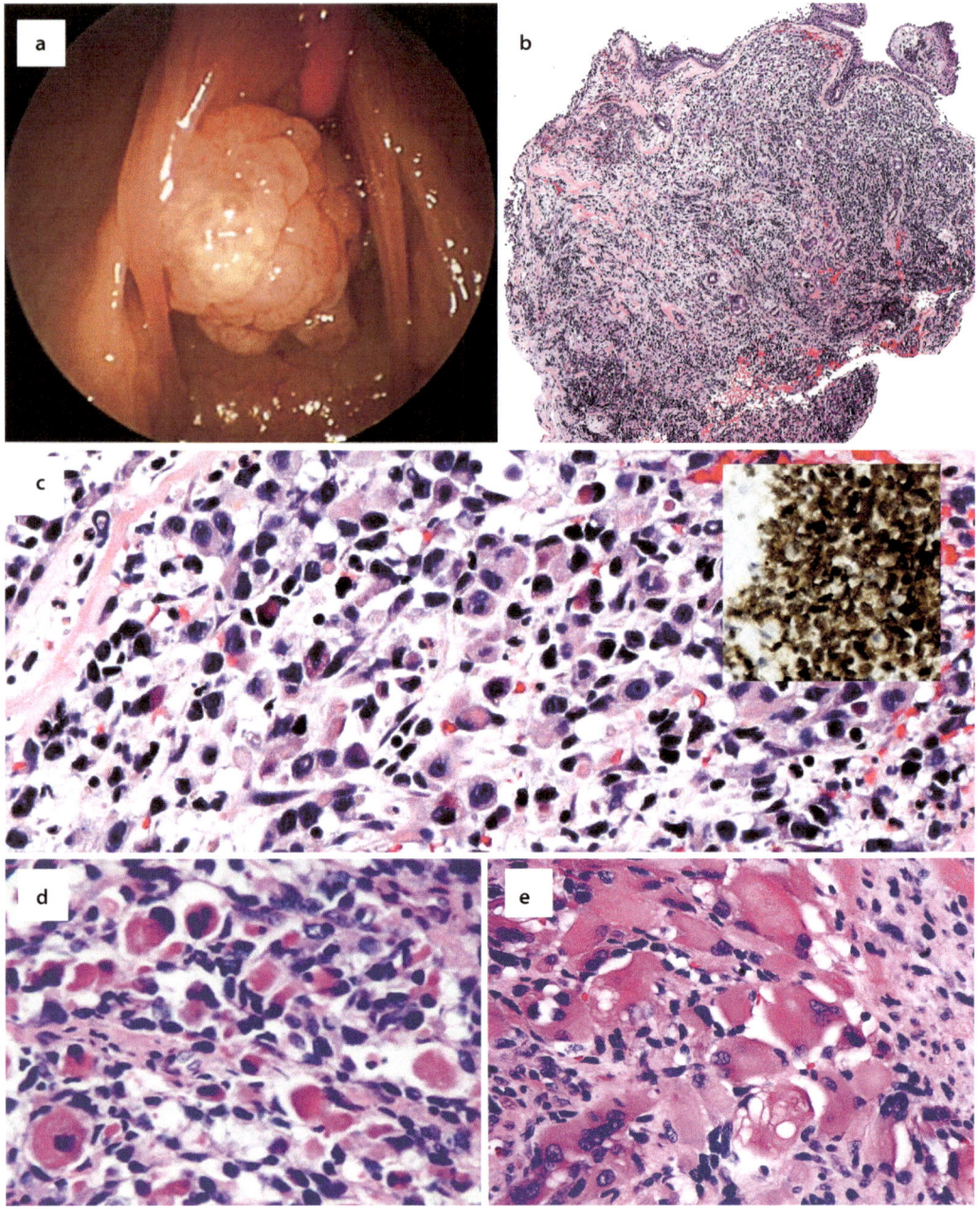

■ **Fig. 4.15** Rhabdomyosarcoma: (**a**) Nasopharyngeal rhabdomyosarcoma in a child, presenting as a papillary polypoid lesion. (**b**, **c**) Pleomorphic rhabdomyosarcoma. *Inset*: Immunohistochemistry for MyoD with nuclear expression. (**d**, **e**) Strap cells

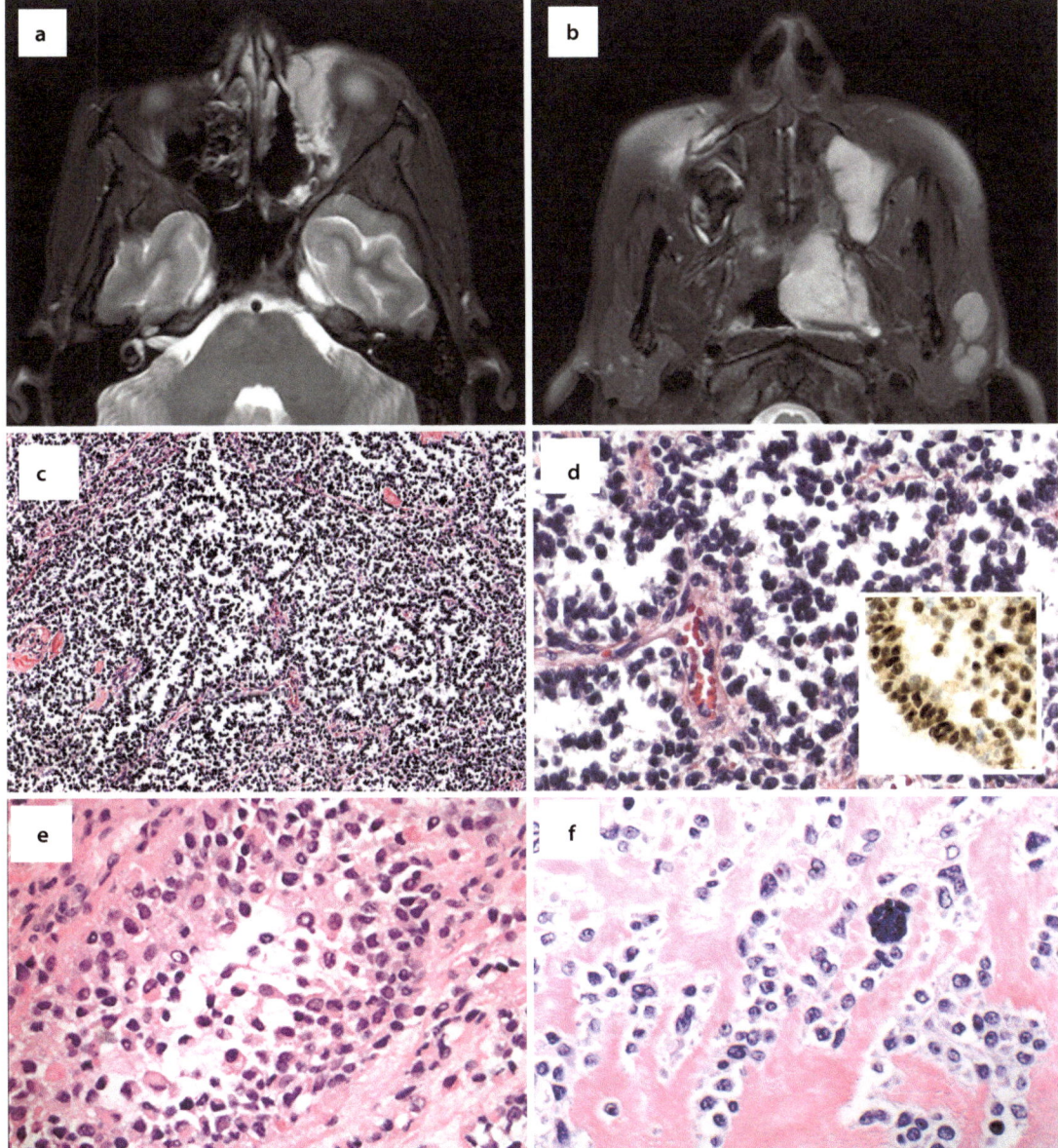

■ **Fig. 4.16** The distinction between **alveolar rhabdomyosarcoma** (ARMS) and embryonal rhabdomyosarcoma (ERMS) has significant therapeutic and prognostic implications. (**a, b**) Axial T2 noncontrast MR scans of a parameningeal ARMS involving orbit, maxilla, and nasopharynx (Courtesy of Dr. Phil Chapman) (**c, d**) Centrally discohesive "small blue round cells" are adherent to fibrous septae. This tumor expressed desmin, myo-D1, myoglobin, and myogenin (*inset*). The PAX3-FOXO01 fusion transcript was detected by PCR, confirming the diagnosis of ARMS. (**e**) Discohesive strap cells forming an alveolar pattern. (**f**) **Sclerosing variant of rhabdomyosarcoma** resembles a "desmoplastic blue round cell tumor"

Immunohistochemistry

Myogenin, nuclear staining:
- ARMS: typically strong and diffuse
- ERMS: typically moderate intensity

- Sclerosing variant ERMS: weak
- Epithelioid variant ERMS: scatteredmyogenin
  MyoD1 (nuclear), desmin (cytoplasmic), INI –
no loss

Cytokeratin expression possible in ARMS [85], epithelioid variant ERMS [89], pleomorphic rhabdomyosarcoma [90].

True rhabdomyoblastic differentiation can also be seen in sinonasal teratocarcinomas, which are extremely rare. It has also been reported in other malignancies (melanoma, malignant peripheral nerve sheath tumor, spindle cell variant of squamous carcinoma) albeit not specific to the sinonasal tract [91, 92].

Rhabdoid features is a histological descriptor of muscle-like morphology (eccentric nucleus, abundant polarized cytoplasmic "tail", filamentous cytoplasmic "rhabdoid" inclusion). Rhabdoid cells show no evidence of skeletal muscle differentiation (Negative for myogenin, MyoD1) (See following section on INI-deficient Sinonasal Carcinoma).

4.3.2 INI-Deficient Sinonasal Carcinoma

This recently described entity is defined by inactivation of tumor suppressor gene *SMARCB1* (*SW1/SNF-related Matrix-associated actin-dependent Regulator of Chromatin subfamily B member 1*) located on chromosome 22q11.2. The SMARCB1 protein (also known as INI-1) is a member of the switch/sucrose nonfermenting (SW1/SNF) chromatin-remodeling complex, which regulates transcription of proliferation and differentiation pathways [93]. Loss of *SMARCB1* is been associated with a diverse group of malignancies (malignant rhabdoid tumor of kidney, renal medullary carcinoma, CNS rhaboid tumor, extraskeletal myxoidchrondrosarcoma), all unified by the histological finding of rhabdoid morphology (eccentric nuclei, cytoplasmic filamentous "rhabdoid" inclusions). More recently, complete loss of SMARCB1 protein has been identified in 6.4% (9/140) of primary sinonasal carcinomas [94]. Five carcinomas harbored homozygous *SMARCB1* deletions (bi-allelic loss), one carcinoma had a heterozygous *SMARCB1* deletion, while two carcinomas (both misdiagnosed as myoepithelial carcinomas) reveals no *SMARCB1* aberration by FISH. Histologically, these carcinomas are infiltrative, necrotic, mitotically active, and lack overt squamous or glandular differentiation. Significant nuclear pleomorphism was also lacking. The degree of rhabdoid phenotype was variable; most often rhabdoid cells were focal. Most commonly, these tumors were diagnosed as nonkeratinizing squamous cell carcinoma, SNUC, or myoepithelial carcinoma (due to plasmacytoid tumor cells). Another report published at the same time described three sinonasal INI-deficient carcinomas with complete loss of SMARCB1 expression, subtle rhabdoid tumor cell component, and prominent basaloid morphology [95]. Greater experience with this group of tumors is necessary.

4.3.3 Sinonasal Low-Grade Myxoid Neoplasia

Sinonasal myxomas, despite the implication of benignity by existing nosology, do have the potential for recurrence and local aggressive behavior. They are discussed here as they may enter into the differential diagnosis of sinonasal rhabdomyosarcomas [96]. Head and neck myxomas can develop in both pediatric and adult patients. Myxomas of the jaw are much more common than head and neck soft tissue myxomas. Mandibular myxomas are more common than maxillary/sinonasal myxomas. However, maxillary/sinonasal myxomas predominate over mandibular myxomas in pediatric patients [97]. The tendency to refer to jaw myxomas as "odontogenic myxomas" is unjustifiable for tumors arising in non-tooth bearing areas and lacking odontogenic epithelium.

Sinonasal myxomas characteristically present with nasolacrimal or nasobuccal soft tissue swelling; skullbase myxomas may present with occular or sinonasal symptoms [98–106]. Radiographically, they can appear as expansile intraosseous radiolucencies with cystic "soap bubbles" or "honey combs". MRI findings reflect high-water content: intermediate to low-signal intensity on T1-weighted images and high-signal intensity on T2-weighted images. Sinonasal myxomas can be confined to the nasal cavity, or extend into paranasal sinuses, skull base, or central nervous system. Grossly, sinonasal myxomas are described as multinodular, gelatinous, and friable. Treatment consists of wide local resection with negative margins; incomplete surgery may result in local recurrence. No metastatic disease has ever been reported.

■ Histopathology

Grossly, myxomas are nonencapsulated. They are composed of stellate and spindled shaped tumor cells embedded in paucicellular mucoid/myxoid matrix (■ Fig. 4.17). Tumor nuclei are long, bland, and hyperchromatic; cytoplasm is basophilic and vacuolated. Tumor cellularity may predict recurrence [107, 108]. Blood vessels can be numerous. Bony invasion may be seen. Mitotic activity is low and necrosis is not pres-

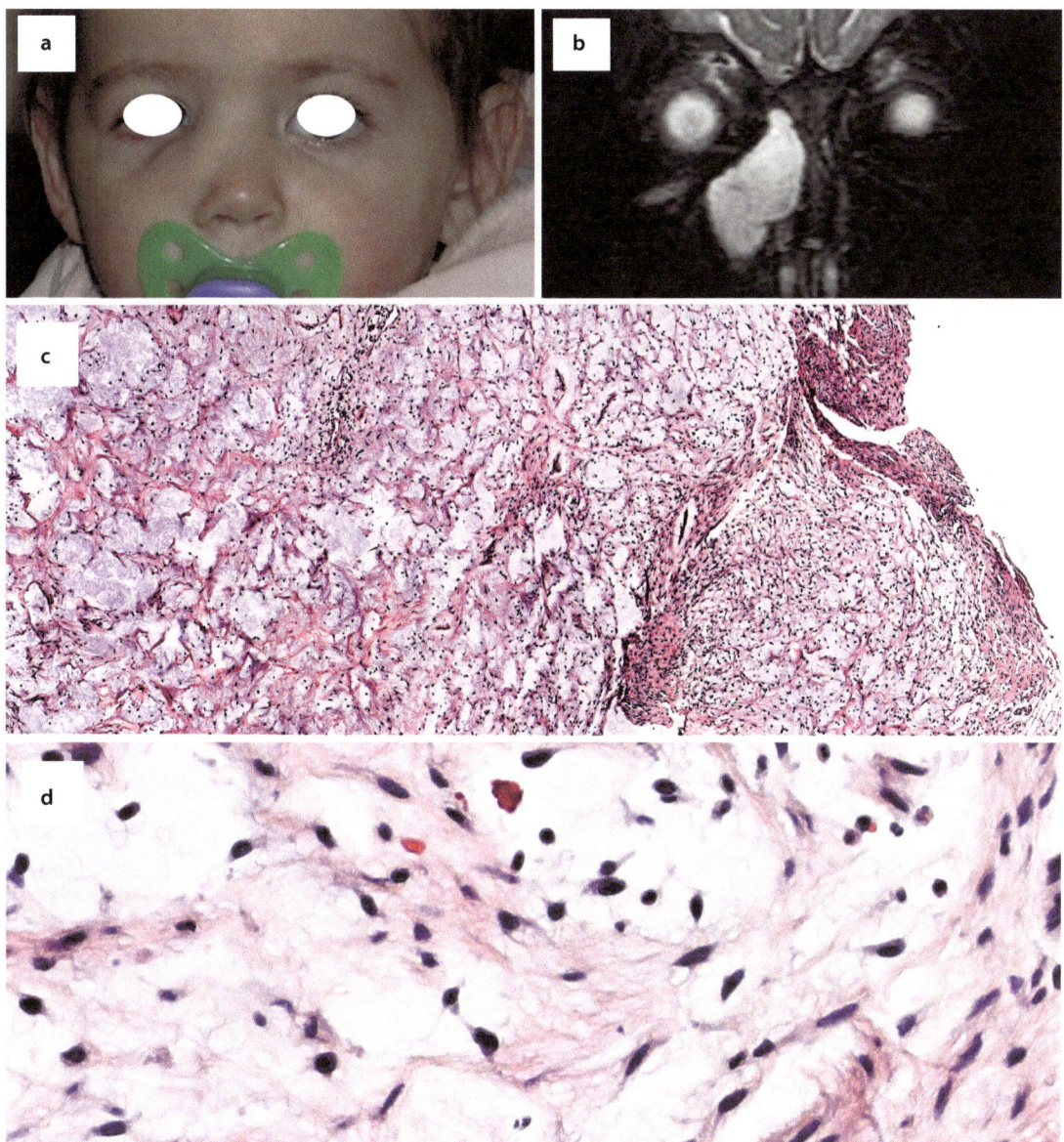

■ **Fig. 4.17**   Sinonasal low-grade myxoid neoplasm may clinically mimic rhabdomyosarcoma. (**a, b**) A periorbital mass and polypoid sinonasal tumor in a 1-year-old girl makes for an alarming presentation. (**c, d**) Low-grade myxoid neoplasm composed of bland stellate tumor cells with condensed dark chromatin. This is from a 13-year old girl who developed local recurrence 3 years after initial excision

ent. Odontogenic epithelium should not be seen. The mucoid/myxoid matrixis composed of mucopolysaccharides (glycosaminoglycans, GAG); the nature of these glycosaminoglycans is reflected it its tinctorial properties on hematoxylin and eosin staining. Sulfated GAG appear basophilic. Nonsulfated GAG is only faintly basophilic. Mesenchymalmucins are glycoproteins which appear variably eosinophilic. The immunohistochemical profile is vimentin+, and negative for S100, smooth muscle actin, desmin, and CD34.

> Glycosaminoglycans = Alcian blue+, Hale's colloidal iron+
>
> Mesenchymal mucin = Faint PAS+, Alcian blue+, Hale's colloidal iron+

- If prominent fibrous or osseous stroma present, then consider other diagnoses such as ossifying fibroma, etc.
- Be aware: small biopsies of sinonasal myxoma may be misdiagnosed as "polyp"
- If prominent fibrous/osseous stroma present, then consider other diagnoses (e.g. ossifying fibroma)

4.4   Small Blue Round Cell Neuronal/Neuroendocrine

4.4.1   Olfactory Neuroblastoma

Olfactory neuroblastoma (ONB, esthesioneuroblastoma) is a neoplasm of **neuronal/neural crest** origin arising from the olfactory mucosa of the superior nasal cavity. Genetically, they are entirely unrelated to PNET (Primitive Nerve Sheath Tumors)/ES (Ewings' sarcomas) (see below) [109–113]. ONB occurs over a wide age range with a peak incidence in the sixth decade. Small, polypoid ONB are limited to the superior nasal cavity and may cause nasal obstruction, epistaxis, and rhinorrhea. Larger ONB can invade adjacent paranasal sinuses, orbit, and skull base, causing orbital symptoms, middle ear symptoms, and pain. The Kadish staging system is based the anatomic extent of primary site disease (Kadish A: nasal cavity only, Kadish B: paranasal sinus involvement, Kadish C: beyond paranasal sinuses). Subsequent modifications to the Kadish system included lymph node status, intracranial extension, and resectability. Histopathologically, the Hyams' four-tiered grading system remains a standard prognosticator and is summarized in Table 4.8 [114–117]. It is commonly collapsed as a two tiered schema (Hyams I/II versus III/IV).

◼ **Table 4.8**   Rhabdomyosarcoma – risk groups

	AJCC stage	Histology	Clinical group
Low-risk group	1	ERMS	I, II, III
	2 or 3	ERMS	I, II
Intermediate-risk group	2 or 3	ERMS	III
	1, 2, 3	ARMS	
High-risk group	4	ERMS or ARMS	IV

Reproduced with permission from AJCC Cancer Staging Manual 8th edition, 2016

The surgical mainstay for ONB is anterior craniofacial resection and Kadish A tumors can be treated by primary surgery alone. Multimodality treatment is indicated for more extensive disease, with the addition of either neoadjuvant or postoperative chemoradiotherapy. The rates of disease progression, manifesting as local recurrence, regional metastasis, or distant metastasis, are around 50%; progression can develop up to two decades after initial treatment. Disease progression is associated with the acquisition of new gene mutations [118].

Outcome analyses for ONB are limited by the rarity of this tumor; historical and SEER data are of little use as they lack pathological re-review in the light of current nosology. An excellent study of 121 ONB by Bell and colleagues demonstrated that collapsed two-tiered Hyam's grading was significantly predictively of disease-free survival on Kaplan Meier analysis, thus justifying its use in guiding adjuvant therapies [114]. They also demonstrated that patient age at presentation, and stage, did not impact disease-specific outcome.

■ **Histopathology**

ONB is composed of relatively uniform cells with scanty cytoplasm that are slightly larger than lymphocytes. ONB nuclei are round to oval with minimal pleomorphism, occasional prominent nucleoli, and either fine chromatin ("salt and pepper") or coarse chromatin. Fibrillary matrix is a general feature of ONB; it corresponds to the neurofibrillary processes of neuronal differentiation. Psammomatoid, lamellated calcifications are another feature, occasionally these calcifications are confluent. Ganglionic differentiation extremely rare [117].

> Homer-Wright pseudorosettes: tumor cells aligned around neurofibrillary processes
> Flexner-Wintersteiner rosettes: glandular structures formed by columnar/cuboidal cells, evidence of true olfactory differentiation.

◘ Table 4.9 discusses the histologic grading features. Grade I ONB is characterized by a lobular and organoid growth pattern and abundant Homer-Wright pseudorosettes (◘ Figs. 4.18 and 4.19). On the other end of the spectrum, grade IV ONB are characterized by sheet-like growth pattern, necrosis, and brisk mitotic activity. The degree of nuclear pleomorphism in Hyams III/IV ONB is still less than that seen in other high-grade malignancies, e.g. sinonasal undifferentiated carcinoma (SNUC), sinonasal neuroendocrine carcinoma (SNEC). If pronounced nuclear pleomorphism is seen, then consider other diagnoses.

Unusual ONB features include divergent differentiation (glandular or squamous) and melanin containing tumor cells [114]. Hyperplastic, invaginated surface respiratory epithelium ("Glandular hyperplasia") juxtaposed to ONB: associated with better prognosis [116].

◘ **Table 4.9** Hyams' grading for ONB

	Architecture	Rosettes	Mitoses	Necrosis	Pleomorphism
I	Organoid lobules, abundant neurofibrillary stroma	May be abundant	None	None	None, uniform cells
II	Organoid lobules and more solid areas	Occasional	Can be seen	None	Moderate
III	Limited neurofibrillary stroma	Occasional	Abundant	Apoptotic cells	Yes
IV	No neurofibrillary stroma	None	Abundant	Yes	Yes

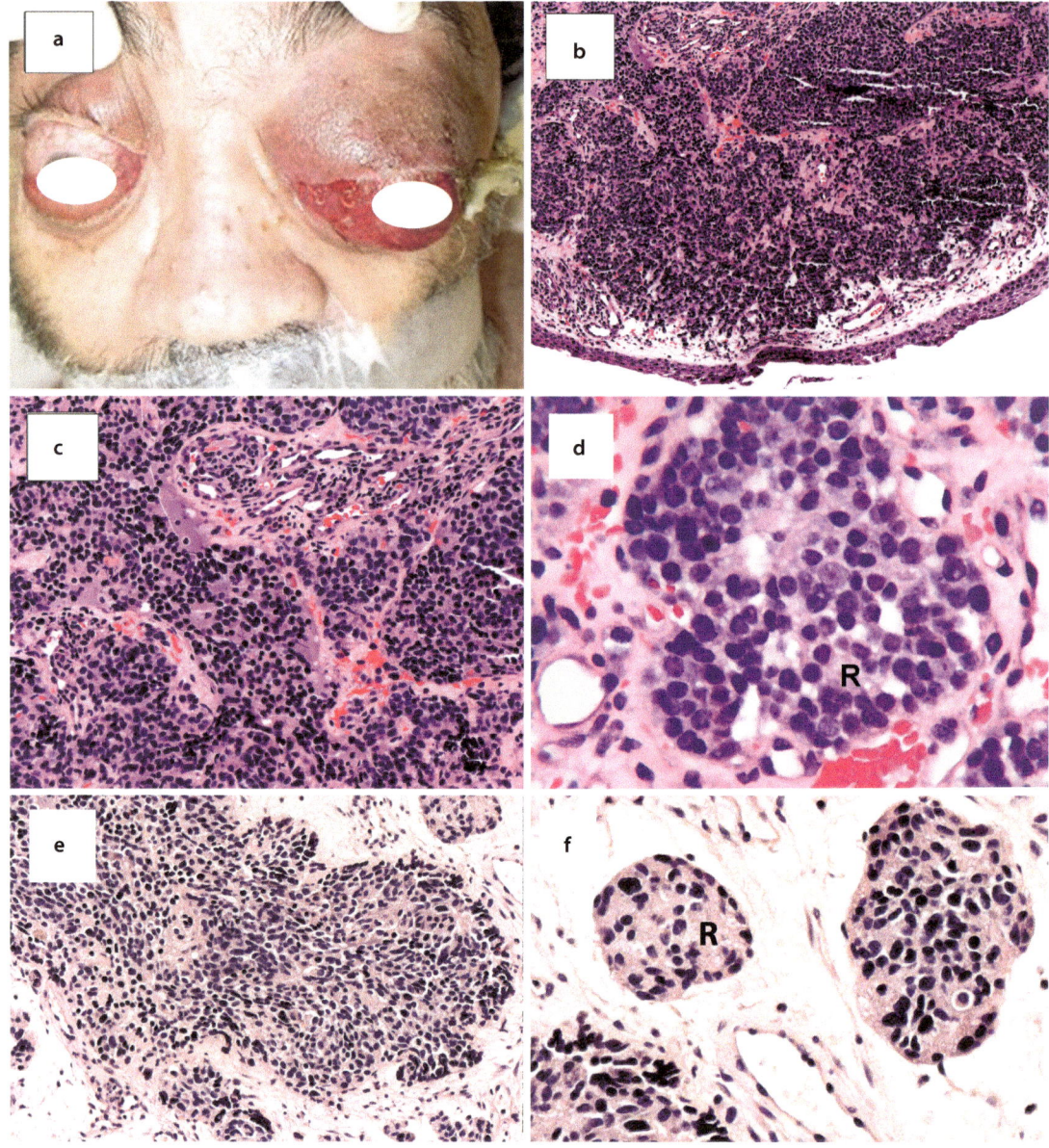

🔹 **Fig. 4.18**   Olfactory neuroblastoma (ONB): (**a**) Massive bilateral proptosis (Courtesy of Dr. Pearl Rosenbaum). (**b–f**) Well-differentiated ONB with lobular/organoid pattern. Homer-Wright rosettes with neurofibrillary deposition (**d**, **f**, *arrows*)

Immunohistochemistry
- **Synaptophysin** +, **chromogranin** +
- **Calretinin** + [119]
- **p63 and p40**: negative or focal [120]

- **S100+** corresponds to sustentacular cells, which directly correlates with differentiation
- Variable expression of cytokeratins, GFAP, neurofibrillary protein, CD57, CD56, EMA

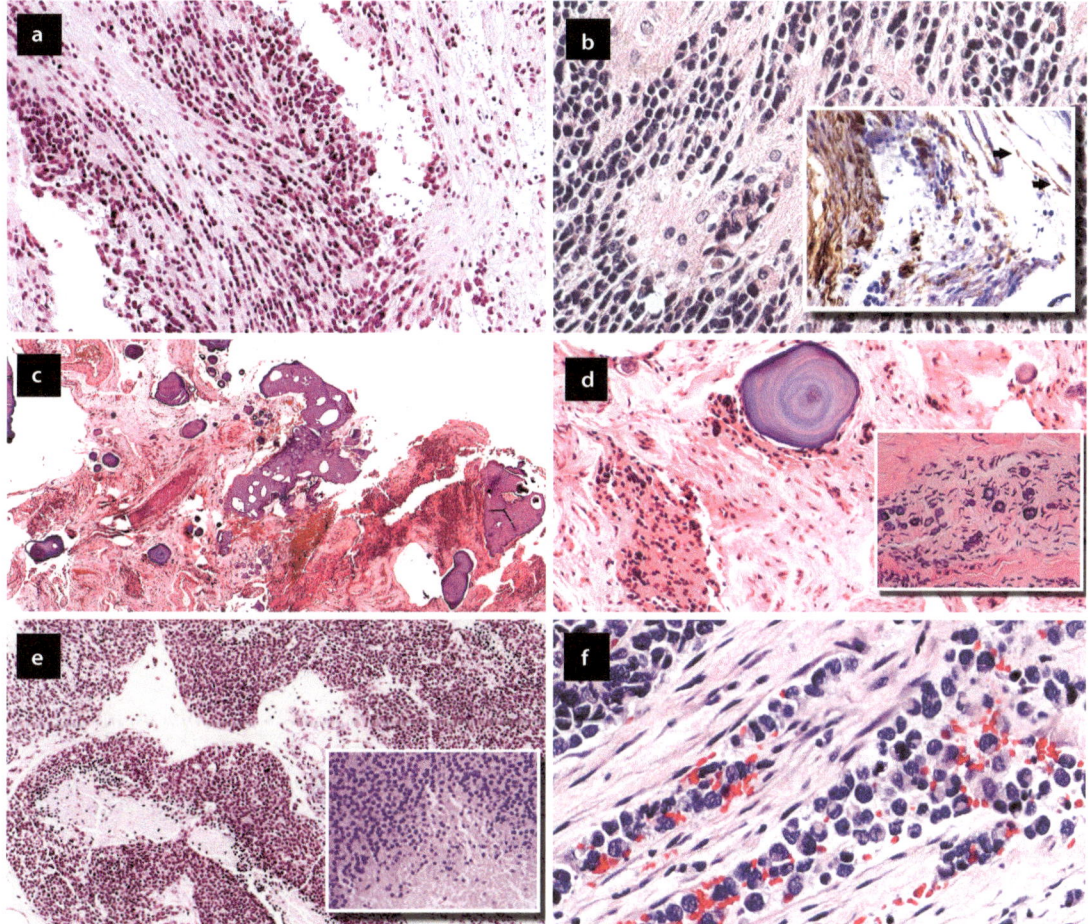

Fig. 4.19 ONB: (**a**) Neurofibrillary background, which can best be appreciated by dropping down the microscope condenser. *Inset*: S100 accentuates neurofibrillary processes. (**c**, **d**) Intratumoral calcifications can be especially helpful in limited biopsies. Here we see confluent psammomatoid concretions. The differential diagnosis includes meningioma and psammomatoid ossifying fibroma. *Inset*: Calcifications are normally present in the olfactory nerves. (**e**) Frank necrosis in a Grade IV ONB. (**f**) The cytologic pleomorphism seen in a Grade IV ONB is still much less that that seen in a SNUC or a basaloid SCC

4.4.2 PNET (Primitive Nerve Sheath Tumor)/ES (Ewings' Sarcoma) or EFT (Ewing Family of Tumors)

EFT refers to a group of primitive tumors defined by their well-characterized gene translocations. Historically, ES was first recognized as a primary osseous "small blue round cell tumor". PNET was subsequently described as a much rarer soft tissue counterpart (the "P" connoted either peripheral or primitive). The characteristic translocation, t(11;22)(q24;q12), generates fusion of *EWS* (Ewings sarcoma breakpoint region 1) and transcription factor *FLI1* (Friend leukemia virus integration 1). The *EWS-FLI1* fusion is present in 90–95 % of EFT; it blocks differentiation of pluripotential marrow stromal cells. *ERG* is a less common *EWS* fusion partner; rarer fusion partners are *ETV1*, *E1AF*, and *FEV*.

The peak incidence of EFT is in the second decade; there is a known male predominance. EFT most commonly affects the long bones and pelvis; about 4 % of EFT involves the head and neck, usually jaws [121]. Sinonasal EFT usually includes the maxillary bone and should not be considered as extraskeletal [122, 123]. Adamantinoma-like EFT represents a rare EFT histological variant characterized by epithelial differentiation and keratin expression which can represent a major diagnostic challenge; it is discussed below [124, 125].

EFT is considered a systemic disease, even if no metastases are found on preoperative studies. Standard therapy includes induction multi-agent chemotherapy (vincristine, doxorubicin, and cyclophosphamide, alternating with ifosfamide and etoposide) [126]. The primary tumor site is treated by radiotherapy, or surgery, or both, depending upon anatomic site, tumor size, response to chemotherapy, and resection margin status. The chemotherapeutic regiment is completed post-operatively for a total of 48 weeks of therapy. Positive prognosticators include presentation with localized disease, axial tumor site, and age under 15 years [127].

Hafezi and colleagues reported 14 sinonasal EFT cases, and reviewed the English language literature for cases of interest with outcome data, for a total of 29 sinonasal EFT patients [122]. The average age of this group was 24 years; the average follow-up period was 51 months. Twenty-one patients remained progression-free; eight patients developed locoregional or distant metastases. Of this latter subgroup, two patients, both with late treatment failures (30 and 192 months) were salvaged and remained disease-free at 207 and 122 months, respectively.

▪ Histopathology

Conventional EFT is composed of monotonous, homogenous tumor cells with round, bland, nuclei showing little or no pleomorphism; thus it can resemble ONB. Nucleoli are absent or small. Cytoplasm is usually minimal, cytoplasmic clearing can be seen (◘ Fig. 4.20). Conventional EFT can grow in diffuse, nesting, cords, or filigreed patterns. The tumor may exhibit a perivascular distribution of viable cells. A common finding is that of interspersed apoptotic tumor cells ("dark cells"). Frank necrosis can be seen. High mitotic count is associated with disseminated disease at presentation [128]. Though distinguishing between Ewing's sarcoma and PNET is of no practical significance, an iconic finding of Ewings sarcoma is cytoplasmic glycogen: **PAS +/DPAS–**. The finding of Homer-Wright rosettes indicates neuronal differentiation and warrants tumor classification as **PNET**.

Approximately 20 % of EFT are variants (**Atypical EFT**), which may be associated with poorer prognosis [128]. Confirmation of *EWS-FLI1* fusion can be especially useful for this group below:

Large cell/anaplastic EFT is composed of tumor cells with large nuclei, prominent nucleoli, anaplasia, abundant pink cytoplasm, and binucleate cells.

Spindled variant EFT contains greater degree of spindling and well-developed vasculature.

Sclerosing variant EFT contains abundant, hyalinized, eosinophilic stroma.

Hemangioendothelial variant EFT has abundant vascular-like spaces and erythrocytes-filled lacunae.

Adamantinoma-like EFT exhibits a nested growth pattern with peripherally pallisading tumor cells, which are epithelioid with moderate pleomorphism. Overt squamous differentiation can be seen. Hyaline-like stromal desmoplasia may be present. IHC for keratins are usually positive either diffusely, or focally.

Immunohistochemically, EFT typically show diffuse expression of **CD99** and **FLI1**, however, this lacks specificity. The following markers can be expressed, which might become cause confusion: keratins (focal), neuroendocrine markers, S100 (no sustentacular pattern), desmin (focal), p63, and p40. Molecular confirmation of the *EWS-FLI1* fusion is not a diagnostic pre-requisite for conventional EFT. When necessary, the *EWS-FLI1* fusion can be confirmed by FISH using dual color break-apart probe that span common breakpoints on EWS, or RT-PCR for EWS-FLI1 fusion transcript.

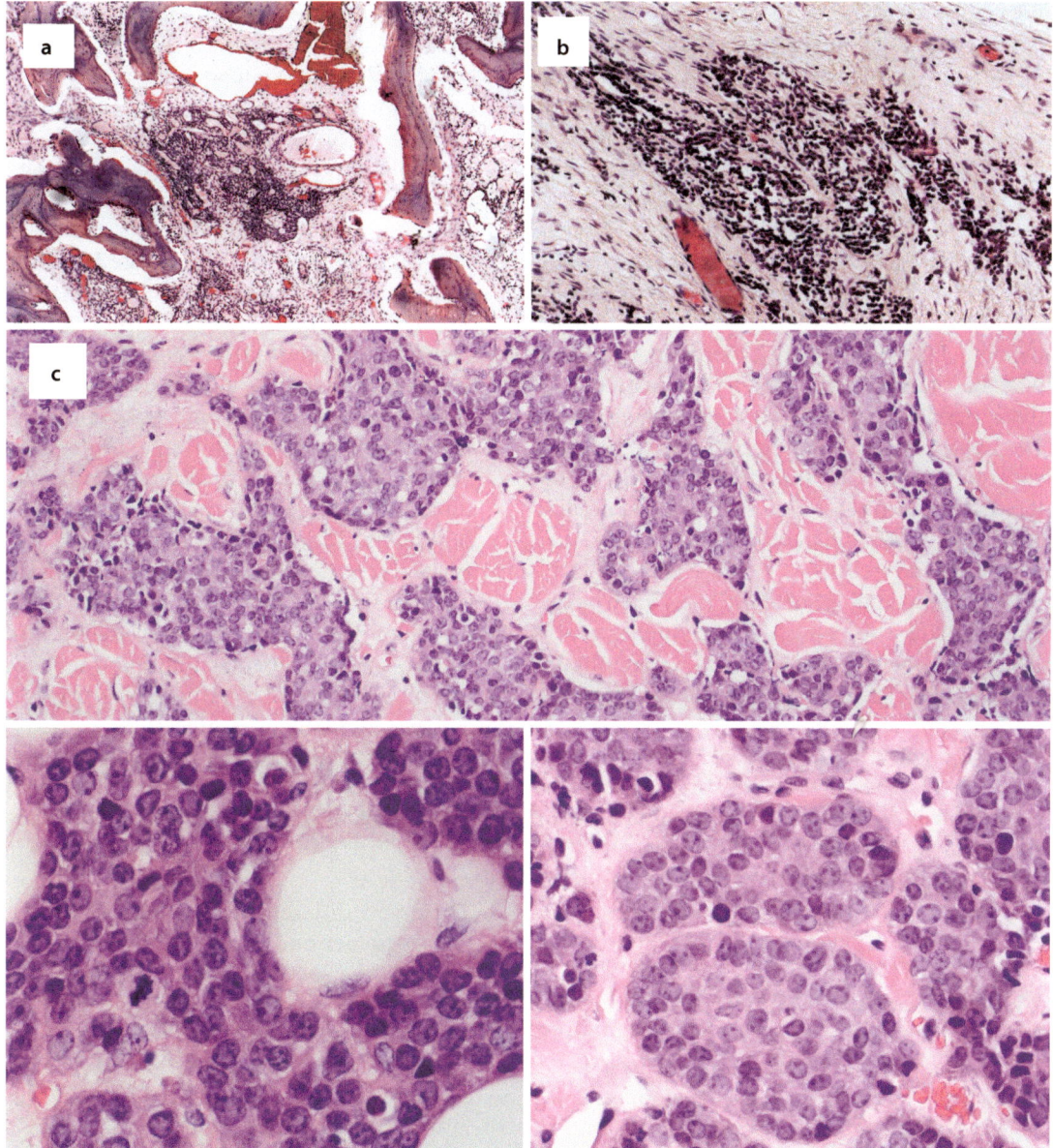

◼ **Fig. 4.20** (**a**, **b**) This **PNET** is composed of monotonous small blue forming vague rosettes. (**c**) **Adamantinoma-like EFT**: This tumor infiltrates in discreet islands. (**d**) Unlike conventional EFT, tumor cells are epithelioid, with prominent nucleoli, and moderate pleomorphism. (**e**) Peripheral pallisading (Courtesy of Drs Claudia Velosa and Shahid Bokhari)

4.4.3 Sinonasal Neuroendocrine Carcinoma (SNEC)

The most common head and neck site for primary neuroendocrine carcinoma is the larynx. By contrast, neuroendocrine carcinomas of the sinonasal tract are extremely uncommon [5, 129–133].

Contemporary case series focusing solely on these tumors are limited [134]. The presenting sinonasal symptoms are usually nonspecific and most patients have Stage IV disease at diagnosis. Some SNEC patients present with SIADH (Syndrome Inappropriate Antidiuretic Hormone) which is also associated with pulmonary small cell neuroendocrine carcinomas, squamous carcinomas of the head and neck, and ONB [135, 136]. SNEC is among the head and neck malignancies diagnosed in young patients post-treatment for retinoblastoma [137].

SNEC is graded analogous to pulmonary and laryngeal neuroendocrine carcinomas (see below); most diagnosed SNEC are either moderately- or poorly-differentiated (atypical carcinoid, and small cell, respectively). The standard of care includes resection, if feasible, plus multimodality therapy. Likhacheva and colleagues published outcomes for 20 SNEC patients; roughly half of them developed locoregional recurrence [134]. The impact of tumor grade could be seen in the subgroup of patients treated with surgery plus RT. The mean disease-free survivals for moderately-, and poorly-differentiated NEC were 63 and 16 months, respectively.

The histopathology of SNEC is outlined below. The following two points deserve emphasize: (1) IHC for neuroendocrine markers (synaptophysin, chromogranin) should *always* be included in the workup of sinonasal "small blue round cell tumors" even in the absence of neuroendocrine patterns (2) mixed histologies (e.g. neuroendocrine differentiation plus adenocarcinoma, or squamous carcinoma) are not uncommon [138–141]. Once you arrive at your first diagnosis, don't stop looking for a potential second diagnosis.

- **Histopathology** (Figs. 4.21 and 4.22)

Well-differentiated SNEC (Grade I, Carcinoid) is composed of epithelioid tumor cells with round nuclei, fine chromatin, inconspicuous nucleoli, and amphophilic, eosinophilic, or occasionally oncocytic cytoplasm. Grade I tumors are well vascularized and characterized by the lack of pleomorphism, mitotic activity, or necrosis. Specific neuroendocrine growth patterns (nested, ribbons, trabeculae, cords, "Zell-ballen") are seen. True glandular differentiation can be seen. No ONB features (Homer-Wright pseudorosettes, neurofibrillary background) should be present.

Moderately-differentiated SNEC (Grade II, Atypical Carcinoid) demonstrate the usual neuroendocrine growth patterns (as above) or solid, sheet-like, or pattern-less architecture. True gland formation, or interspersed goblet cells may be present. The carcinoma is composed of epithelioid or spindle tumor cells with round to oval nuclei, stippled or vesicular chromatin, prominent nucleoli, and some pleomorphism. Distinguishing features include increased mitotic activity (2–10 mitoses/10 HPF) and/or necrosis.

Poorly-differentiated SNEC (Grade III, Small cell carcinoma) can be subclassified as Small- and Large-Cell Types. The small cell variant is composed of cells smaller than three resting lymphocytes; nuclei are oval, or round, and cytoplasm is minimal. If the cells are slightly larger, with minimal to moderate amount of cytoplasm, then the tumor is classified as intermediate *variant* of small cell carcinoma. Tumor cells of the large cell variant are very rare, they larger than small cell variant and contain more cytoplasm. Tumor nuclei are vesicular with fine to coarse chromatin and frequent, multiple nucleoli. Pleomorphism and necrosis are prominent, and mitotic activity is high (>10/10 HPFs). Grade III tumors form sheets and interconnecting ribbons of undifferentiated tumor cells. DNA coating blood vessels walls and "crush artifact" (Azzopardi phenomenon) can be seen.

Divergent differentiation is not an uncommon phenomenon. Different combinations have been described such as poorly-differentiated (small cell carcinoma) or moderately-differentiated neuroendocrine carcinoma plus squamous carcinoma, or intestinal-type adenocarcinoma, or adenocarcinoma-not-otherwise-specified.

SNEC expresses both epithelial and neuroendocrine proteins
Synapto + (50%), **Chromo** + (50%),
CD56 + (89%), **SOX2** + (89%)
S100 and CD99 usually negative
Pankeratin +, **AE1/AE3** +, **EpCAM** +
Be aware, sinonasal melanomas may also express neuroendocrine markers [142]

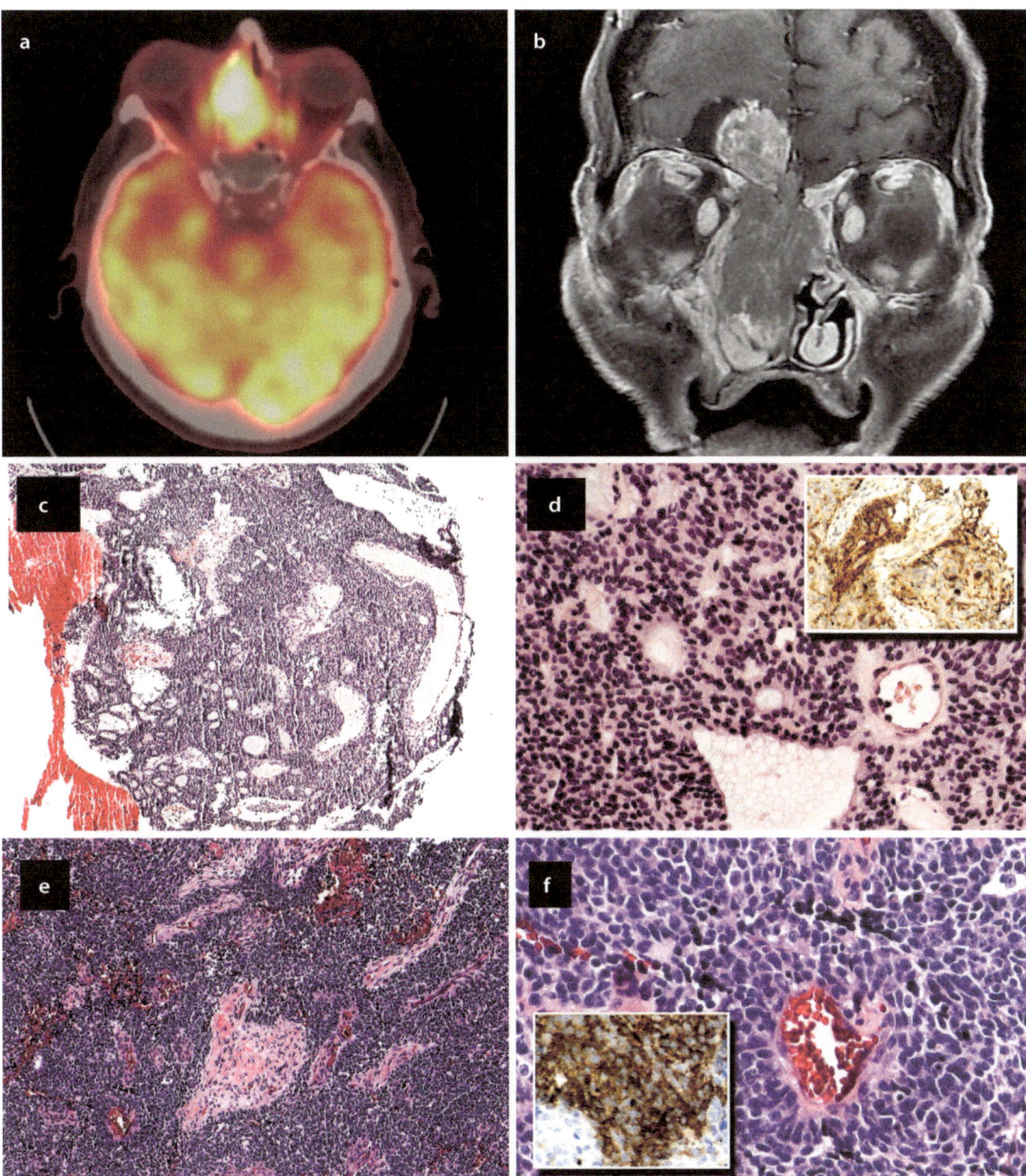

◼ **Fig. 4.21** Sinonasal neuroendocrine carcinoma (SNEC). (**a**) Enhancing sinonasal tumor on PET CT. (**b**) Massive sinonasal tumor with intracranial extension on coronal MRI T2 weighted (Courtesy of Dr. Phil Chapman). (**c–f**) These two SNECs appear as nondescript uniform small blue cell tumors. The diagnoses were established by confirming epithelial and neuroendocrine differentiation (*Both insets*: synaptophysin). Remember to exclude the possibility of pituitary macroadenoma, which can present as an intranasal tumor with the same expression profile (See Sect. 5.7)

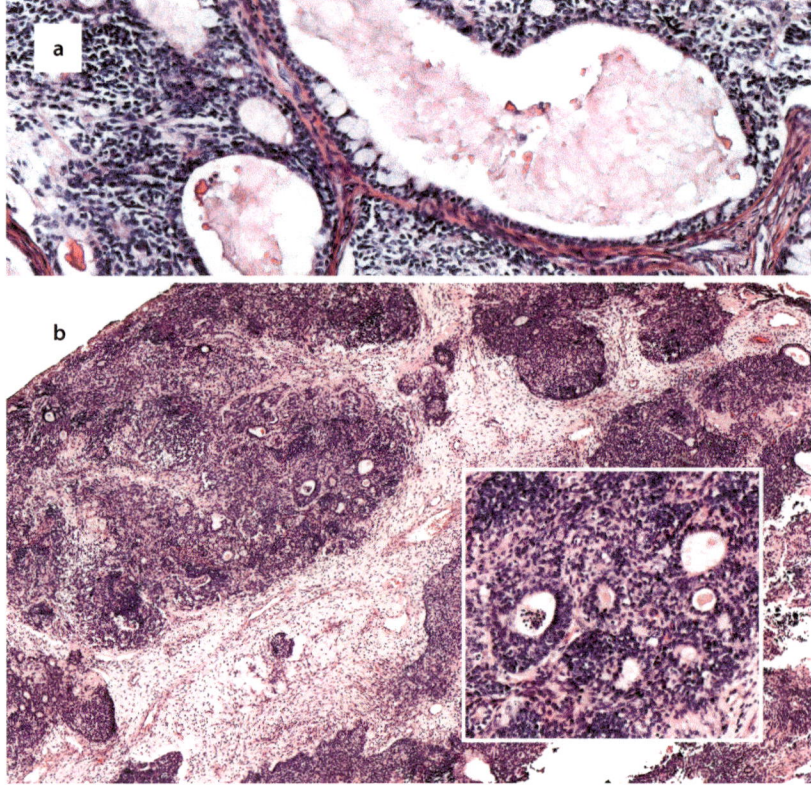

4.5   Glandular

4.5.1   Intestinal Type Adenocarcinoma (ITAC)

ITAC was first recognized as a heterogenous group of sinonasal glandular malignancies resembling gastrointestinal adenocarcinomas, especially in the context of occupational exposures among woodworkers and shoemakers [143–146]. The established risk is dose-related, with a latency period of at least 10 years [147]. *TP53* mutations, usually missense base substitutions, are common to ITAC; their likelihood is significantly increased with duration of wood exposure greater than 24 years [150, 151]. Of note, the histology of exposure-related sinonasal cancers is not limited to ITAC [148, 149]. Furthermore, ITAC also develops in the absence of occupational exposures. Sporadic tumors are more common in the maxilla, whereas exposure-related ITACs are more common to the nasal cavity and ethmoids. Exposure-associated ITACs are more likely to be symptomatic and diagnosed at an earlier stage than sporadic ITAC [145].

Treatment consists of primary surgery +/− adjuvant radiotherapy depending upon individual patient factors. Contemporary reports of ITAC patients and outcome are limited, and may require a leap of faith when the diagnostic requisites are not detailed [152]. Having said that, local recurrence and distant metastatic rates of 38 % and 13 %, respectively, were reported by a group in Belgium [152]. The most common metastatic sites were bone, lung, and liver. Five- and 10-year disease-specific and recurrence-free survival rates were 82 % and 62 %, 74 % and 45 %, respectively [152]. Another group reported similar rates for local recurrence and distant metastases, 26 % and 11 %, respectively [153].

■ **Histopathology**

Grossly, ITAC often appear exophytic. ITACs are classified as low-, intermediate-, or high-grade, based on cytological grade and presence of aggressive histologic features. The five described growth patterns are papillary, colonic (tubular), solid, mucinous, and mixed. The "tubular" descriptor refers to the long tubular shaped glands of colonic adenocarcinoma [143]. Prognostically, the papillary pattern is noteworthy in that low-grade papillary ITAC may be entirely noninvasive. The solid pattern is usually associated with necrosis, invasion, and high-grade.

Low-grade ITAC is characterized by slender papillae; secondary or tertiary arborizing papillae may be seen but are not diagnostically requisite. The papillae are lined by single layers of columnar tumor cells with little or no pleomorphism and only minor cellular crowding. The nuclei are cigar-shaped and polarity is maintained. Goblet and Paneth-type cells may be seen. Long "tubular" gland formation may also be present (◘ Fig. 4.23).

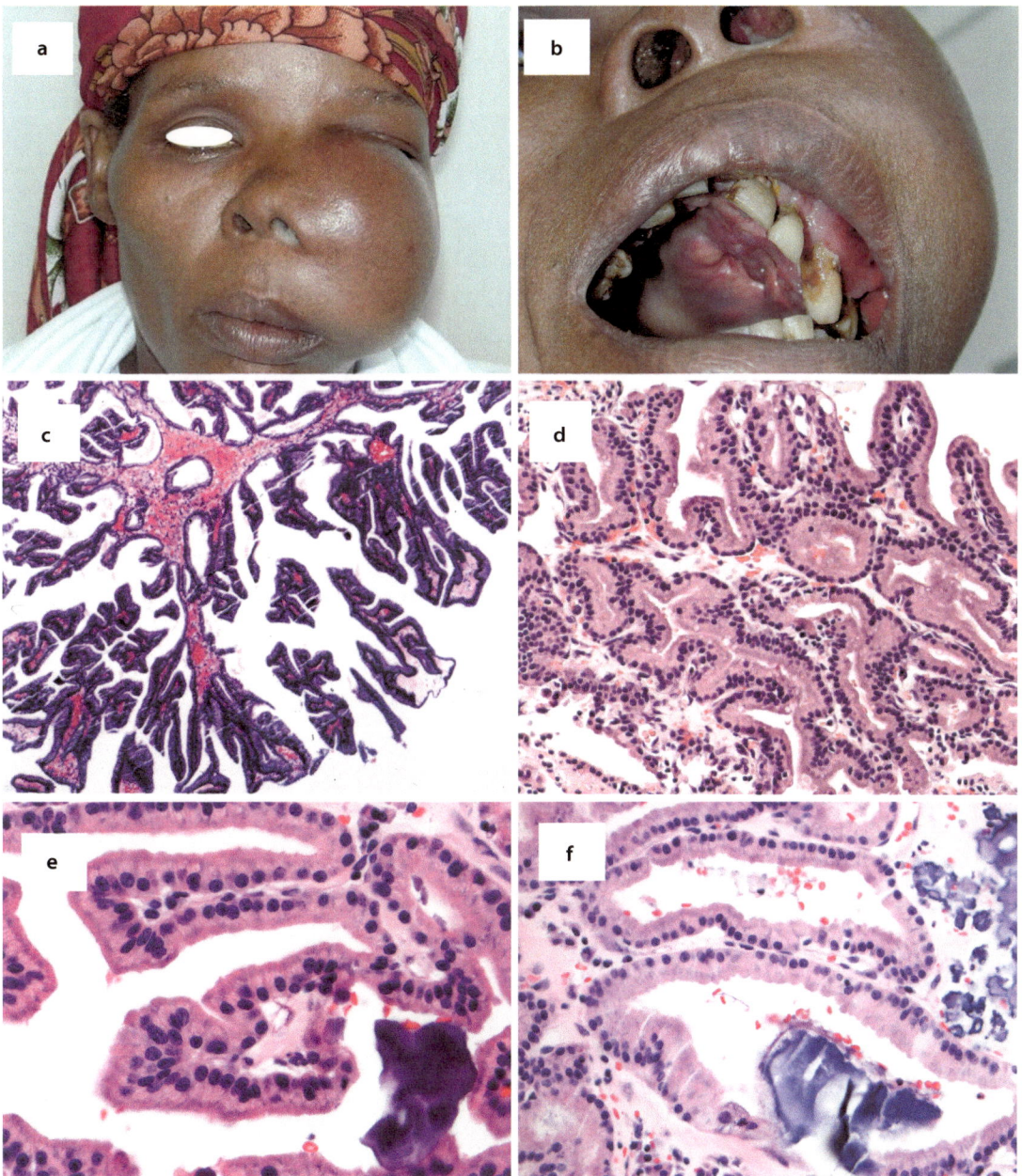

◘ **Fig. 4.23** Intestinal type adenocarcinoma (ITAC) (**a**, **b**): a neglected massive ITAC. (**c**) Low-grade papillary ITAC with thin papillae and secondary arborization. (**d**) Long "tubular" glands. (**e**, **f**) Columnar tumor cells without atypia and only minor cell crowding. Nuclear polarity is maintained

Intermediate-grade ITAC resembles colonic tubulovillous adenoma. There is usually both papillary and glandular (colonic, tubular) growth patterns, with invasion into underlying tissues. Tumor nuclei are larger, pseudo stratified, with loss of polarity (◘ Fig. 4.24). Increased mitotic activity is present.

High-grade ITAC is invasive, and characterized by a greater degree of cytological pleomorphism and more loss of nuclear polarity. Solid growth patterns, necrosis, brisk mitotic activity, signet ring cells, goblet cells, and pleomorphic columnar cells can be seen in high-grade ITAC.

Mucosal intestinal metaplasia with aberrant biomarker expression, +/− dysplasia, can be observed adjacent to ITAC (◘ Fig. 4.25) [154, 155]. Characteristically, ITAC expresses gastrointestinal biomarkers: **CDX2 + (87 %)**, **MUC2 + (92 %)**, **CK20 + (87 %)**. **CDX2/CK20** expression is important in distinguishing ITAC from sinonasal non-intestinal adenocarcinomas. However, CDX2 expression is not specific for ITAC and can also be expressed in sinonasal salivary adenocarcinomas [156].

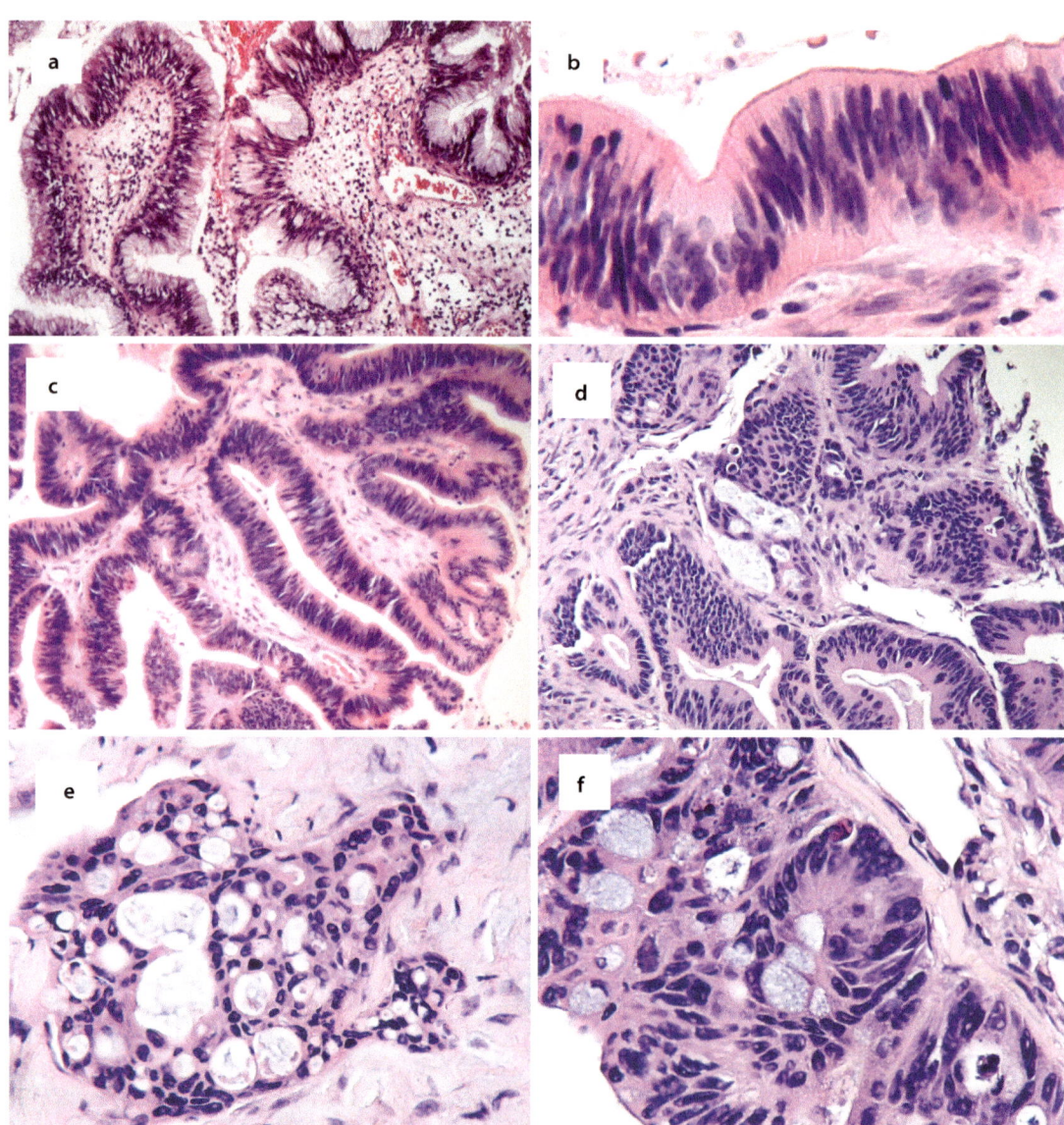

◘ Fig. 4.24 (**a–d**) **Intermediate-grade ITAC** resembles colonic tubulovillous adenoma. (**b**) Pseudostratified columnar cells with long nuclei and loss of nuclear polarity. (**e, f**) **High-grade ITAC** reveals more extreme pleomorphism. The majority of ITAC express CDX-2, MUC2, and CK20

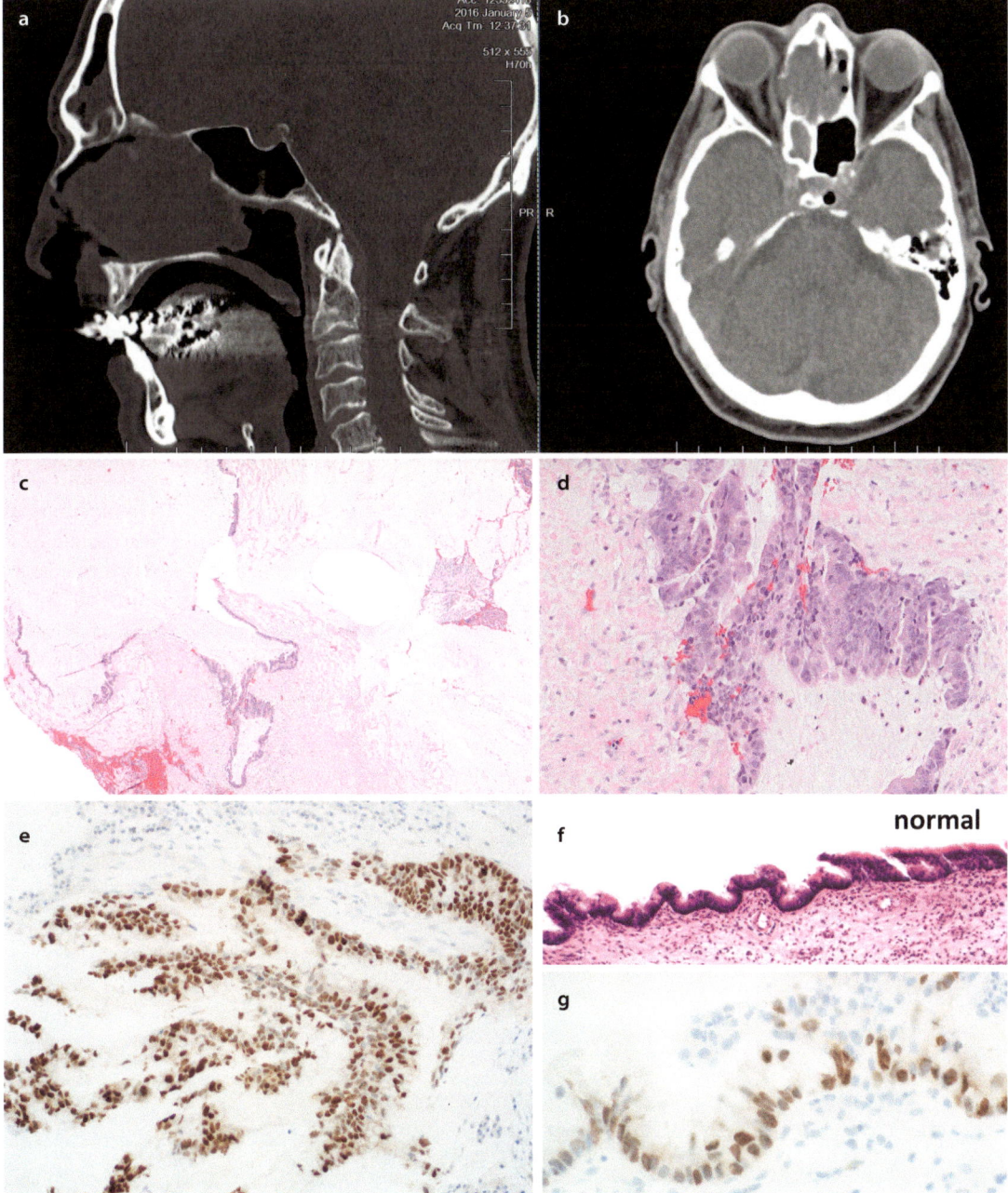

Fig. 4.25 Mucinous ITAC: this man's vocation was refinishing wood floors. (**a**) Sagital view of nasal cavity mass extending to skull base. (**b**) Coronal view at the level of the ethmoid sinuses reveals tumor extension into the right orbit. (**c**) Low-power view of a mucinous polyp with strands of tumor cells. (**d**) The columnar tumor cells demonstrate loss of nuclear polarity and nuclear pleomorphism. This is a Grade 2 ITAC. (**e**) Tumor expression of CDX-2. (**f**) Carcinoma-*in-situ* (*left*) with pseudostratified mucinous columnar cells with some loss of nuclear polarity. The adjacent normal mucosa retains the orderly appearance of stratified respiratory epithelium. (**g**) CDX-2 expression in carcinoma-in-situ. Adjacent normal mucosa is CDX-2 negative (not shown)

– Differential diagnosis
  • Oncocytic Schneiderian papilloma is lined by stratified columnar oncocytes. ITAC is lined by simple columnar cells.
  • Papillary sinusitis has thicker papillae with dense inflammation. Papillary sinusitis may be quite florid, in which case radiographic correlation will aid in distinguishing it from low-grade ITAC.

4.5.2 Sinonasal Adenocarcinoma, (SNAC) Non Intestinal Type (Not Otherwise Specified)

Sinonasal adenocarcinomas which cannot be classified according to a specific histology (e.g. ITAC, salivary-type, neuroendocrine) can broadly be grouped as Sinonasal Adenocarcinoma (SNAC). Within this category, a subgroup of low-grade, surface mucosal-derived adenocarcinomas have been described which resemble ITAC, but lack CDX2/CK20 expression [157–162]. One unusual case expressed TTF-1 [160]. However, a more systematic institutional review revealed that intermediate/high-grade non-intestinal SNAC can be as common as low-grade non-intestinal SNAC [162].

■ **Histology** (◘ Figs. 4.26 and 4.27)

Grading can be assigned based on traditional cytology and presence of aggressive features. Low-grade SNAC is comprised of small, monomorphic, evenly spaced nuclei, smooth nuclear membranes, small nucleoli, with a tubulopapillary or glandular growth pattern. Mucinous differentiation may be seen. A sinonasal serous hamartoma-like (SSH-like, minimal deviation) neoplasm has been described which demonstrates a lobular arrangement of small tubules lined by cuboidal cells with rounded borders. Unlike SSH, these tumors also manifest solid, cribriform, and papillary growth patterns and/or infiltration. Intermediate-grade SNAC have larger nuclei, some nuclear overlapping, pleomorphism, prominent nucleoli, mitotic rate < 5 mitoses/10 high power fields, and individual cell apoptosis. High-grade SNAC had prominent nuclear pleomorphism, mitotic rate

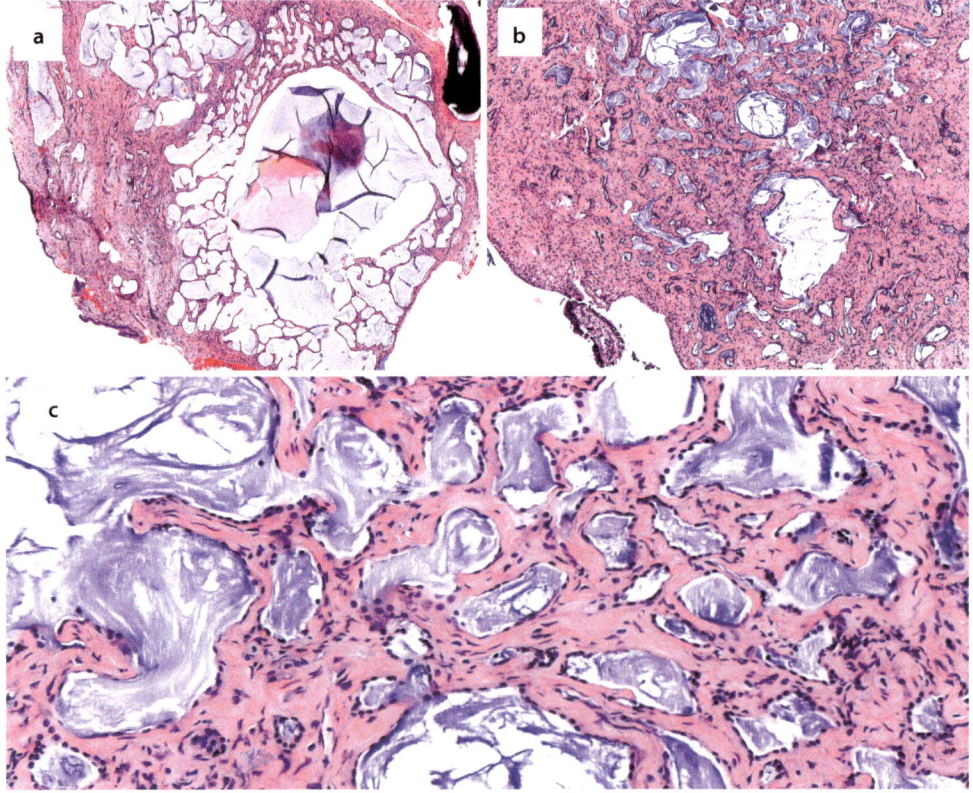

◘ **Fig. 4.26** Sinonasal adenocarcinoma NOS (SNAC) – this is an exclusionary diagnosis. (**a, b**) Low-power view of infiltrating mucinous glandular neoplasm. (**c**) This neoplasm is histologically bland and negative for CDX-2 and CK20

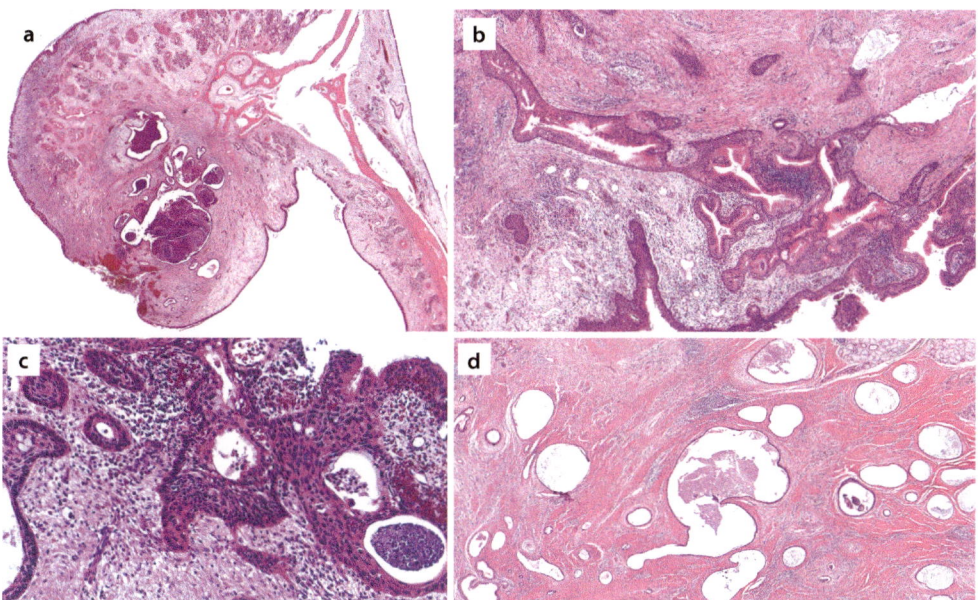

■ **Fig. 4.27** This **SNAC** was associated with occupation exposure. (**a**) Low-power view of turbinate reveals expansile tumor with superficial erosion. (**b**) Complex ductoglandular hyperplasia. (**c**) *In-situ* carcinoma. (**d**) Low-power view of well differential adenocarcinoma infiltrating palatal tissue. This carcinoma was also **CDX**-2- and **CK20**-

greater ≥ 5/10 high power fields, solid growth pattern, and necrosis.

Characteristically, and by definition, **SNAC expresses CK7, but not CK20, MUC2 or CDX2**.

4.5.3 Sinonasal Renal Cell-Like Adenocarcinoma

This rare, low-grade neoplasm bears no resemblance to any other sinonasal primary tumor [163–165]. Currently, 16 patients with SNRCLA have been reported in total [166]. Epistaxis is a common presenting symptom, although nonspecific. Most tumors arise in the nasal cavity; two originated in the nasopharynx. A number of reports specifically document no pre-existing, synchronous, or subsequentthe clear cell variant of renal cell carcinoma. Although classified as a carcinoma, thus far SNRCLA appears to have no malignant potential. No patient presented with positive lymph nodes. No patient to date has developed metastatic disease or local recurrence [166]. Therefore, adjuvant radiotherapy and cervical neck dissection do not appear to be warranted.

■ **Histology**

SNRCLA is composed of monomorphous, cuboidal to columnar glycogen-rich clear cells lacking mucin. The cellular cytoplasm may be "crystal clear" or slightly eosinophilic. Occasionally, tumor cells with basophilic and oncocytoid cytoplasm can be intermixed with tumor clear cells. Tumor nuclei are typically small, round or condensed, and may have a single prominent nucleolus; intranuclear holes may also be seen. The glandular structures are composed of simple back-to-back glands with a microfollicular pattern (■ Fig. 4.28). Larger, longer, tubular glands can be present, containing eosinophilic secretory material and mimicking thyroid follicular carcinoma, clear cell variant. Nested, solid, or papillary patterns may also be seen. No necrosis, hyalinized stroma or myoepithelial differentiation is seen. Nuclear pleomorphism and mitotic activity are usually limited.

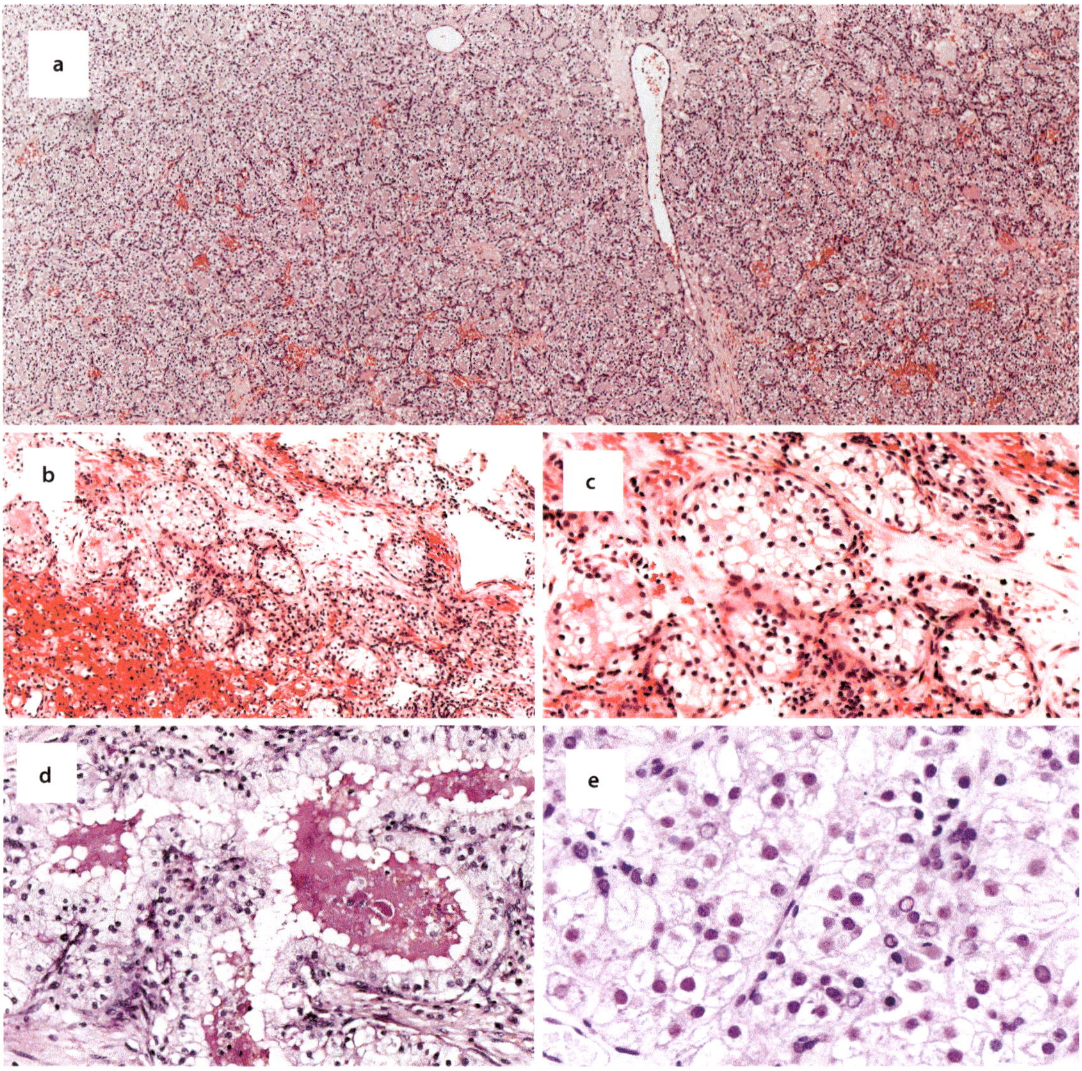

■ **Fig. 4.28** Sinonasal renal cell like adenocarcinoma (SNRCLC) (**a–c**): a clear cell neoplasm with a hemorrhagic background brings to mind metastatic renal cell carcinoma. (**d**) Follicular and glandular structures. (**e**) Cuboidal tumor cells with rounded nuclei, fine chromatin, prominent nucleoli and occasional intranuclear holes

Some tumors are described as infiltrating. Dilated vascular spaces are seen. Overall, SNRCLA is less vascular and pleomorphic, compared to the clear cell variant of renal cell carcinoma.

The immunohistochemical profile demonstrates keratin expression (cytokeratin +, CK7+, variable CK20 expression), EMA expression, and variable S100 expression. With respect to renal markers, CAIX expression has been recently described; (■ Fig. 4.29) SNRCLA does not express other renal markers such as RCC or Pax8 [166].

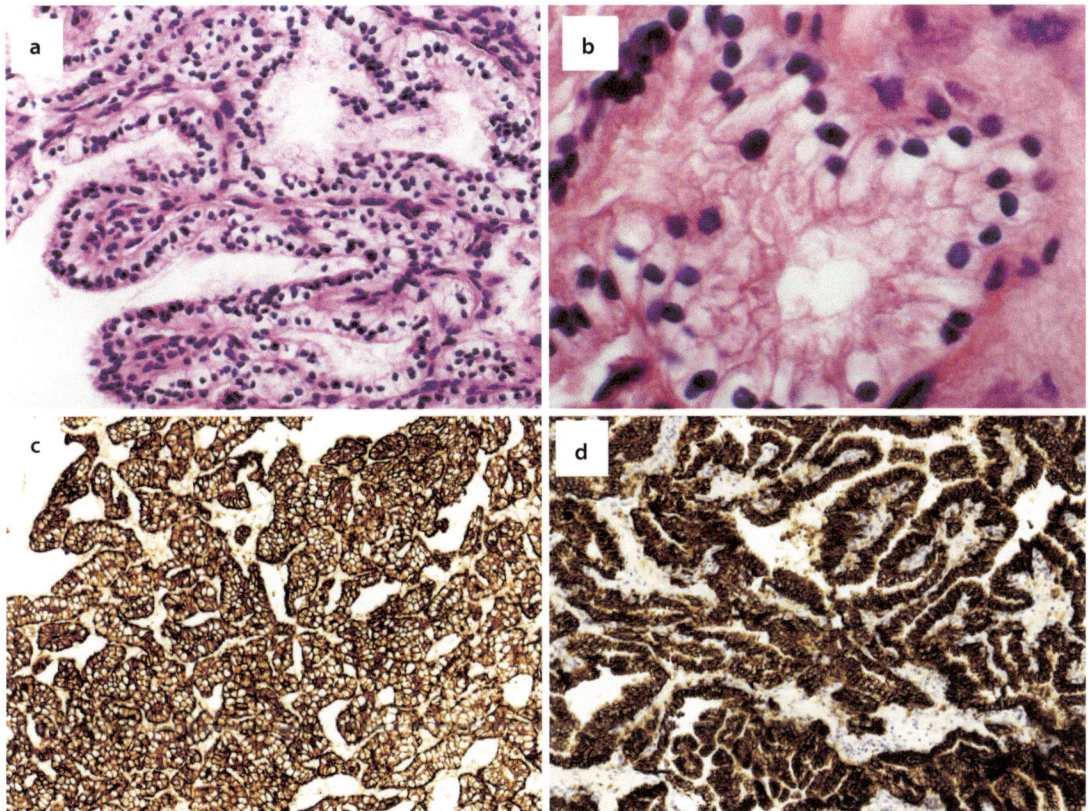

Fig. 4.29 (**a, b**) This **sinonasal renal cell like adenocarcinoma** has a prominent papillary architecture reminiscent of endolymphatic sac tumor (Case courtesy of Dr. Lester Thompson). (**c, d**) Another "renal-cell-like" feature of SNRCLC is robust CA-IX expression

4.5.4 Sinonasal Teratocarcinosarcoma (Malignant Teratoma, Teratocarcinoma)

Sinonasal teratocarcinosarcoma represents a rare, highly aggressive malignancy arising from pluripotential cells that differentiate into ectodermal, mesenchymal, and endodermal tissues [167–176]. There is a pronounced male predominance (male/female = 7:1) and a reported wide age range, usually from third to seventh decades. Patients complain of nasal obstruction, headache and epistaxis. Syndrome of inappropriate anti-diuretic hormone secretion (SIADH) has also been reported with sinonasal teratocarcinosarcoma. The nasal cavity is most commonly affected. On nasal examination, the tumor has been described as firm, red, reddish-purple, friable, and necrotic; it may protrude from the nares.

Sinonasal teratocarcinosarcoma is uniformly an aggressive malignancy. Most reported patients have received multimodality therapy (surgery and adjuvant radiotherapy) due to advanced T stage. Unfortunately, local recurrence, which can be rapid, and/or regional metastases (dura, brain) are common. Distant metastases (e.g. lung) are less common. The 3- and 5-year survival rates are low (30 % and 20 %, respectively).

▪ Histology

Tumor heterogeneity usually leads to misdiagnosis especially with limited sampling. Many of the cases reported by Heffner were initially misdiagnosed as adenocarcinoma, olfactory neuroblastoma, fibrosarcoma, and rhabdomyosarcoma [167]. Sinonasal teratocarcinosarcoma is characterized by a complex mixture of epithelial, mesenchymal, and neuroepithelial tissues which appear benign, atypical, and frankly malignant (☐ Figs. 4.30 and 4.31).

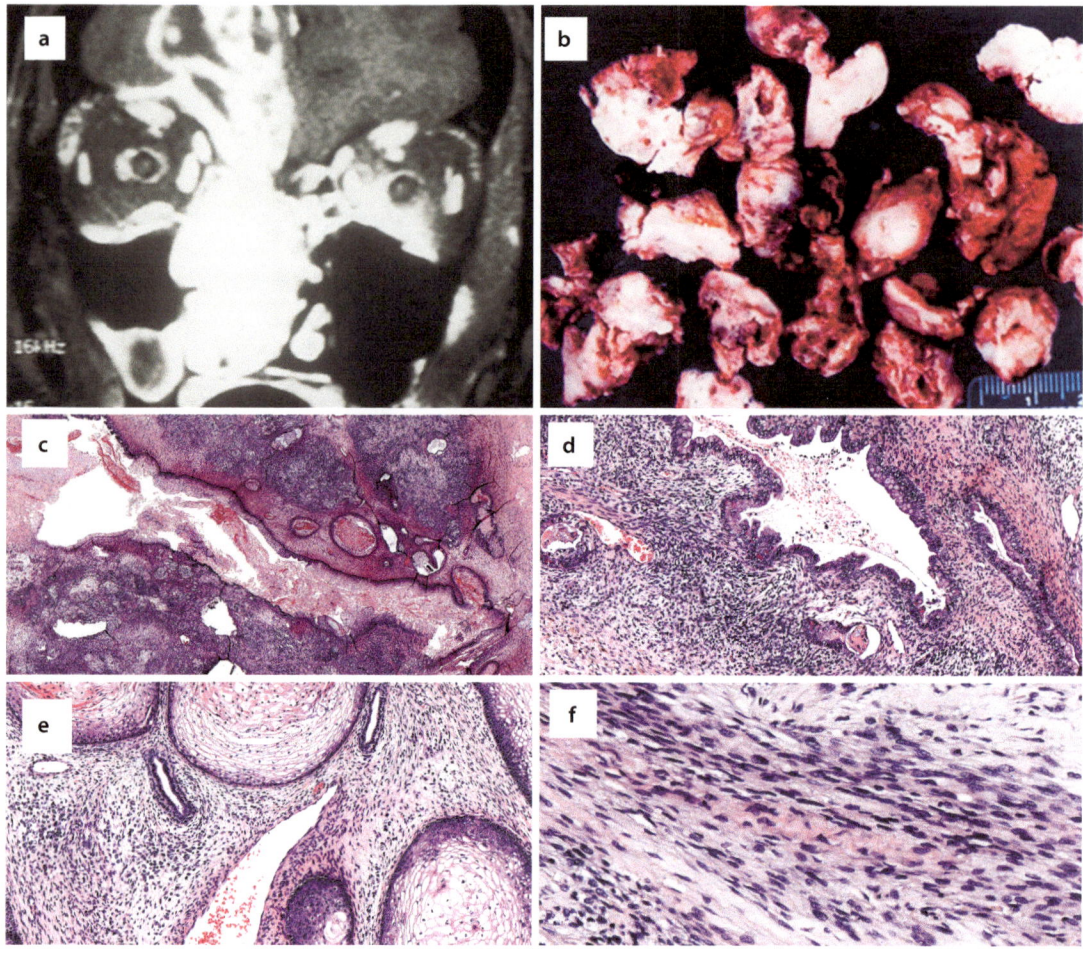

◘ Fig. 4.30   Sinonasal teratocarcinosarcoma is composed of benign and malignant elements of variable maturation derived from ectodermal, endodermal and mesodermal origins. (**a**) Sinonasal teratocarcinoma with massive intracranial extension. (**b**) Tumor fragments with variegated color and texture. (**c–f**) Keratinizing squamous cysts, gastrointestinal differentiation, and background of undifferentiated spindle cells

Benign epithelial elements: Immature glycogen-rich squamous epithelium (fetal squamous), glands lined by ciliated, columnar, or mucinous epithelium. The benign tissues can assemble to form multi-tissue "organoid structures" (e.g. bronchi, intestine)

Malignant epithelial elements: Adenocarcinoma, squamous carcinoma

Benign mesenchymal elements: Cartilage, fibroblastic, myxomatous, skeletal muscle, smooth muscle

Malignant mesenchymal elements: Rhabdomyosarcoma, osteosarcoma, chondrosarcoma, rhabdoid cells with juxtanuclear eosinophilic hyaline inclusions [174]

Neuroepithelial elements: Differentiated neuronal cells (pseudorosettes, neuropil, ganglionic differentiation) collections of small, primitive blastemal neuronal cells (**CD99**+)

Germ cell elements are not typically present, but can occur rarely. Yolk sac elements (Schiller Duval bodies, **AFP**+) in conjunction with germ cell features (isochromosome 12p amplification (i12P0)) have been reported [175]. Primary sinonasal germ cell malignancies are rare and contain no teratocarcinosarcomatous elements [177].

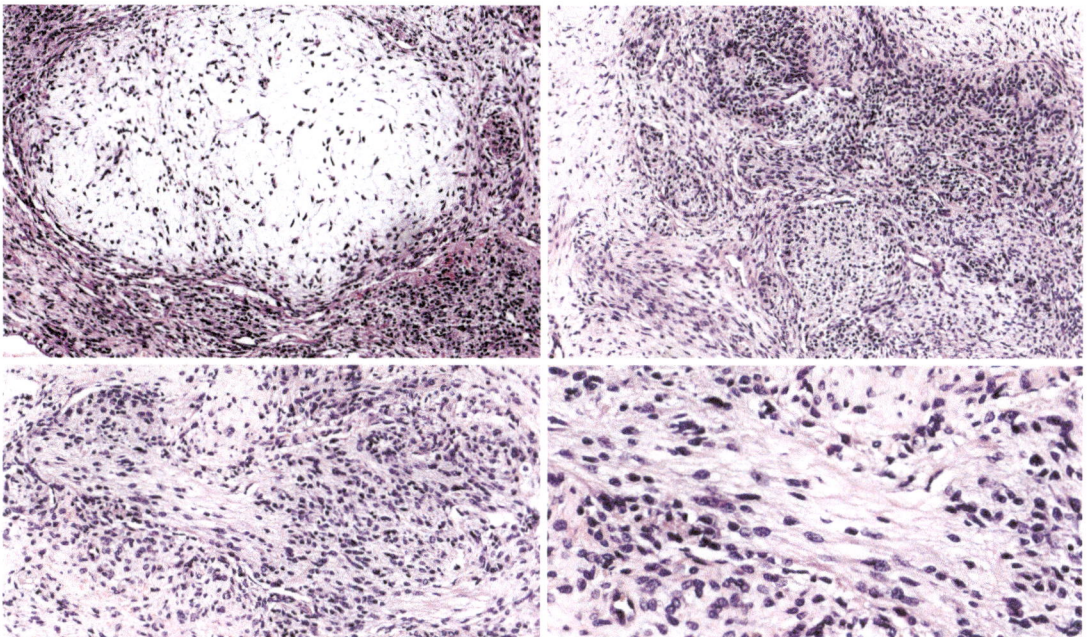

> **Fig. 4.31** Sinonasal teratocarcinosarcoma: *Top left*: pleomorphic myxoid cells. *Top right and bottom panels*: Primitive neuronal differentiation – Homer Wright pseudorosettes and neurofibrillary background similar to olfactory neuroblastoma

- Sinonasal spindled neoplasia are generally uncommon. Benign and borderline spindle cell entities (hemangiopericytoma/ glomangiopericytoma, solitary fibrous tumor) are discussed below, and in Chap. 3 (plexiform neurofibroma, schwannoma, meningioma).
- Squamous carcinoma, spindle-cell variant should top the differential diagnoses list for sinonasal spindled *malignancies*.
- True sinonasal *sarcomas* are rare. Rhabdomysarcomas are the most common and the two variants to consider are embryonal rhabdomyosarcoma, spindle variant, and pleomorphic rhabdomyosarcoma, adult-type.
- Given the emerging data on biphenotypic sinonasal sarcoma and its association with tPAX3-MAML3, tPAX3-FOXO1, or PAX3-NCOA1, and given the few

contemporary reports on sinonasal fibrosarcomas, there appears to be a spectrum of low-grade sinonasal fibrosarcomas with varying additional mesenchymal phenotype. These entities are grouped together in the last chapter section.

4.6 Spindle Cell

4.6.1 Sinonasal Hemangiopericytoma (Glomangiopericytoma)

Stout and Murray coined the term "hemangiopericytoma" to describe vascular tumors purportedly derived from "Zimmermann's pericyte" [178] – a perivascular smooth muscle cell which normally regulates capillary blood flow [179]. Compagno and Hyams first used the term "hemangiopericytoma-*like*" to describe a group of sinonasal vascular spindle cell tumors which differed from their soft tissue namesakes by the overall association with a better prognosis [180]. The diagnostic category of *soft tissue hemangiopericytoma* had long been derided as a "wastebasket" category and this designation has been dropped from soft tissue tumor classifications [181]. It is now appreciated that most tumors formerly designated as soft tissue hemangiopericytomas represent the *cellular variant of solitary fibrous tumors*. True hemangiopericytomas are related to glomus tumors, the designation "glomangiopericytoma" is another preferred designation. It is ironic that the sinonasal tumors designated as hemangiopericytoma-*like* represent a homogenous group of *bona fide* glomangiopericytomas/hemangiopericytomas; the seterms being diagnostically synonymous.

An Armed Forces Institute of Pathology review of 104 sinonasal hemangiopericytoma (SNHPC) demonstrated a wide age range at presentation (5–86 years, mean 62 years) [182]. Most patients complained of nasal obstruction and bleeding. The majority of SNHPC involved the nasal cavity, whereas sole involvement of the maxillary or ethmoid sinuses or the nasopharynx was relatively uncommon [182].

SNHPC are treated by primary surgery and most patients have an excellent outcome. The local recurrence rate is 17–18%; metastatic disease and disease-related mortality is extremely rare, approximately 3% [182, 183].

■ **Histology**

Sinonasal hemangiopericytomas are polypoid and rimmed by a border of superficially spared stroma and respiratory epithelium. They may have pushing and/or locally infiltrative borders. Tumor nuclei are short, bland, uniform, and evenly spaced. The tumor cells have a moderate amount of eosinophilic cytoplasm with *indistinct* cell membranes imparting a syncitial appearance. The spindled cells form fascicular, storiform, or whorled growth patterns (■ Fig. 4.32). The degree of cellularity can vary within a tumor imparting a "Schwannoma"-like landscape. Tumor vessels are numerous, thin-walled and branching ("staghorn" vessels) and form clefts and gaping spaces. Perivascular hyalinization is a characteristic feature; tumor cells may be seen oriented perpendicular to these hyalinized vessel walls. Generally, there is a low mitotic rate and nuclear pleomorphism is absent or minimal. Unusual reported features include keloid-like collagen deposition and lipomatous change [182].

Immunohistochemically, sinonasal hemangiopericytomas express vimentin, smooth muscle actin, muscle specific actin, and factor XIIIa [184–186]. Recently, recurrent exon three missense mutations in *CTNNB1* have been identified and associated with nuclear overexpression of β-catenin [187, 188]. STAT6, desmin, CD34, bcl-2, factor VIII, and S100 protein are usually negative.

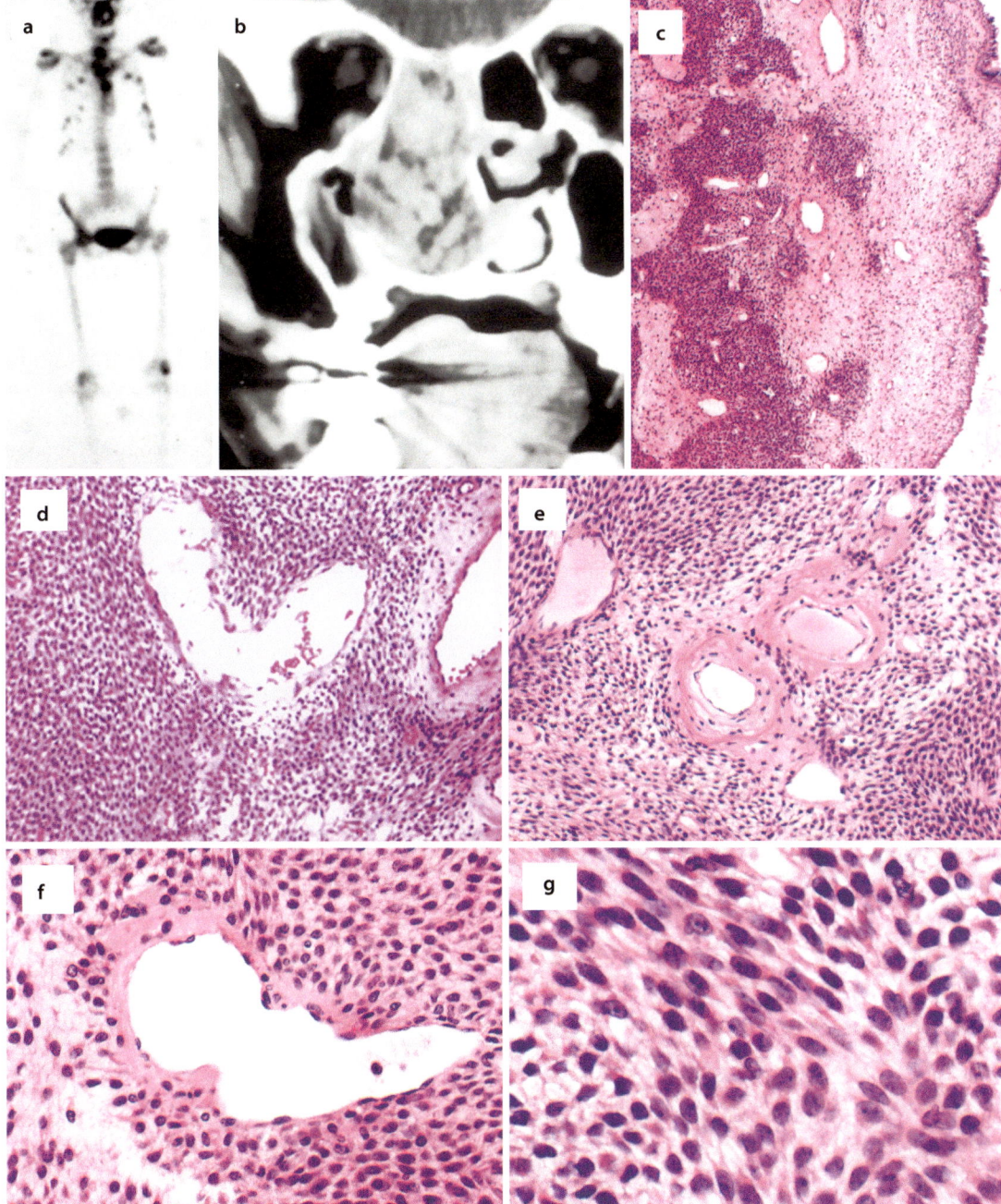

■ **Fig. 4.32** (**a**) Sixty six-year-old Russian female presented with profound immobilizing weakness and diffuse bone pain. This bone scan disclosed multiple lytic lesions throughout the skeleton with a fairly symmetrical distribution. A rib biopsy was unremarkable and investigations for multiple myeloma (urine and serum immmunoglobulin) and hyperparathyroidism (serum PTH on two occasions) were negative. The patient's daughter was informed that her mother probably had widespread metastatic disease from an unknown primary. (**b**) Incidentally, she also complained of epistaxis, frontal headaches, and nasal obstruction "for years". A CT scan showed a sinonasal mass involving the right maxillary and ethmoid sinus up to the cribriform plate. This is an example of **sinonasal hemangiopericytoma** associated with tumor-induced rickets. (**c–g**) Cellular neoplasm composed of short, relatively bland spindle cells. Perivascular hyalinization is common. "Staghorn vessels" are neither sensitive nor specific to hemangiopericytoma. (**f**) Characteristic short spindled cells perpendicularly oriented to the hyalinized vessels.

4.6.2 Solitary Fibrous Tumor

Many soft tissue "hemangiopericytomas" are now reclassified as solitary fibrous tumor-cellular variant. Sinonasalsolitary fibrous tumors are less common than sinonasal hemangiopericytomas and are usually the subject of case reports [189–197]. Solitary fibrous tumorsare categorized as either benign, atypical, or malignant; 10–20 % of tumors can develop local recurrence and/or distant metastasis.

NAB2-STAT6 is a recurrent gene fusion transcript that has been identified in solitary fibrous tumors. The NAB2-STAT6 fusion leads to EGR1 activation and transcriptional deregulation of EGR1-dependent target genes [198]. The fusion transcript is associated with strong and consistent nuclear STAT6 overexpression, a feature which distinguishes solitary fibrous tumor from sinonasal hemangiopericytomas [198, 199].

■ **Histology**

The descriptor of "pattern less pattern" is usually applied to solitary fibrous tumor. In practice, the solitary fibrous tumor-fibrous variant lesions are predominantly dense spindle cell proliferation with regions of amorphous keloid-like collagen deposition, haphazardly arranged cells, and alternating hypercellular and hypocellular regions. Tumor cells can form fascicular and storiform patterns. Vascularity is prominent with perivascular hyalinization (■ Fig. 4.33). There is a morphological continuum between solitary fibrous tumor-fibrous variant and solitary fibrous tumor-cellular variant, the latter contains numerous medium-sized ramifying vessels. Most solitary fibrous tumor appear cytologically benign. Tumor nuclei are typically bland with an open, vesicular, chromatin pattern and occasional nuclear pseudoinclusions. Tumor nuclei are longer and larger as compared with sinonasal hemangiopericytomas, with greater overlapping.

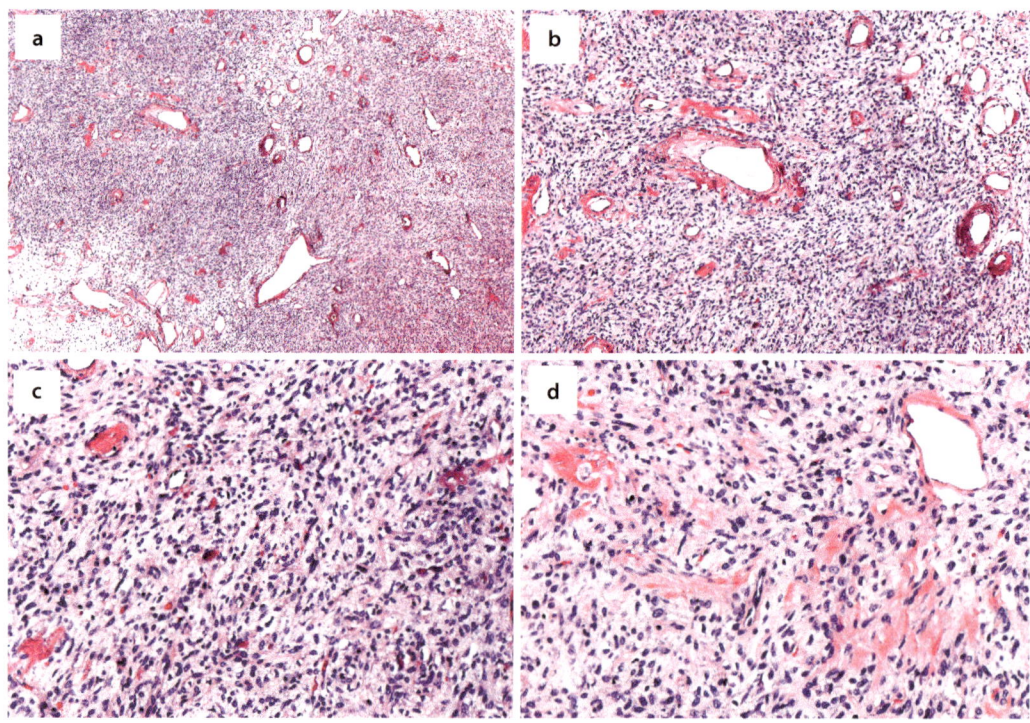

■ **Fig. 4.33**   Solitary fibrous tumor (**a–d**): this bland spindle cell tumor with prominent vessels histologically resembles sinonasal hemangiopericytoma but for the haphazard arrangement of spindle cells and haphazard collagen deposition

Histological features of malignancy include tumor spindling, increased cellularity, increased nuclear/cytoplasmic ratio, pleomorphism, vesicular nuclei with large nucleoli, increased mitotic rate (>4/10 HPF), hemorrhage and necrosis (◘ Fig. 4.34). If one or two of these features are present, the tumor can be classified as atypical solitary fibrous tumor. In addition to the above features, large size (>15 cm) and positive resection margins suggest a more aggressive course.

CD34 expression is characteristic of SFT-fibrous variant, but is less frequent in SFT-cellular variant. CD34 expression is also diminished in malignant SFT. Smooth muscle actin expression is limited or negative (◘ Fig. 4.35). Nuclear β-catenin expression in SFT is variable [200].

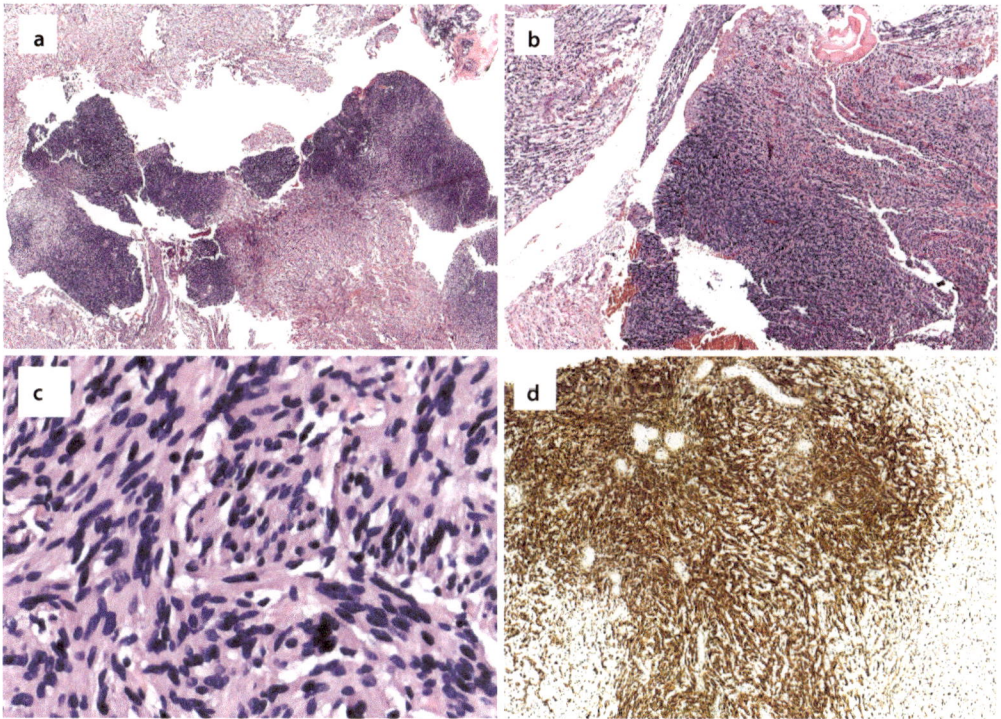

◘ **Fig. 4.34** Sinonasal atypical solitary fibrous tumor. (**a–c**) Greater cellularity and pleomorphism present. (**d**) Characteristic CD34

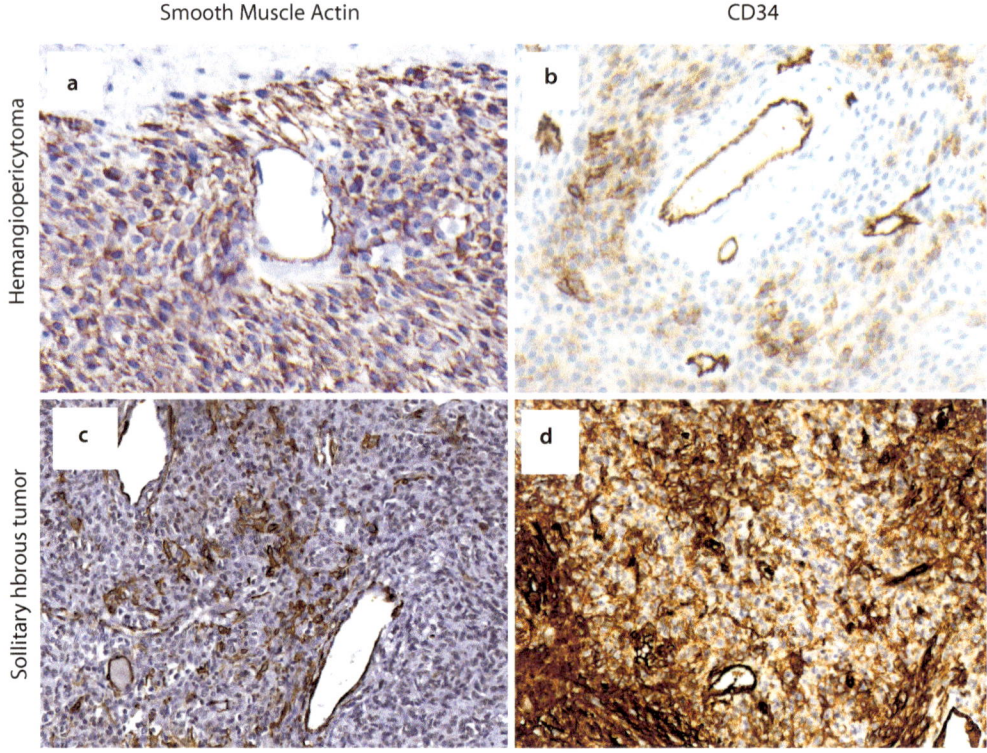

Smooth Muscle Actin   CD34

Hemangiopericytoma

Solitary hbrous tumor

◘ Fig. 4.35 (**a**) **Sinonasal hemangiopericytoma**: diffuse SMA +. (**b**) Sinonasal hemangiopericytoma: focal CD34 expression. The converse expression patterns are seen in solitary fibrous tumor. (**c**) SMA highlights vessels within solitary fibrous tumor, but is negative in the cells of interest. (**d**) Strong CD34 expression in solitary fibrous tumor

4.6.3 Fibrosarcoma/ Myofibrosarcoma/ Biphenotypic Sinonasal Sarcoma/Low-Grade Sinonasal Sarcoma with Neural and Myogenic Features

Contemporary reports on sinonasal fibrosarcomas with confirmatory modern studies are limited to a few case reports, with all due respect to prior publications [201, 202]. One reported sinonasal "low-grade fibrosarcoma" was **Vim**+/**CD34** and**SMA** (smooth muscle actin) weakly focally +/**S00**– and **desmin**–. That patient was disease free after 2 years [203]. A report of sinonasal myofibroblastic sarcoma was **Vim** +, **SMA**+, **αSMA**+ (alpha smooth muscle antigen)/**S100 focally** +. That patient was disease-free after 14 months [204]. Another sinonasal low-grade fibrosarcoma illustrated inverted papilloma-like invaginations; it was **Vim**+/**S100**–, **CD34**–, **desmin**–, **MSA**–, and **αSMA**– [205]. Lewis and colleagues published 28 patients with "low-grade

sinonasal sarcoma with neural and myogenic features", which began to "connect the dots" [206]. All tumors were composed of low-grade fibrosarcoma-like spindle cells; 70 % demonstrated proliferating and invaginating Schneiderian mucosa which mimicked inverted papilloma. S100 was expressed in all cases, but was focal in two tumors. Smooth muscle differentiation was seen in all cases, but was focal in two tumors. Three tumors also demonstrated focal rhabdomyoblastic differentiation. No synovial sarcoma fusion transcripts, SS18-SSX were identified in any tumor. A subsequent case report described a similar low-grade sarcoma with invaginating Schneiderian mucosa [207]. More recently, PAX3-MAML-3 translocation was demonstrated in six bi-phenotypic sinonasal sarcomas [208, 209]. Other translocations, PAX3-NCOA1 (nuclear receptor coactivator-1) [209] and PAX3-FOX01 [210] have been identified, which relate to focal rhabdomyoblastic differentiation. Taken together, the term "bi-phenotypic sinonasal sarcomas" for this entity is quite appropriate,

Fig. 4.36 Bi-phenotypic sinonasal sarcomas (**a–c**): densely hypercellular spindle cell neoplasm with embedded proliferating hyperplastic Schneiderian mucosa

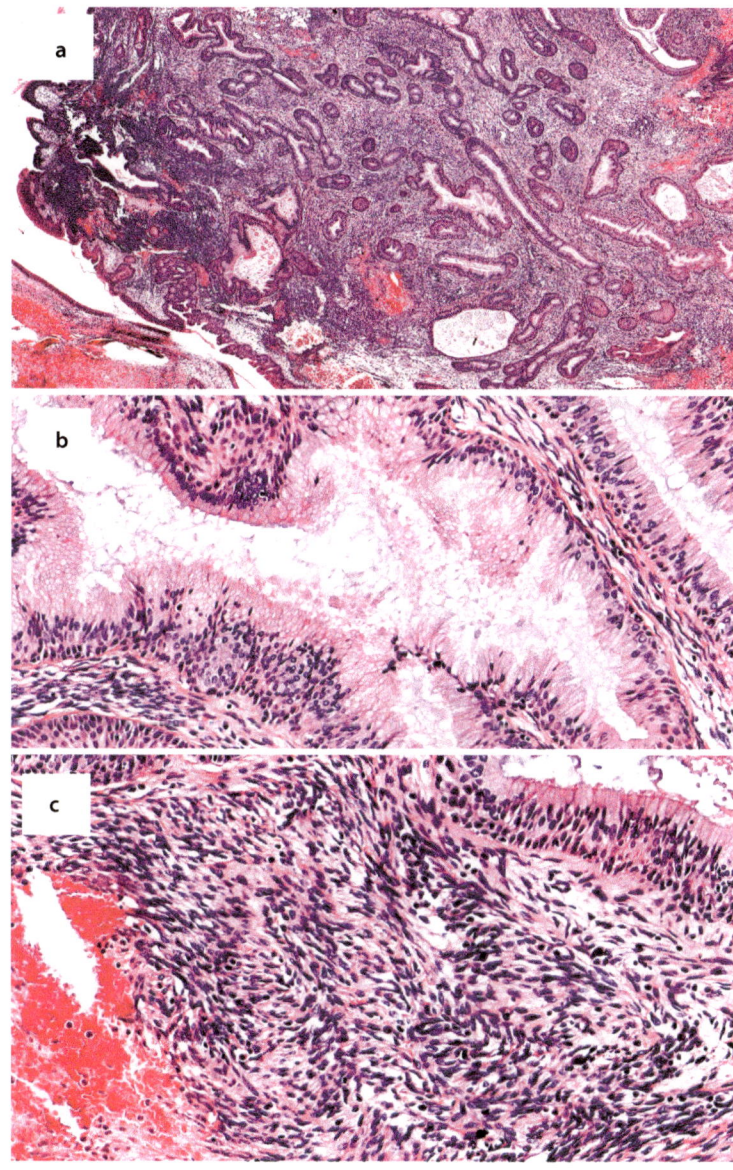

given the variability of the additional mesenchymal phenotype and Schneiderian proliferation.

Local recurrences up to 9 years after treatment, are reported in 44 % of patients with bi-phenotypic sinonasal sarcomas [206]. Metastatic disease or disease-specific mortality have not been reported thus far.

■ Histology

Bi-phenotypic sinonasal sarcomas are characterized as highly cellular spindle cell tumors forming intersecting fascicles, and "herringbone" or "chevron" growth patterns, with variable collagen deposition (■ Fig. 4.36). Nuclear pallisading can be present mimicking peripheral nerve sheath tumor. The tumor cells have elongated bland nuclei and mild to moderate pleomorphism. Mitotic activity is low. Bony invasion is common. Necrosis is not seen. A few cases demonstrate focal rhabdomyoblastic differentiation, which may related to alternate fusion partners (NCOA1 and FOX01). Proliferating hyperplastic Schneiderian ductule structures are embedded within the spindle cell infiltrate. These ductular structures are haphazardly arranged, not confined to any lobular arrangement. Parabasal cell and goblet cell hyperplasia is present; no atypia is seen.

Self Study

1. Which of the following statements is/are correct regarding the sinonasal tumor depicted in ◘ Fig. 4.37?
    (a) This tumor is mediated by high-risk HPV.
    (b) The smooth contours are indicative of diffuse carcinoma-in-situ.
    (c) **CDX2+/CK20+**
    (d) All are correct.
    (e) None are correct.

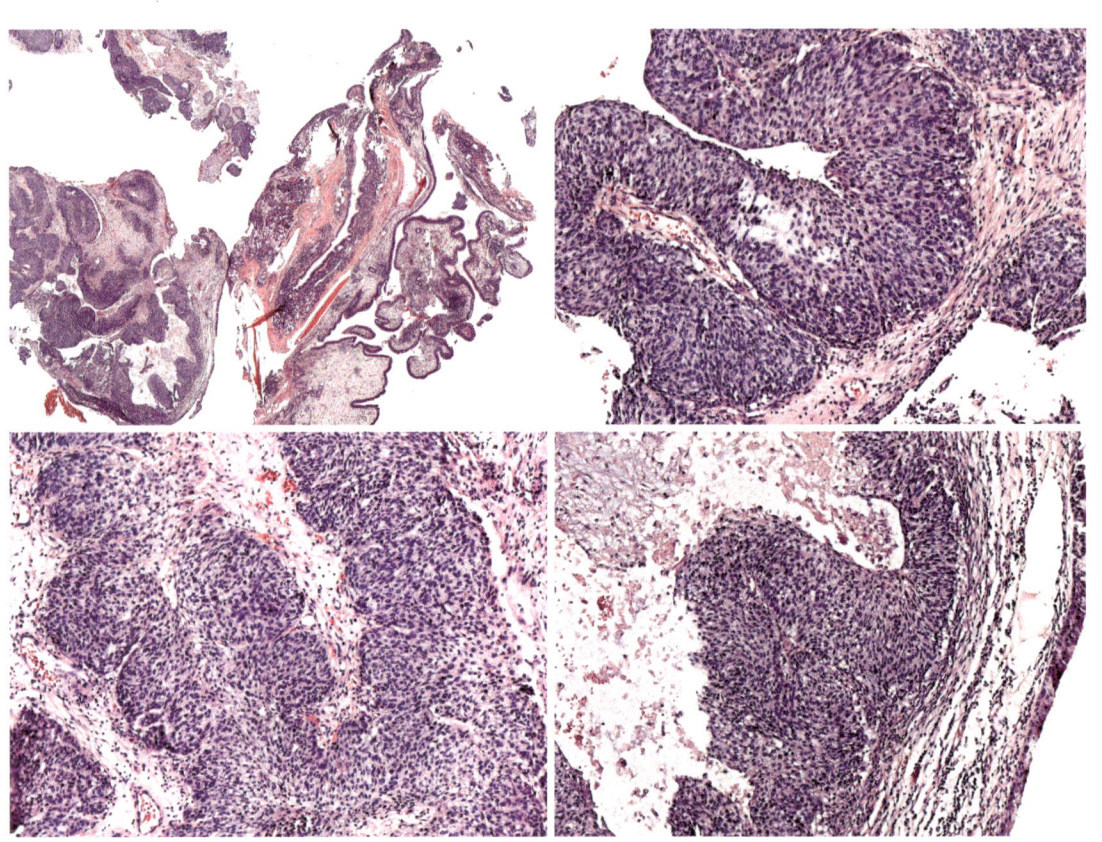

◘ **Fig. 4.37**   Self study

2. Which statement is true regarding
   the sinonasal tumor depicted in
   ◘ Fig. 4.38?
   (a) If **S100+/chromogranin+/
       synaptophysin+/keratins–/CD99–/
       FLI1–/MyoD1–** then this is Hyams II/IV.
   (b) If **S100+/HMB45+** then likely sensitive to
       BRAFV600E inhibitors.

   (c) If **MyoD1+/desmin+/FISH neg** with
       EWS and **FOX01** break-apart probes,
       then this is classic alveolar
       rhabdomyosarcoma.
   (d) If **keratins+/vimentin+/NSE+/
       chromogranin–/synaptophysin–** and no
       evidence of squamous differentiation,
       then this is SNUC.

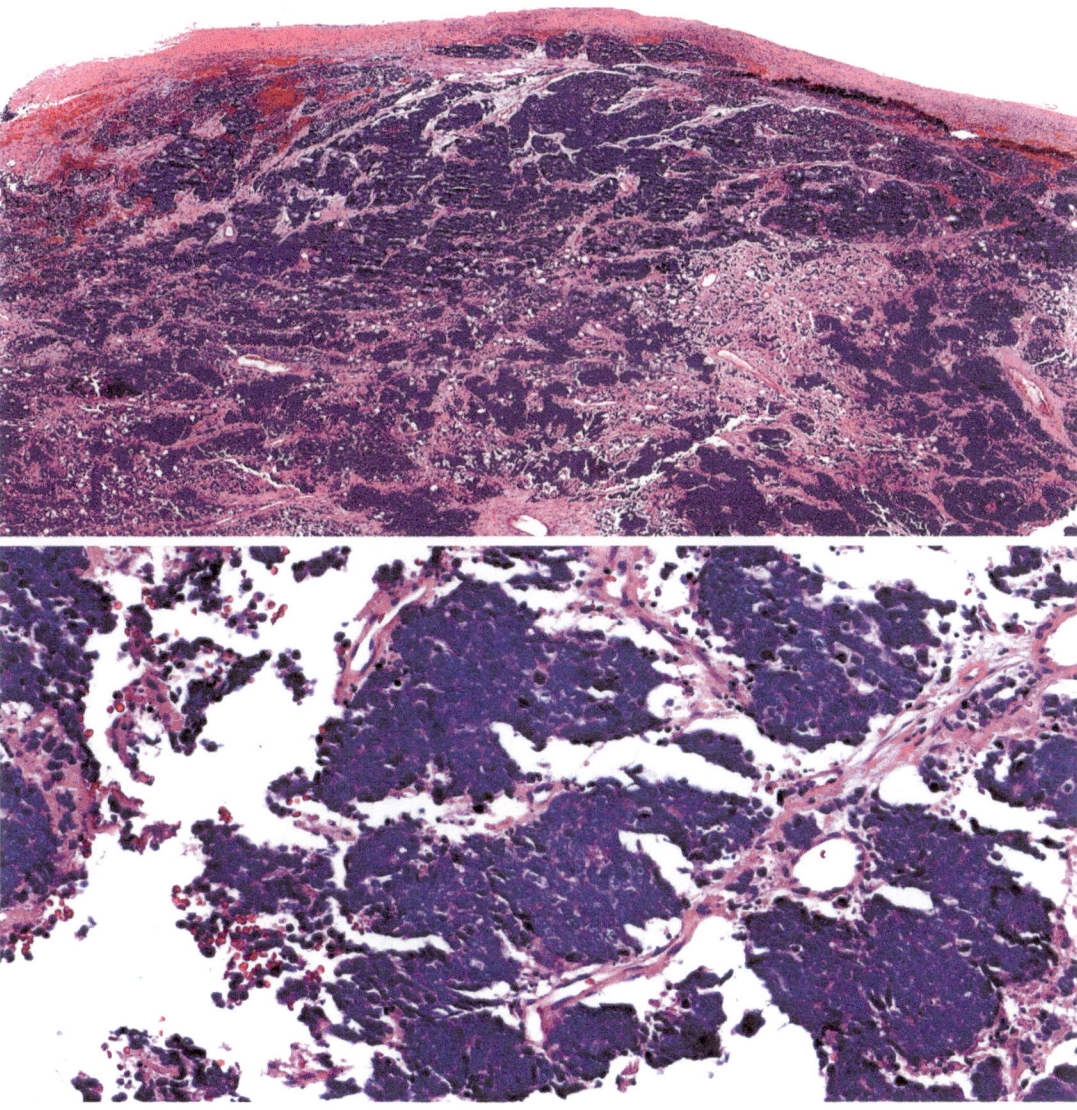

◘ **Fig. 4.38**   Self study

3. Which statement is correct regarding
   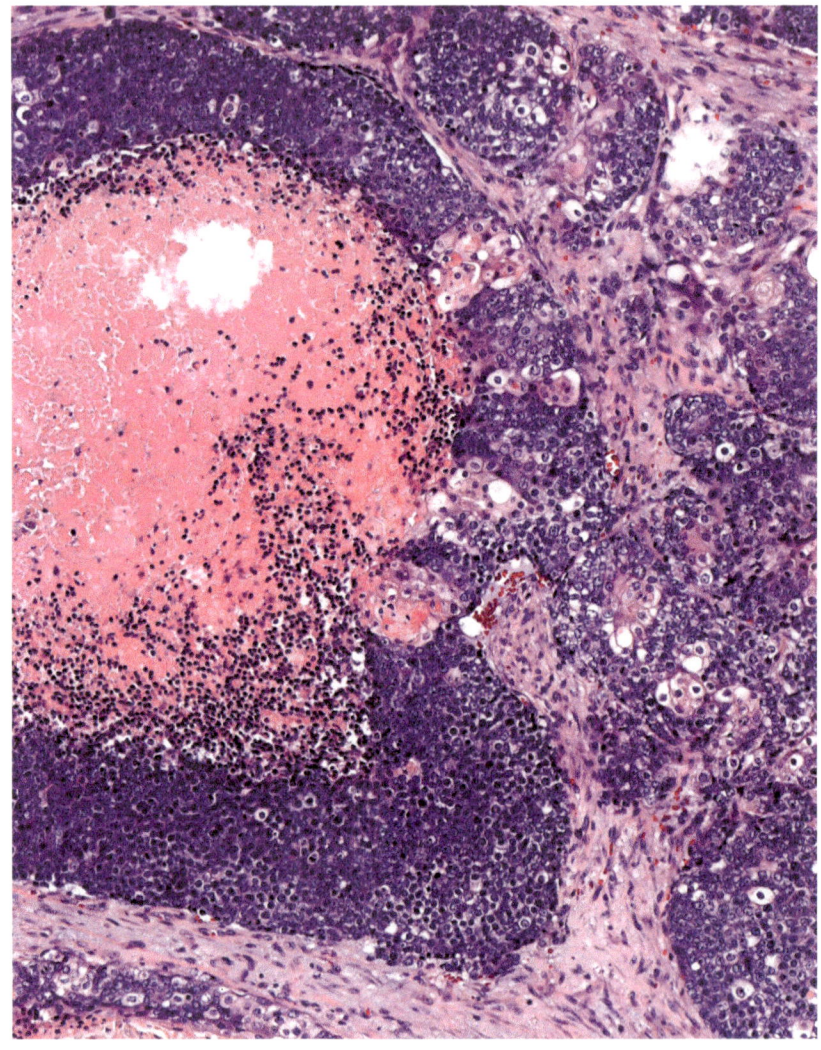 Fig. 4.39?
   (a) Neuroendocrine markers are negative; this is a sinonasal undifferentiated carcinoma (SNUC).
   (b) This tumor is not responsive to cisplatin, 5 FU, cetuximab protocols.
   (c) This Grade III adenoid cystic carcinoma is associated with a poor prognosis.
   (d) This is an EBV-mediated malignancy.

■ **Fig. 4.39**   Self study

4. Which of the following is correct regarding the sinonasal tumor depicted in 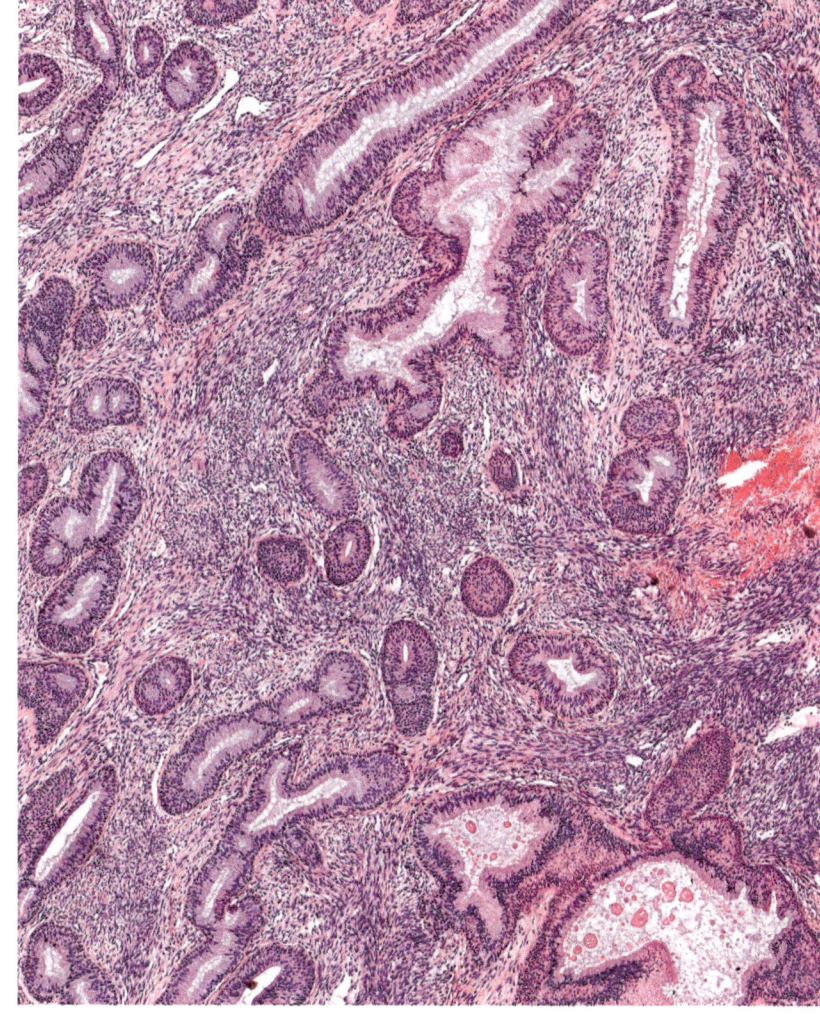 Fig. 4.40?
   (a) Associated with *SS18-SSX* translocation
   (b) Likely, fetal-type squamous epithelium can be found elsewhere within this tumor.
   (c) This represents a sarcoma-ex-inverted papilloma
   (d) This is a hamatomatous process
   (e) None of the above correct

Fig. 4.40 Self study

5. Which of the following is correct regarding the sinonasal tumor depicted in
   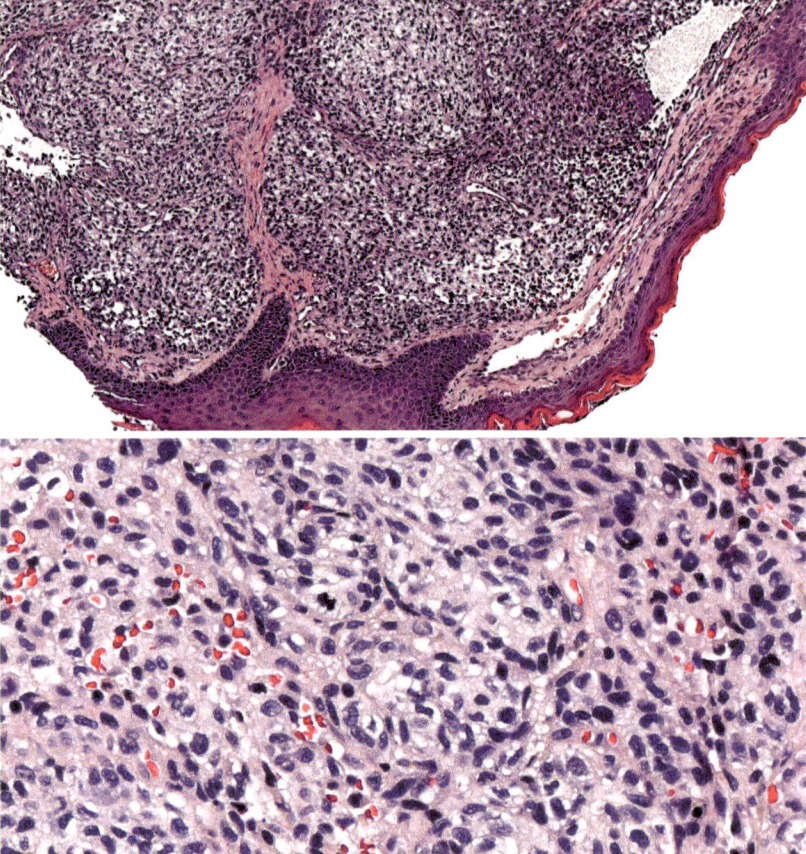 Fig. 4.41?
   (a) This tumor is likely to be sensitive to BRAFV600E inhibitors.
   (b) Although this is a single sinonasal mass, it is more like to be metastasis from a dermal primary rather than a sinonasal primary.
   (c) Molecular testing for *PAX-FOX01* and *EWS-FLI1* will establish the correct diagnosis,
   (d) It should be staged according to histology-specific staging criteria.

 Fig. 4.41   Self study

6. A young man with significant indoor exposure to wood dust was diagnosed with a sinonasal tumor depicted in 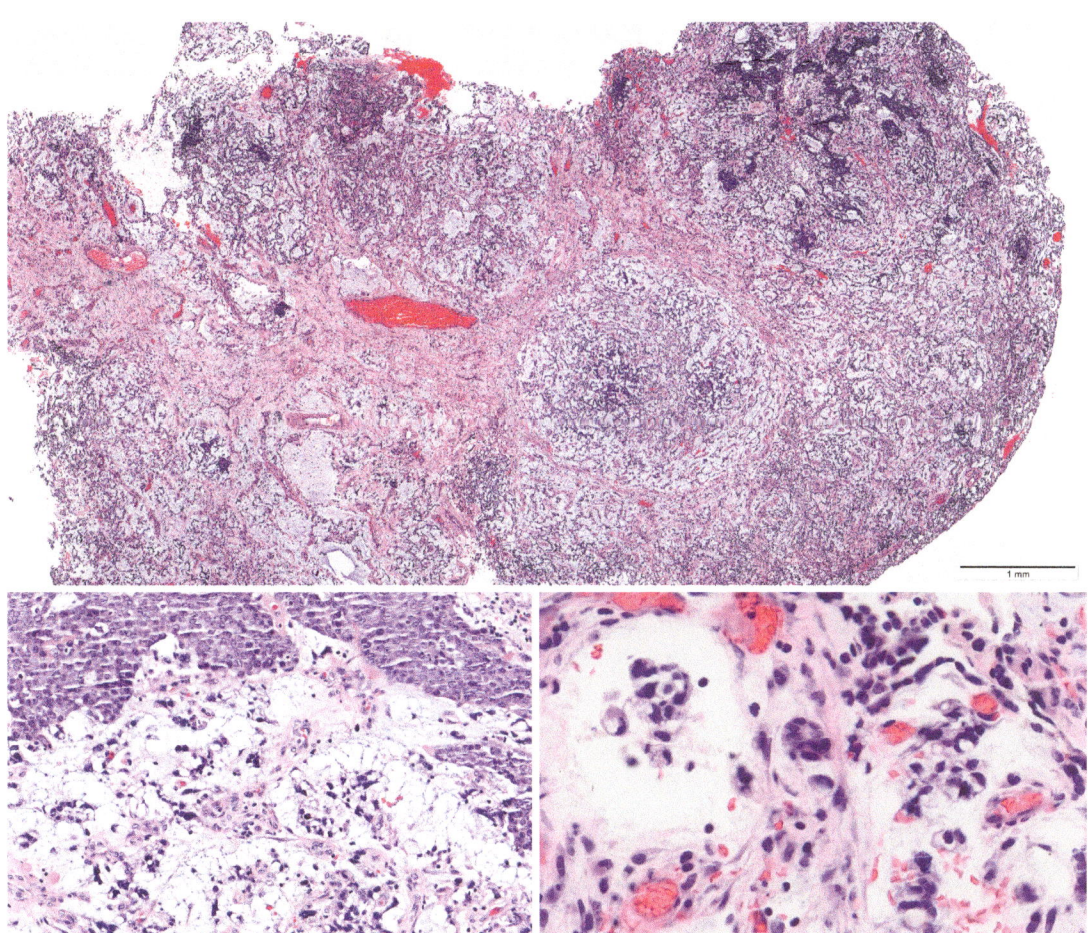 Fig. 4.42. Which of the following statements is most likely to be true?

 (a) It is **CK20+/CDX2+** and represents a low-grade ITAC.

 (b) It is **CK7+/CDX2–** and likely represents colonic metastasis.

 (c) It is **CRTC1/MAML2 fusion gene** + and represents sinonasal low-grade mucoepidermoid carcinoma.

 (d) It is **CK7+/CDX2+** and represents a high-grade ITAC.

◻ **Fig. 4.42**   Self study

Answers

1. Which of the following statements is/are correct regarding the sinonasal tumor depicted ▣ Fig. 4.37?

   This is a squamous carcinoma, transitional variant.

   (a) This tumor is mediated by high-risk HPV. **No**. *Perhaps you were thinking carcinoma-ex-inverted papilloma. If you look carefully, there is no evidence of benign inverted papilloma in these images.*

   (b) The smooth contours are indicative of diffuse carcinoma-in-situ. **No, which is the point of this question. Many a time, residents will apply the criteria for invasion in the urinary bladder to the upper airway. Different context, different criteria. This transitional pattern represents a non-aggressive pattern of invasion.*

   (c) **CDX2+/CK20+ No**. *This could not be ITAC, which is CDX2+/CK20+. Look at the ribbons of carcinoma. You can recognize that it's recapitulating mucosa by noticing the proliferating basal side and the maturing side, which shows flattening of the tumor cells. This morphology excludes the possibility of an adenocarcinoma.*

   (d) All are correct. **No**

   (e) None are correct. **CORRECT**

2. Which statement is true regarding the sinonasal tumor depicted in ▣ Fig. 4.38?

   This is a SNUC, and this question if about recognizing IHC and translocation profiles.

   (a) If **S100+/chromogranin+/ synaptophysin+/keratins–/CD99–/ FLI1–/MyoD1–** then this is Hyams II/IV. **No**. *This IHC profile is consistent with olfactory neuroblastoma (ONB). In case you weren't certain, the reference to Hyam's grading is a big hint. But Hyams II ONB would have rossettes and neuropil, and not demonstrate any necrosis. The presence of necrosis negates the possibility of Hyams II ONB.*

   (b) If **S100+/HMB45+** then likely sensitive to BRAFV600E inhibitors. **No**. *This IHC profile is consistent with sinonasal melanoma. However the BRAFV600E*

   mutation has not been detected in sinonasal melanoma.

   (c) If **MyoD1+/desmin+/FISH neg** with **EWS** and **FOX01** break-apart probes, then this is classic alveolar rhabdomyosarcoma. **No**. *This IHC profile MyoD1+/desmin+ is consistent with sinonasal rhabdomyosarcoma. EWS break-apart probe results exclude Ewing family tumor. FOX01 break-apart probes results exclude alveolar rhabdomyosarcoma. Solid alveolar rhabdomyosarcoma may be fusion negative. That's why I specific "classic" alveolar rhabdomyosarcoma.*

   (d) If **keratins+/vimentin+/NSE+/ chromogranin-/synaptophysin–** and no evidence of squamous differentiation, then this is SNUC. **CORRECT. Any evidence of differentiation (keratin pearls, glandular spaces) excludes SNUC.**

3. Which statement is correct regarding ▣ Fig. 4.39?

   This is a BRD4-NUT Translocation Midline Carcinoma. Multiple foci of abrupt keratinization are seen in the right side of the panel.

   (a) Neuroendocrine markers are negative; this is a sinonasal undifferentiated carcinoma (SNUC). **No**. *Any evidence of differentiation, such as keratinization, rules out SNUC.*

   (b) This tumor is not responsive to cisplatin, 5FU, cetuximab protocols. **CORRECT**. *Diffuse speckled nuclear expression of NUT protein is diagnostic. These tumors are unresponsive to the usual chemotherapy protocols. Patients should be referred for clinical trials using bromodomain inhibitors (BETi) and histone deacetylase inhibitors (HDACi).*

   (c) This Grade III adenoid cystic carcinoma is associated with a poor prognosis. **No**. *The solid areas and necrosis might bring this diagnosis to mind. However, the abrupt keratinization rules out this possibility.*

   (d) This is an EBV-mediated malignancy. **No**. *EBER testing is part of the work-up protocol, which should be negative.*

4. Which of the following is correct regarding the sinonasal tumor depicted in ◩ Fig. 4.40?

   This represents a biphenotypic sinonasal sarcoma, which has been associated with following translocations: PAX3-MAML-3, PAX3-NCOA1, and PAX3-FOX01.

   (a) Associated with *SS18-SSX* translocation. **No.** *Biphenotypic sinonasal sarcomas are negative for synovial sarcoma fusion transcripts* [206].

   (b) Likely, fetal-type squamous epithelium can be found elsewhere within this tumor. **No.** *Fetal-type squamous epithelium is common to sinonasal teratocarcinosarcoma.*

   (c) This represents a sarcoma-ex-inverted papilloma. **No.** *The proliferating Schneiderian mucosa can be mistaken for inverted papilloma. Inverted papilloma is composed of stratified squamous epithelium, which is nonkeratinizing and glycogenated. Here we see hyperplastic respiratory epithelium. Furthermore, there is no such entity as sarcoma-ex-inverted papilloma.*

   (d) This is a hamatomatous process. **No.** *This is a tumor process.*

   (e) None of the above correct. **CORRECT.**

5. Which of the following is correct regarding the sinonasal tumor depicted in ◩ Fig. 4.41?

   This is a sinonasal melanoma, clear cell variant.

   (a) This tumor is likely to be sensitive to BRAFV600E inhibitors. **No.** *The BRAFV600E mutation has not been detected in sinonasal melanoma.*

   (b) Although this is a single sinonasal mass, it is more like to be metastasis from a dermal primary rather than a sinonasal primary. **No.** *Metastatic melanoma to upper airway mucosa is usually part of widely disseminated disease, and rarely an isolated event from cutaneous melanoma.*

   (c) Molecular testing for *PAX-FOX01* and *EWS-FLI1* will establish the correct diagnosis. **No.** *Those tests are for rhabdomyosarcoma and Ewing's family tumor.*

   (d) It should be staged according to histology-specific staging criteria. **CORRECT.** *Sinonasal melanomas are staged as mucosal melanomas. There is no T1 or T2. If the melanoma is a polypoid intranasal mass involving submucosa, but not bony structures, then it is T3. Any tumor beyond this is T4.*

6. A young man with significant indoor exposure to wood dust was diagnosed with a sinonasal tumor depicted in ◩ Fig. 4.42. Which of the following statements is most likely to be true?

   (a) It is **CK20+/CDX2 +** and represents a low-grade ITAC. **No.** *The lower images demonstrate a high-grade neoplasm.*

   (b) It is **CK20−/CDX2−** and likely represents colonic metastasis. **No.** *Colonic adenocarcinoma and sinonasal intestinal type adenocarcinoma (ITAC) are both **CK20+/CDX2 +**. The exposure history suggests ITAC.*

   (c) It is **CRTC1/MAML2 fusion gene +** and represents sinonasal low-grade mucoepidermoid carcinoma. **No.** *More than half of mucoepidermoid carcinomas harbor the CRTC1/MAML2 fusion gene, which is more often seen in low- and intermediate-grade mucoepidermoid carcinomas. However, this is clearly a high-grade neoplasm.*

   (d) It is **CK7+/CDX2+** and represents a high-grade ITAC. **CORRECT.** This is an invasive, mucinous adenocarcinoma with signet-ring cells. The tumor cells are morphologically high-grade. ITAC are uniformly **CK20+/CDX2+; CK7** expression is variable.

References

1. Frierson Jr HF, Mills SE, Fechner RE, Taxy JB, Levine PA. Sinonasal undifferentiated carcinoma. An aggressive neoplasm derived from Schneiderian epithelium and distinct from olfactory neuroblastoma. Am J Surg Pathol. 1986;10:771–9.

2. Levine PA, Frierson Jr HF, Stewart FM, Mills SE, Fechner RE, Cantrell RW. Sinonasal undifferentiated carcinoma: a distinctive and highly aggressive neoplasm. Laryngoscope. 1987;97:905–8.

3. Gallo O, Graziani P, Fini-Storchi O. Undifferentiated carcinoma of the nose and paranasal sinuses. An immunohistochemical and clinical study. Ear Nose Throat J. 1993;72:588–90, 593–5.

4. Houston GD. Sinonasal undifferentiated carcinoma: report of two cases and review of the literature. Oral Surg Oral Med Oral Pathol Oral Radiol Endod. 1998;85:185–8.

5. Smith SR, Som P, Fahmy A, Lawson W, Sacks S, Brandwein M. A clinicopathological study of sinonasal neuroendocrine carcinoma and sinonasal undifferentiated carcinoma. Laryngoscope. 2000;110:1617–22.

6. Cerilli LA, Holst VA, Brandwein MS, Stoler MH, Mills SE. Sinonasal undifferentiated carcinoma: immunohistochemical profile and lack of EBV association. Am J Surg Pathol. 2001;25:156–63.

7. Kumar R, Chandra A, Rastogi A. Intracranial sinonasal undifferentiated carcinoma (SNUC) in a child. Childs Nerv Syst. 2006;22:1208–11.

8. Sobota A, Pena M, Santi M, Ali AA. Undifferentiated sinonasal carcinoma in a patient with nevoid basal cell carcinoma syndrome. Int J Surg Pathol. 2007;15: 303–6.

9. Tetzlaff MT, Liu P, O'Malley Jr BW, LiVolsi VA, Elder D. Report of a case of sinonasal undifferentiated carcinoma arising in a background of extensive nasal gliomatosis. Head Neck. 2008;30:549–55.

10. Reiersen DA, Pahilan ME, Devaiah AK. Meta-analysis of treatment outcomes for sinonasal undifferentiated carcinoma. Otolaryngol Head Neck Surg. 2012;147:7–14.

11. Bourne TD, Bellizzi AM, Stelow EB, Loy AH, Levine PA, Wick MR, Mills SE. p63 Expression in olfactory neuroblastoma and other small cell tumors of the sinonasal tract. Am J Clin Pathol. 2008;130:213–8.

12. Wadsworth B, Bumpous JM, Martin AW, Nowacki MR, Jenson AB, Farghaly H. Expression of p16 in sinonasal undifferentiated carcinoma (SNUC) without associated human papillomavirus (HPV). Head Neck Pathol. 2011;5:349–54.

13. Yoshida E, Aouad R, Fragoso R, Farwell DG, Gandour-Edwards R, Donald PJ, Chen AM. Improved clinical outcomes with multi-modality therapy for sinonasal undifferentiated carcinoma of the head and neck. Am J Otolaryngol. 2013;34:658–63.

14. Lin EM, Sparano A, Spalding A, Eisbruch A, Worden FP, Heth J, Sullivan SE, Thompson BG, Marentette LJ. Sinonasal undifferentiated carcinoma: a 13-year experience at a single institution. Skull Base. 2010;20:61–7.

15. Bauer DE, Mitchell CM, Strait KM, Lathan CS, Stelow EB, Lüer SC, Muhammed S, Evans AG, Sholl LM, Rosai J, Giraldi E, Oakley RP, Rodriguez-Galindo C, London WB, Sallan SE, Bradner JE, French CA. Clinicopathologic features and long-term outcomes of NUT midline carcinoma. Clin Cancer Res. 2012;18:5773–9.

16. French CA, Kutok JL, Faquin WC, Toretsky JA, Antonescu CR, Griffin CA, Nose V, Vargas SO, Moschovi M, Tzortzatou-Stathopoulou F, Miyoshi I, Perez-Atayde AR, Aster JC, Fletcher JA. Midline carcinoma of children and young adults with NUT rearrangement. J Clin Oncol. 2004;22:4135–9.

17. French CA. The importance of diagnosing NUT midline carcinoma. Head Neck Pathol. 2013;7:11–6.

18. French C. NUT midline carcinoma. Nat Rev Cancer. 2014;14:149–50.

19. Mills AF, Lanfranchi M, Wein RO, Mukand-Cerro I, Pilichowska M, Cowan J, Bedi H. NUT midline carcinoma: a case report with a novel translocation and review of the literature. Head Neck Pathol. 2014;8:182–6.

20. Grayson AR, Walsh EM, Cameron MJ, Godec J, Ashworth T, Ambrose JM, Aserlind AB, Wang H, Evan GI, Kluk MJ, Bradner JE, Aster JC, French CA. MYC, a

21. Ziai J, French CA, Zambrano E. NUT gene rearrangement in a poorly-differentiated carcinoma of the submandibular gland. Head Neck Pathol. 2010;4:163–8.

22. Bakker MA, Beverloo BH, van den Heuvel-Eibrink MM, Meeuwis CA, Tan LM, Johnson LA, French CA, van Leenders GJ. NUT midline carcinoma of the parotid gland with mesenchymal differentiation. Am J Surg Pathol. 2009;33:1253–8.

23. Salles PG, Moura Rde D, Menezes LM, Bacchi CE. Expression of P16 in NUT carcinomas with no association with human papillomavirus (HPV). Appl Immunohistochem Mol Morphol. 2014;22:262–5.

24. Bishop JA, Ogawa T, Stelow EB, Moskaluk CA, Koch WM, Pai SI, Westra WH. Human papillomavirus-related carcinoma with adenoid cystic-like features: a peculiar variant of head and neck cancer restricted to the sinonasal tract. Am J Surg Pathol. 2013;37:836–44.

25. Hwang SJ, Ok S, Lee HM, Lee E, Park IH. Human papillomavirus-related carcinoma with adenoid cystic-like features of the inferior turbinate: a case report. Auris Nasus Larynx. 2015;42:53–5.

26. Wenig BM. Recently described sinonasal tract lesions/neoplasms: considerations for the new World Health Organization book. Head Neck Pathol. 2014;8:33–41.

27. Bishop JA, Guo TW, Smith DF, Wang H, Ogawa T, Pai SI, Westra WH. Humanpapillomavirus-related carcinomas of the sinonasal tract. Am J Surg Pathol. 2013;37:185–92.

28. Brill 2nd LB, Kanner WA, Fehr A, Andrén Y, Moskaluk CA, Löning T, Stenman G, Frierson Jr HF. Analysis of MYB expression and MYB-NFIB gene fusions in adenoid cystic carcinoma and other salivary neoplasms. Mod Pathol. 2011;24:1169–76.

29. West RB, Kong C, Clarke N, Gilks T, Lipsick JS, Cao H, Kwok S, Montgomery KD, Varma S, Le QT. MYB expression and translocation in adenoid cystic carcinomas and other salivary gland tumors with clinicopathologic correlation. Am J Surg Pathol. 2011;35:92–9.

30. Boland JM, McPhail ED, García JJ, Lewis JE, Schembri-Wismayer DJ. Detection of human papilloma virus and p16 expression in high-grade adenoid cystic carcinoma of the head and neck. Mod Pathol. 2012;25:529–36.

31. Isayeva T, Xing D, Brandwein-Gensler M. Transcriptionally active HPV infection and salivary adenoid cystic carcinomas. Mod Pathol. 2013;26:S2,307A.

32. Chang AE, Karnell LH, Menck HR. The national cancer data base report on cutaneous and noncutaneous melanoma: a summary of 84,836 cases from the past decade. The American College of Surgeons Commission on Cancer and the American Cancer Society. Cancer. 1998;83:1664–78.

33. Gal TJ, Silver N, Huang B. Demographics and treatment trends in sinonasal mucosal melanoma. Laryngoscope. 2011;121:2026–33.

34. Brandwein M, Rothstein A, Lawson W, Bodian C, Urken ML. Sinonasal melanoma – a clinicopathologic study of 25 cases and literature meta-analysis. Arch Otolaryngol Head Neck Surg. 1997;123:290–6.

35. Prasad ML, Busam KJ, Patel SG, Hoshaw-Woodard S, Shah JP, Huvos AG. Clinicopathologic differences in

malignant melanoma arising in oral squamous and sino-nasal respiratory mucosa of the upper aerodigestive tract. Arch Pathol Lab Med. 2003;127:997–1002.

36. Jayaraj SM, Hern JD, Mochloulis G, Porter GC. Malignant melanoma arising in the frontal sinuses. J Laryngol Otol. 1997;111:376–8.

37. Thompson LDR, Wieneke JA, Mienttinen M. Sinonasal tract and nasopharyngeal melanoma. A clinicopatho-logic study of 115 cases with a proposed staging system. Am J Surg Pathol. 2003;27:594–611.

38. Edge SB, Byrd DR, Compton CC, Fritz AG, Greene FL, Trotti A, editors. American Joint Cancer Committee can-cer staging handbook. 7th ed. New York: Springer; 2010. p.123.

39. Koivunen P, Bäck L, Pukkila M, Laranne J, Kinnunen I, Grénman R, Mäkitie AA. Accuracy of the current TNM classification in predicting survival in patients with sino-nasal mucosal melanoma. Laryngoscope. 2012;122: 1734–8.

40. American Joint Cancer Committee cancer staging hand-book. 8th ed. (in print).

41. Meng XJ, Ao HF, Huang WT, Chen F, Sun XC, Wang JJ, Liu ZF, Han WW, Fry AN, Wang DH. Impact of different surgical and postoperative adjuvant treatment modali-ties on survival of sinonasal malignant melanoma. BMC Cancer. 2014;14:608. doi:10.1186/1471-2407-14-608.

42. Sun CZ, Li QL, Hu ZD, Jiang YE, Song M, Yang AK. Treatment and prognosis in sinonasal mucosal mela-noma: a retrospective analysis of 65 patients from a sin-gle cancer center. Head Neck. 2014;36:675–81.

43. Zebary A, Jangard M, Omholt K, Ragnarsson-Olding B, Hansson J. KIT, NRAS and BRAF mutations in sinonasal mucosal melanoma: a study of 56 cases. Br J Cancer. 2013;109:559–64.

44. Turri-Zanoni M, Medicina D, Lombardi D, Ungari M, Balzarini P, Rossini C, Pellegrini W, Battaglia P, Capella C, Castelnuovo P, Palmedo G, Facchetti F, Kutzner H, Nicolai P, Vermi W. Sinonasal mucosal melanoma: molecular profile and therapeutic implications from a series of 32 cases. Head Neck. 2013;35:1066–77.

45. Chraybi M, Abd Alsamad I, Copie-Bergman C, Baia M, André J, Dumaz N, Ortonne N. Oncogene abnormalities in a series of primary melanomas of the sinonasal tract: NRAS mutations and cyclin D1 amplification are more frequent than KIT or BRAF mutations. Hum Pathol. 2013;44:1902–11.

46. Colombino M, Lissia A, Franco R, Botti G, Ascierto PA, Manca A, Sini MC, Pisano M, Paliogiannis P, Tanda F, Palmieri G, Cossu A. Unexpected distribu-tion of cKIT and BRAF mutations among southern Italian patients with sinonasal melanoma. Dermatology. 2013;226:279–84.

47. Feeley C, Theaker J. Epithelial markers in primary sinonasal mucosal melanoma. Histopathology. 2004; 45:96–8.

48. Smith SM, Schmitt AC, Carrau RL, Iwenofu OH. Primary sinonasal mucosal melanoma with aberrant diffuse and strong desmin reactivity: a potential diagnostic pitfall! Head Neck Pathol. 2015;9(1):165–71.

49. Mochel MC, Duncan LM, Piris A, Kraft S. Primary mucosal melanoma of the sinonasal tract: a clinicopath-ologic and immunohistochemical study of thirty-two cases. Head Neck Pathol. 2015;9:236–43.

50. Shuman AG, Light E, Olsen SH, Pynnonen MA, Taylor JM, Johnson TM, Bradford CR. Mucosal melanoma of the head and neck: predictors of prognosis. Arch Otolaryngol Head Neck Surg. 2011;137:331–7.

51. Moreno MA, Roberts DB, Kupferman ME, DeMonte F, El-Naggar AK, Williams M, Rosenthal DS, Hanna EY. Mucosal melanoma of the nose and paranasal sinuses, a contemporary experience from the M. D Anderson Cancer Center Cancer. 2010;116:2215–23.

52. Chan JK, Fletcher CD, Nayler SJ, Cooper K. Follicular dendritic cell sarcoma. Clinicopathologic analysis of 17 cases suggesting a malignant potential higher than cur-rently recognized. Cancer. 1997;79:294–313.

53. Shia J, Chen W, Tang LH, Carlson DL, Qin J, Guillem JG, Nobrega J, Wong WD, Klimstra DS. Extranodal follicular dendritic cell sarcoma: clinical, pathologic, and histoge-netic characteristics of an underrecognized disease entity. Virchows Arch. 2006;449:148–58.

54. Dalia S, Jaglal M, Chervenick P, Cualing H, Sokol L. Clinicopathologic characteristics and outcomes of his-tiocytic and dendritic cell neoplasms: the Moffitt cancer center experience over the last twenty five years. Cancers (Basel). 2014;6:2275–95.

55. Perez-Ordonez B, Erlandson RA, Rosai J. Follicular den-dritic cell tumor: report of 13 additional cases of a dis-tinctive entity. Am J Surg Pathol. 1996;20:944–55.

56. Ohtake H, Yamakawa M. Interdigitating dendritic cell sarcoma and folliculardendritic cell sarcoma: histopath-ological findings for differential diagnosis. J Clin Exp Hematop. 2013;53:179–84.

57. Saygin C, Uzunaslan D, Ozguroglu M, Senocak M, Tuzuner N. Dendritic cell sarcoma: a pooled analysis including 462 cases with presentation of our case series. Crit Rev Oncol Hematol. 2013;88:253–71.

58. Pokuri VK, Merzianu M, Gandhi S, Baqai J, Loree TR, Bhat S. Interdigitating dendritic cell sarcoma. J Natl Compr Canc Netw. 2015;13:128–32.

59. Yu L, Yang SJ. Primary follicular dendritic cell sarcoma of the thyroid gland coexisting with Hashimoto's thy-roiditis. Int J Surg Pathol. 2011;19:502–5.

60. Choe JY, Go H, Jeon YK, Yun JY, Kim YA, Kim HJ, Huh J, Lee H, Shin DH, Kim JE. Inflammatory pseudotumor-like follicular dendritic cell sarcoma of the spleen: a report of six cases with increased IgG4-positive plasma cells. Pathol Int. 2013;63:245–51.

61. Lee SY, Lee SR, Chang WJ, Kim HS, Kim BS, Kim IS. Successful treatment of disseminated interdigitating dendritic cell sarcoma with adriamycin, bleomycin, vin-blastine, and dacarbazine chemotherapy. Korean J Hematol. 2012;47:150–3.

62. Shi Y, Wang E. Blastic plasmacytoid dendritic cell neo-plasm: a clinicopathologic review. Arch Pathol Lab Med. 2014;138(4):564–9.

63. Parada D, Peña KB, Gil I, Queralt R, Garcia A, Alos L. Interdigitating dendritic cell sarcoma presenting in the nasal region. Pathol Res Pract. 2012;208:368–71.

64. Karabulut B, Orhan KS, Guldiken Y, Dogan O. Follicular dendritic cell sarcoma of the nasopharynx. Int J Oral Maxillofac Surg. 2012;41:218–20.

65. Horton WB, Joyner DA, Daley WP, Pitman KT, Khan MA. Nasopharyngeal dendritic cell sarcoma, not other-wise specified, in a 34-year-old man. Ear Nose Throat J. 2011;90:E7–10.

66. Lee EJ, Hyun DW, Cho HJ, Lee JG. A rare case of interdigitating dendritic cell sarcoma in the nasal cavity. Case Rep Otolaryngol. 2013;2013:913157. doi:10.1155/2013/913157.

67. Bachar G, Goldstein D, Brown D, Tsang R, Lockwood G, Perez-Ordonez B, Irish J. Solitary extramedullary plasmacytoma of the head and neck – long-term outcome analysis of 68 cases. Head Neck. 2008;30(8):1012–9.

68. Ashraf MJ, Azarpira N, Khademi B, Abedi E, Hakimzadeh A, Valibeigi B. Extramedullary plasmacytoma of the nasal cavity report of three cases with review of the literature. Iran Red Crescent Med J. 2013;15:363–6.

69. Patel TD, Vázquez A, Choudhary MM, Kam D, Baredes S, Eloy JA. Sinonasal extramedullary plasmacytoma: a population-based incidence and survival analysis. Int Forum Allergy Rhinol. 2015. doi:10.1002/alr.21544.

70. D'Aguillo C, Soni RS, Gordhan C, Liu JK, Baredes S, Eloy JA. Sinonasal extramedullary plasmacytoma: a systematic review of 175 patients. Int Forum Allergy Rhinol. 2014;4:156–63.

71. Lezzoni JC, Mills SE. "Undifferentiated" small round cell tumors of the sinonasal tract: differential diagnosis update. Am J Clin Pathol. 2005;124 Suppl:S110–21.

72. Chang YL, Chen PY, Hung SH. Extramedullary plasmacytoma of the nasopharynx: a case report and review of the literature. Oncol Lett. 2014;7(2):458–60.

73. Sodhi KS, Khandelwal N, Virmani V, Das A, Panda N. Solitary extramedullary plasmacytoma of the nasal tract: an unusual cause of epistaxis. Ear Nose Throat J. 2013;92:E51.

74. Chen SW, Chang ST, Lu CL, Hwang WS, Tsao CJ, Huang WT, Chang KY, Chuang SS. Upper aerodigestive tract lymphoma in Taiwan. J Clin Pathol. 2010;63:888–93.

75. Dubal PM, Dutta R, Vazquez A, Patel TD, Baredes S, Eloy JA. A comparative population-based analysis of sinonasal diffuse large B-cell and extranodal NK/T-cell lymphomas. Laryngoscope. 2015;125:1077–83.

76. Vazquez A, Khan MN, Blake DM, Sanghvi S, Baredes S, Eloy JA. Extranodal natural killer/T-cell lymphoma: a population-based comparison of sinonasal and extranasal disease. Laryngoscope. 2014;124:888–95.

77. Kanumuri VV, Khan MN, Vazquez A, Govindaraj S, Baredes S, Eloy JA. Diffuse large B-cell lymphoma of the sinonasal tract: analysis of survival in 852 cases. Am J Otolaryngol. 2014;35:154–8.

78. Termote K, Dierickx D, Verhoef G, Jorissen M, Tousseyn T, Mombaerts I. Series of extranodal natural killer/T-cell lymphoma, nasal type, with periorbital involvement. Orbit. 2014;33:245–51.

79. Peng KA, Kita AE, Suh JD, Bhuta SM, Wang MB. Sinonasal lymphoma: case series and review of the literature. Int Forum Allergy Rhinol. 2014;4:670–4.

80. Lee GW, Go SI, Kim SH, Hong J, Kim YR, Oh S, Kim SY, Do YR, Lee H, Lee SI, Bae SH, Oh SY, Song MK, Lee WS, Lee B, Kim JS, Kim MK, Kang HJ, Ahn JS, Yhim HY, Kim HJ, Kim SJ, Kim WS, Suh C, Consortium for Improving Survival of Lymphoma (CISL) study group. Clinical outcome and prognosis of patients with primary sinonasal tract diffuse large B-cell lymphoma treated with rituximab-cyclophosphamide, doxorubicin, vincristine and prednisone chemotherapy: a study by the consortium for improving survival of lymphoma. Leuk Lymphoma. 2015;56:1020–6.

81. Sanghvi S, Misra P, Patel NR, Kalyoussef E, Baredes S, Eloy JA. Incidence trends and long-term survival analysis of sinonasal rhabdomyosarcoma. Am J Otolaryngol. 2013;34:682–9.

82. Gerth DJ, Tashiro J, Thaller SR. Pediatric sinonasal tumors in the United States: incidence and outcomes. J Surg Res J. 2014;190:214–20.

83. Thompson CF, Kim BJ, Lai C, Grogan T, Elashoff D, St John MA, Wang MB. Sinonasal rhabdomyosarcoma: prognostic factors and treatment outcomes. Int Forum Allergy Rhinol. 2013;3:678–83.

84. Szablewski V, Neuville A, Terrier P, Laé M, Schaub R, Garrel R, Coindre JM, Costes V. Adult sinonasal soft tissue sarcoma: analysis of 48 cases from the French Sarcoma Group database. Laryngoscope. 2015;125:615–23.

85. Montone KT, Barr FG, Zhang PJ, Feldman MD, LiVolsi VA. Embryonal and alveolar rhabdomyosarcoma of parameningeal sites in adults: a report of 13 cases. Int J Surg Pathol. 2009;17:22–30.

86. Skapek SX, Anderson J, Barr FG, Bridge JA, Gastier-Foster JM, Parham DM, Rudzinski ER, Triche T, Hawkins DS. PAX-FOXO1 fusion status drives unfavorable outcome for children with rhabdomyosarcoma: a children's oncology group report. Pediatr Blood Cancer. 2013;60:1411–7.

87. Parham DM, Qualman SJ, Teot L, Barr FG, Morotti R, Sorensen PH, Triche TJ, Meyer WH, Soft Tissue Sarcoma Committee of the Children's Oncology Group. Correlation between histology and PAX/FKHR fusion status in alveolar rhabdomyosarcoma: a report from the Children's Oncology Group. Am J Surg Pathol. 2007;31:895–901.

88. Rudzinski ER, Teot LA, Anderson JR, Moore J, Bridge JA, Barr FG, Gastier-Foster JM, Skapek SX, Hawkins DS, Parham DM. Dense pattern of embryonal rhabdomyosarcoma, a lesion easily confused with alveolar rhabdomyosarcoma: a report from the Soft Tissue Sarcoma Committee of the Children's Oncology Group. Am J Clin Pathol. 2013;140:82–90.

89. Zin A, Bertorelle R, Dall'Igna P, Manzitti C, Gambini C, Bisogno G, Rosolen A, Alaggio R. Epithelioid rhabdomyosarcoma: a clinicopathologic and molecular study. Am J Surg Pathol. 2014;38:273–8.

90. Stock N, Chibon F, Binh MB, Terrier P, Michels JJ, Valo I, Robin YM, Guillou L, Ranchère-Vince D, Decouvelaere AV, Collin F, Birtwisle-Peyrottes I, Gregoire F, Aurias A, Coindre JM. Adult-type rhabdomyosarcoma: analysis of 57 cases with clinicopathologic description, identification of 3 morphologic patterns and prognosis. Am J Surg Pathol. 2009;33:1850–9.

91. Bishop JA, Thompson LD, Cardesa A, Barnes L, Lewis Jr JS, Triantafyllou A, Hellquist H, Stenman G, Hunt JL, Williams MD, Slootweg PJ, Devaney KO, Gnepp DR, Wenig BM, Rinaldo A, Ferlito A. Rhabdomyoblastic differentiation in head and neck malignancies other than rhabdomyosarcoma. Head Neck Pathol. 2015;9(4):507–18.

92. Shenjere P, Fisher C, Rajab R, Patnaik L, Hazell S, Thway K. Melanoma with rhabdomyosarcomatous differentiation: two further cases of a rare pathologic pitfall. Int J Surg Pathol. 2014;22:512–9.

93. Agaimy A. The expanding family of SMARCB1(INI1)-deficient neoplasia: implications of phenotypic, biological,

and molecular heterogeneity. Adv Anat Pathol. 2014; 21:394–410.

94. Bishop JA, Antonescu CR, Westra WH. SMARCB1 (INI-1)-deficient carcinomas of the sinonasal tract. Am J Surg Pathol. 2014;38:1282–9.

95. Agaimy A, Koch M, Lell M, Semrau S, Dudek W, Wachter DL, Knöll A, Iro H, Haller F, Hartmann A. SMARCB1(INI1)-deficient sinonasal basaloid carcinoma: a novel member of the expanding family of SMARCB1-deficient neoplasms. Am J Surg Pathol. 2014;38: 1274–81.

96. Leiberman A, Forte V, Thorner P, Crysdale W. Maxillary myxoma in children. Int J Pediatr Otorhinolaryngol. 1990;18:277–84.

97. Fu YS, Perzin KH. Non-epithelial tumors of the nasal cavity, paranasal sinuses and nasopharynx: a clinico-pathologic study. VII. Myxomas. Cancer. 1977; 39:195–203.

98. Safadi A, Fliss DM, Issakov J, Kaplan I. Infantile sinonasal myxoma: a unique variant of maxillofacial myxoma. J Oral Maxillofac Surg. 2011;69:553–8.

99. Chen HH, Streubel SO, Durairaj VD. Odontogenic myxoma with orbital involvement. Ophthal Plast Reconstr Surg. 2013;29:e47–9.

100. King TJ, Lewis J, Orvidas L, Kademani D. Pediatric maxillary odontogenic myxoma: a report of 2 cases and review of management. J Oral Maxillofac Surg. 2008;66:1057–62.

101. Iatrou IA, Theologie-Lygidakis N, Leventis MD, Michail-Strantzia C. Sinonasal myxoma in an infant. J Craniofac Surg. 2010;21:1649–51.

102. Prasannan L, Warren L, Herzog CE, Lopez-Camarillo L, Frankel L, Goepfert H. Sinonasal myxoma: a pediatric case. J Pediatr Hematol Oncol. 2005;27:90–2.

103. Zhang L, Zhang M, Zhang J, Luo L, Xu Z, Li G, Tian Y, Wang Y, Wu Z, Wang Z. Myxoma of the cranial base. Surg Neurol. 2007;68 Suppl 2:S22–8.

104. Yılmaz S, Edizer DT, Yağız C, Sar M, Cansız H. Maxillary sinus nonodontogenic myxoma extending into the sphenoid sinus and pterygopalatine fossa: case report. Ear Nose Throat J. 2011;90:E28–30.

105. Yin H, Cai BW, An HM, You C. Huge primary myxoma of skull base: a report of an uncommon case. Acta Neurochir (Wien). 2007;149:713–7.

106. Sato H, Gyo K, Tomidokoro Y, Honda N. Myxoma of the sphenoidal sinus. Otolaryngol Head Neck Surg. 2004;130:378–80.

107. Heffner DK. Sinonasal myxomas and fibromyxomas in children. Ear Nose Throat J. 1993;72:365–8.

108. Hyams VJ, Batsakis JG, Micheals L. Tumors of the upper respiratory tract and ear. In: Atlas of tumor pathology, vol. 2. Washington, DC: Armed Forces Institute of Pathology; 1988. p. 240–8.

109. Saade RE, Hanna EY, Bell D. Prognosis and biology in esthesioneuroblastoma: the emerging role of Hyams grading system. Curr Oncol Rep. 2015;17:423–8.

110. Argani P, Perez-Ordoñez B, Xiao H, Caruana SM, Huvos AG, Ladanyi M. Olfactory neuroblastoma is not related to the Ewing family of tumors: absence of EWS/FLI1 gene fusion and MIC2 expression. Am J Surg Pathol. 1998;22:391–8.

111. Mezzelani A, Tornielli S, Minoletti F, Pierotti MA, Sozzi G, Pilotti S. Esthesioneuroblastoma is not a member of the primitive peripheral neuroectodermal tumour-Ewing's group. Br J Cancer. 1999;81:586–91.

112. Kumar S, Perlman E, Pack S, Davis M, Zhang H, Meltzer P, Tsokos M. Absence of EWS/FLI1 fusion in olfactory neuroblastomas indicates these tumors do not belong to the Ewing's sarcoma family. Hum Pathol. 1999;30: 1356–60.

113. Holland H, Koschny R, Krupp W, Meixensberger J, Bauer M, Kirsten H, Ahnert P. Comprehensive cytogenetic characterization of an esthesioneuroblastoma. Cancer Genet Cytogenet. 2007;173:89–96.

114. Bell D, Saade R, Roberts D, Ow TJ, Kupferman M, DeMonte F, Hanna EY. Prognostic utility of Hyams histological grading and Kadish-Morita staging systems for esthesioneuroblastoma outcomes. Head Neck Pathol. 2015;9:51–9.

115. Ow TJ, Bell D, Kupferman ME, Demonte F, Hanna EY. Esthesioneuroblastoma. Neurosurg Clin N Am. 2013;24:51–65.

116. Gallagher KK, Spector ME, Pepper JP, McKean EL, Marentette LJ, McHugh JB. Esthesioneuroblastoma: updating histologic grading as it relates to prognosis. Ann Otol Rhinol Laryngol. 2014;123:353–8.

117. Bates T, Plessis DD, Polvikoski T, Sloan P, McQueen A, Meikle D, Kelly C, Robinson M. Ganglioneuroblastic transformation in olfactory neuroblastoma. Head Neck Pathol. 2012;6:150–5.

118. Weiss GJ, Liang WS, Izatt T, Arora S, Cherni I, Raju RN, Hostetter G, Kurdoglu A, Christoforides A, Sinari S, Baker AS, Metpally R, Tembe WD, Phillips L, Von Hoff DD, Craig DW, Carpten JD. Paired tumor and normal whole genome sequencing of metastatic olfactory neuroblastoma. PLoS One. 2012;7:e37029.

119. Wooff JC, Weinreb I, Perez-Ordonez B, Magee JF, Bullock MJ. Calretinin staining facilitates differentiation of olfactory neuroblastoma from other small round blue cell tumors in the sinonasal tract. Am J Surg Pathol. 2011;35:1786–93.

120. Tilson MP, Bishop JA. Utility of p40 in the differential diagnosis of small round blue cell tumors of the sinonasal tract. Head Neck Pathol. 2014;8:141–5.

121. Siegal GP, Oliver WR, Reinus WR, Gilula LA, Foulkes MA, Kissane JM, Askin FB. Primary Ewing's sarcoma involving the bones of the head and neck. Cancer. 1987;60:2829–40.

122. Hafezi S, Seethala RR, Stelow EB, Mills SE, Leong IT, MacDuff E, Hunt JL, Perez-Ordoñez B, Weinreb I. Ewing's family of tumors of the sinonasal tract and maxillary bone. Head Neck Pathol. 2011;5:8–16.

123. Yeshvanth SK, Ninan K, Bhandary SK, Lakshinarayana KP, Shetty JK, Makannavar JH. Rare case of extraskeletal Ewings sarcoma of the sinonasal tract. J Cancer Res Ther. 2012;8:142–4.

124. Bishop JA, Alaggio R, Zhang L, Seethala RR, Antonescu CR. Adamantinoma-like ewing family tumors of the head and neck: a pitfall in the differential diagnosis of basaloid and myoepithelial carcinomas. Am J Surg Pathol. 2015;9:1267–74.

125. Folpe AL, Goldblum JR, Rubin BP, Shehata BM, Liu W, Dei Tos AP, Weiss SW. Morphologic and immuno-phenotypic diversity in Ewing family tumors: a study of 66 genetically confirmed cases. Am J Surg Pathol. 2005;29:1025–33.

126. Paulussen M, Craft AW, Lewis I, Hackshaw A, Douglas C, Dunst J, Schuck A, Winkelmann W, Köhler G, Poremba C, Zoubek A, Ladenstein R, van den Berg H, Hunold A, Cassoni A, Spooner D, Grimer R, Whelan J, McTiernan A, Jürgens H, EuropeanIntergroup Cooperative Ewing's Sarcoma Study-92. Results of the EICESS-92 Study: two randomized trials of Ewing's sarcoma treatment – cyclophosphamide compared with ifosfamide in standard-risk patients and assessment of benefit of etoposide added to standard treatment in high-risk patients. J Clin Oncol. 2008;26:4385–93.

127. Cotterill SJ, Ahrens S, Paulussen M, Jürgens HF, Voûte PA, Gadner H, Craft AW. Prognostic factors in Ewing's tumor of bone: analysis of 975 patients from the European Intergroup Cooperative Ewing's Sarcoma Study Group. J Clin Oncol. 2000;18:3108–14.

128. Llombart-Bosch A, Machado I, Navarro S, Bertoni F, Bacchini P, Alberghini M, Karzeladze A, Savelov N, Petrov S, Alvarado-Cabrero I, Mihaila D, Terrier P, Lopez-Guerrero JA, Picci P. Histological heterogeneity of Ewing's sarcoma/PNET: an immunohistochemical analysis of 415 genetically confirmed cases with clinical support. Vichows Arch. 2009;455:397–411.

129. Silva EG, Butler JJ, Mackay B, Goepfert H. Neuroblastomas and neuroendocrine carcinomas of the nasal cavity. Cancer. 1982;50:2388–405.

130. Perez-Ordonez B, Caruana SM, Huvos AG, Shah JP. Small cell neuroendocrine carcinoma of the nasal cavity and paranasal sinuses. Hum Pathol. 1998;29:826–32.

131. Mills SE. Neuroectodermal neoplasms of the head and neck with emphasis on neuroendocrine carcinomas. Mod Pathol. 2002;15:264–78.

132. Babin E, Rouleau V, Vedrine PO, Toussaint B, de Raucourt D, Malard O, Cosmidis A, Makaeieff M, Dehesdin D. Small cell neuroendocrine carcinoma of the nasal cavity and paranasal sinuses. J Laryngol Otol. 2006;120:289–97.

133. Weinreb I, Perez-Ordoñez B. Non-small cell neuroendocrine carcinoma of the sinonasal tract and nasopharynx. Report of 2 cases and review of the literature. Head Neck Pathol. 2007;1:21–6.

134. Likhacheva A, Rosenthal DI, Hanna E, Kupferman M, Demonte F, El-Naggar AK. Sinonasal neuroendocrine carcinoma: impact of differentiation status on response and outcome. Head Neck Oncol. 2011;3:32. doi:10.1186/1758-3284-3-32.

135. Vasan NR, Medina JE, Canfield VA, Gillies EM. Sinonasal neuroendocrine carcinoma in association with SIADH. Head Neck. 2004;26:89–93.

136. Kayakabe M, Takahashi K, Okamiya T, Segawa A, Oyama T, Chikamatsu K. Combined small cell carcinoma of the sinonasal tract associated with syndrome of inappropriate secretion of antidiuretic hormone: a case report. Oncol Lett. 2014;7:1253–6.

137. Franchi A, Sardi I, Cetica V, Buccoliero A, Giordano F, Mussa F, Genitori L, Oliveri G, Miracco C. Pediatric sinonasal neuroendocrine carcinoma after treatment of retinoblastoma. Hum Pathol. 2009;40:750–5.

138. La Rosa S, Furlan D, Franzi F, Battaglia P, Frattini M, Zanellato E, Marando A, Sahnane N, Turri-Zanoni M, Castelnuovo P, Capella C. Mixedexocrine-neuroendocrine carcinoma of the nasal cavity: clinico-pathologic and molecular study of a case and review of the literature. Head Neck Pathol. 2013;7:76–84.

139. Jain R, Gramigna V, Sanchez-Marull R, Perez-Ordoñez B. Composite intestinal-type adenocarcinoma and small cell carcinoma of sinonasal tract. J Clin Pathol. 2009;62:634–7.

140. Franchi A, Rocchetta D, Palomba A, Degli Innocenti DR, Castiglione F, Spinelli G. Primary combined neuroendocrine and squamous cell carcinoma of the maxillary sinus: report of a case with immunohistochemical and molecular characterization. Head Neck Pathol. 2015;9:107–13.

141. Barham HP, Said S, Ramakrishnan VR. Colliding tumor of the paranasal sinus. Allergy Rhinol (Providence). 2013;4:e13–6.

142. Lee H, Torres FX, McLean SA, Chen R, Lee MW. Immunophenotypic heterogeneity of primary sinonasal melanoma with aberrant expression of neuroendocrine markers and calponin. Appl Immunohistochem Mol Morphol. 2011;19:48–53.

143. Kleinsasser O, Schroeder HG. Adenocarcinomas of the inner nose after exposure to wood dust. Morphological findings and relationships between histopathology and clinical behavior in 79 cases. Arch Otorhinolaryngol. 1988;245:1–15.

144. Franquemont DW, Fechner RE, Mills SE. Histologic classification of sinonasal intestinal-type adenocarcinoma. Am J Surg Pathol. 1991;15:368–75.

145. Barnes L. Intestinal-type adenocarcinoma of the nasal cavity and paranasal sinuses. Am J Surg Pathol. 1986;10:192–202.

146. Alonso-Sardón M, Chamorro AJ, Hernández-García I, Iglesias-de-Sena H, Martín-Rodero H, Herrera C, Marcos M, Mirón-Canelo JA. Association between occupational exposure to wood dust and cancer: a systematic review and meta-analysis. PLoS One. 2015;10(7):e0133024.

147. IARC monographs on the evaluation of carcinogenic risks to humans. Lyon: IARC Monographs, Volume 100(C). World Health Organization; 2012. p. 414–30.

148. Bonzini M, Battaglia P, Parassoni D, Casa M, Facchinetti N, Turri-Zanoni M, Borchini R, Castelnuovo P, Ferrario MM. Prevalence of occupational hazards in patients with different types of epithelial sinonasal cancers. Rhinology. 2013;51:31–6.

149. Mensi C, Consonni D, Sieno C, De Matteis S, Riboldi L, Bertazzi PA. Sinonasal cancer and occupational exposure in a population-based registry. Int J Otolaryngol. 2013;2013:672621. doi:10.1155/2013/672621.

150. Pérez-Escuredo J, Martínez JG, Vivanco B, Marcos CÁ, Suárez C, Llorente JL, Hermsen MA. Wood dust-related mutational profile of TP53 in intestinal-type sinonasal adenocarcinoma. Hum Pathol. 2012;43:1894–901.

151. Holmila R, Bornholdt J, Heikkilä P, Suitiala T, Févotte J, Cyr D, Hansen J, Snellman SM, Dictor M, Steiniche T, Schlünssen V, Schneider T, Pukkala E, Savolainen K, Wolff H, Wallin H, Luce D, Husgafvel-Pursiainen K. Mutations in TP53 tumor suppressor gene in wood dust-related sinonasal cancer. Int J Cancer. 2010;127:578–88.

152. Camp S, Van Gerven L, Poorten VV, Nuyts S, Hermans R, Hauben E, Jorissen M. Long-term follow-up of 123 patients with adenocarcinoma of the sinonasal tract treated with endoscopic resection and postoperative radiation therapy. Head Neck. 2014. doi:10.1002/hed.23900.

153. Donhuijsen K, Kollecker I, Petersen P, Gaßler N, Schulze J, Schroeder HG. Metastatic behaviour of sinonasal adenocarcinomas of the intestinal type (ITAC). Eur Arch Otorhinolaryngol. 2016;273(3):649–54.

154. Franchi A, Palomba A, Miligi L, Ranucci V, Innocenti DR, Simoni A, Pepi M, Santucci M. Intestinal metaplasia of the sinonasal mucosa adjacent to intestinal-type adenocarcinoma. A morphologic, immunohistochemical, and molecular study. Virchows Arch. 2015;466:161–8.

155. Kennedy MT, Jordan RC, Berean KW, Perez-Ordoñez B. Expression pattern of CK7, CK20, CDX-2, and villin in intestinal-type sinonasal adenocarcinoma. J Clin Pathol. 2004;57:932–7.

156. Tilson MP, Gallia GL, Bishop JA. Among sinonasal tumors, CDX-2 immunoexpression is not restricted to intestinal-type adenocarcinomas. Head Neck Pathol. 2014;8:59–65.

157. Blumberg JM, Escobar-Stein J, Vining EM, Prasad ML. Low-grade, nonintestinal nonsalivary sinonasal adenocarcinoma associated with an exophytic schneiderian papilloma: a case report. Int J Surg Pathol. 2015;23(8):662–6.

158. Bhaijee F, Carron J, Bell D. Low-grade nonintestinal sinonasal adenocarcinoma: a diagnosis of exclusion. Ann Diagn Pathol. 2011;15:181–4.

159. Jo VY, Mills SE, Cathro HP, Carlson DL, Stelow EB. Low-grade sinonasal adenocarcinomas: the association with and distinction from respiratory epithelial adenomatoid hamartomas and other glandular lesions. Am J Surg Pathol. 2009;33:401–8.

160. Bansal A, Pradeep KE, Gumparthy KP. An unusual case of low-grade tubulopapillary adenocarcinoma of the sinonasal tract. World J Surg Oncol. 2008;6:54. doi:10.1186/1477-7819-6-54. PubMed PMID: 18492272.

161. Purgina B, Bastaki JM, Duvvuri U, Seethala RR. A subset of sinonasal non-intestinal type adenocarcinomas are truly seromucinous adenocarcinomas: a morphologic and immunophenotypic assessment and description of a novel pitfall. Head Neck Pathol. 2015;9:436–46.

162. Stelow EB, Jo VY, Mills SE, Carlson DL. A histologic and immunohistochemical study describing the diversity of tumors classified as sinonasal high-grade nonintestinal adenocarcinomas. Am J Surg Pathol. 2011;35:971–80.

163. Zur KB, Brandwein M, Wang B, Som P, Gordon R, Urken ML. Primary description of a new entity, renal cell-like carcinoma of the nasal cavity: van Meegeren in the house of Vermeer. Arch Otolaryngol Head Neck Surg. 2002;128:441–7.

164. Storck K, Hadi UM, Simpson R, Ramer M, Brandwein-Gensler M. Sinonasal renal cell-like adenocarcinoma: a report on four patients. Head Neck Pathol. 2008;2: 75–80.

165. Brandwein-Gensler M, Wei S. Envisioning the next WHO head and neck classification. Head Neck Pathol. 2014;8:1–15.

166. Shen T, Shi Q, Velosa C, Bai S, Thompson L, Simpson R, Wei S, Brandwein-Gensler M. Sinonasal renal cell-like adenocarcinomas: robust carbonic anhydrase expression. Hum Pathol. 2015. pii: S0046-8177(15)00237-3. doi:10.1016/j.humpath.2015.06.017.

167. Heffner DK, Hyams VJ. Teratocarcinosarcoma (malignant teratoma?) of the nasal cavity and paranasal sinuses. A clinicopathologic study of 20 cases. Cancer. 1984;53:2140–54.

168. Fatima SS, Minhas K, Din NU, Fatima S, Ahmed A, Ahmad Z. Sinonasal teratocarcinosarcoma: a clinicopathologic and immunohistochemical study of 6 cases. Ann Diagn Pathol. 2013;17:313–8.

169. Smith SL, Hessel AC, Luna MA, Malpica A, Rosenthal DI, El-Naggar AK. Sinonasal teratocarcinosarcoma of the head and neck: a report of 10 patients treated at a single institution and comparison with reported series. Arch Otolaryngol Head Neck Surg. 2008;134: 592–5.

170. Wei S, Carroll W, Lazenby A, Bell W, Lopez R, Said-Al-Naief N. Sinonasal teratocarcinosarcoma: report of a case with review of literature and treatment outcome. Ann Diagn Pathol. 2008;12:415–25.

171. Yang S, Sun R, Liang J, Zhou Z, Zhou J, Rui J. Sinonasal teratocarcinosarcoma: a clinical and pathological analysis. Int J Surg Pathol. 2013;21:37–43.

172. Yang Z, Uppaluri R, Lewis Jr JS. Ethmoid sinus mass. Sinonasal teratocarcinosarcoma. JAMA Otolaryngol Head Neck Surg. 2015;141:389–90.

173. Su YY, Friedman M, Huang CC, Wilson M, Lin HC. Sinonasal teratocarcinosarcoma. Am J Otolaryngol. 2010;31:300–3.

174. Kim JH, Maeng YH, Lee JS, Jung S, Lim SC, Lee MC. Sinonasal teratocarcinosarcoma with rhabdoid features. Pathol Int. 2011;61:762–7.

175. Thomas J, Adegboyega P, Iloabachie K, Mooring JW, Lian T. Sinonasal teratocarcinosarcoma with yolk sac elements: a neoplasm of somatic or germ cell origin? Ann Diagn Pathol. 2011;15:135–9.

176. Misra P, Husain Q, Svider PF, Sanghvi S, Liu JK, Eloy JA. Management of sinonasal teratocarcinosarcoma: a systematic review. Am J Otolaryngol. 2014;35:5–11.

177. Bell DM, Porras G, Tortoledo ME, Luna MA. Primary sinonasal choriocarcinoma. Ann Diagn Pathol. 2009;13: 96–100.

178. Stout AP, Murray MR. Hemangiopericytoma: a vascular tumor featuring Zimmermann's pericytes. Ann Surg. 1942;116:26–33.

179. Armulik A, Genové G, Betsholtz C. Pericytes: developmental, physiological, and pathological perspectives, problems, and promises. Dev Cell. 2011;21:193–215.

180. Compagno J, Hyams VJ. Hemangiopericytoma-like intranasal tumors. A clinicopathologic study of 23 cases. Am J Clin Pathol. 1976;66:672–83.

181. Fletcher CD. The evolving classification of soft tissue tumours: an update based on the new WHO classification. Histopathology. 2006;48:3–12.

182. Thompson LD, Miettinen M, Wenig BM. Sinonasal-type hemangiopericytoma: a clinicopathologic and immunophenotypic analysis of 104 cases showing perivascular myoid differentiation. Am J Surg Pathol. 2003;27: 737–49.

183. Catalano PJ, Brandwein M, Shah DK, Urken ML, Lawson W, Biller HF. Sinonasal hemangiopericytomas: a clinicopathologic and immunohistochemical study of seven cases. Head Neck. 1996;18:42–53.

184. Dandekar M, McHugh JB. Sinonasal glomangiopericytoma: case report with emphasis on the differential diagnosis. Arch Pathol Lab Med. 2010;134:1444–9.

185. Wilson T, Hellquist HB, Ray S, Pickles J. Intranasal myo-pericytoma. A tumour with perivascular myoid differentiation: the changing nomenclature for haemangiopericytoma. J Laryngol Otol. 2007;121:786–9.

186. Kuo FY, Lin HC, Eng HL, Huang CC. Sinonasal hemangiopericytoma-like tumor with true pericytic myoid differentiation: a clinicopathologic and immuno-histochemical study of five cases. Head Neck. 2005;27:124–9.

187. Haller F, Bieg M, Moskalev EA, Barthelmeß S, Geddert H, Boltze C, Diessl N, Braumandl K, Brors B, Iro H, Hartmann A, Wiemann S, Agaimy A. Recurrent mutations within the amino-terminal region of β-catenin are probable key molecular driver events in sinonasal hemangiopericytoma. Am J Pathol. 2015;185:563–71.

188. Lasota J, Felisiak-Golabek A, Aly FZ, Wang ZF, Thompson LD, Miettinen M. Nuclear expression and gain-of-function β-catenin mutation in glomangioperi-cytoma (sinonasal-type hemangiopericytoma): insight into pathogenesis and a diagnostic marker. Mod Pathol. 2015;28:715–20.

189. Ganly I, Patel SG, Stambuk HE, Coleman M, Ghossein R, Carlson D, Edgar M, Shah JP. Solitary fibrous tumors of the head and neck: a clinicopathologic and radiologic review. Arch Otolaryngol Head Neck Surg. 2006;132:517–25.

190. Papadakis I, Koudounarakis E, Haniotis V, Karatzanis A, Velegrakis G. Atypical solitary fibrous tumor of the nose and maxillary sinus. Head Neck. 2011. doi:10.1002/hed.21909.

191. Nai GA, Ramalho Neto GC. Solitary fibrous tumor of the nasal cavity. Braz J Otorhinolaryngol. 2009;75:769.

192. Takasaki K, Watanabe T, Hayashi T, Kinoshita N, Kumagami H, Takahashi H. Solitary fibrous tumor aris-ing from the sphenoid sinus. Case Report Med. 2009;2009:316042.

193. Furze AD, Peng Y, Myers LL. Pathology case quiz 2. Solitary fibrous tumor of the nasal cavity and ethmoid sinus with intracranial extension. Arch Otolaryngol Head Neck Surg. 2008;134(334):336–7.

194. Corina L, Volante M, Carconi M, Contucci AM. An unusual solitary fibrous tumor after sphenoethmoidec-tomy. Otolaryngol Head Neck Surg. 2006;134:1063–5.

195. Zielińska-Kaźmierska B, Grodecka J, Szyszkowski A. Solitary fibrous tumor of the nasal cavity and paranasal sinuses: a case report. J Oral Biol Craniofac Res. 2015;5(2):112–6.

196. Fujikura T, Ishida M, Sekine K, Aoki H, Okubo K. Solitary fibrous tumor arising from the superior nasal turbinate: a case report. J Nippon Med Sch. 2012;79(5):373–6.

197. Vermeulen S, Ketels P, Salgado R, Creytens D, Vanderveken OM, Claes J. Solitary fibrous tumour of the nasal cavity: a case report and literature review. B-ENT. 2012;8(3):219–23.

198. Vogels RJ, Vlenterie M, Versleijen-Jonkers YM, Ruijter E, Bekers EM, Verdijk MA, Link MM, Bonenkamp JJ, van der Graaf WT, Slootweg PJ, Suurmeijer AJ, Groenen PJ, Flucke U. Solitary fibrous tumor – clinicopathologic, immunohistochemical and molecular analysis of 28 cases. Diagn Pathol. 2014;29:224. doi:10.1186/s13000-014-0224-6.

199. Agaimy A, Barthelmeß S, Geddert H, Boltze C, Moskalev EA, Koch M, Wiemann S, Hartmann A, Haller F. Phenotypical and molecular distinctness of sinonasal haemangiopericytoma compared to solitary fibrous tumour of the sinonasal tract. Histopathology. 2014;65:667–73.

200. Carlson JW, Fletcher CD. Immunohistochemistry for beta-catenin in the differential diagnosis of spindle cell lesions: analysis of a series and review of the literature. Histopathology. 2007;51:509–14.

201. Fu YS, Perzin KH. Nonepithelial tumors of the nasal cavity, paranasal sinuses, and nasopharynx. A clini-copathologic study. VI. Fibrous tissue tumors (fibroma, fibromatosis, fibrosarcoma). Cancer. 1976;37:2912–28.

202. Heffner DK, Gnepp DR. Sinonasal fibrosarcomas, malig-nant schwannomas, and "Triton" tumors. A clinicopath-ologic study of 67 cases. Cancer. 1992;70:1089–101.

203. Bercin S, Muderris T, Kırıs M, Kanmaz A, Kandemir O. A rare sinonasal neoplasm: fibrosarcoma. Ear Nose Throat J. 2011;90:E6–8.

204. Kondo S, Yoshizaki T, Minato H, Horikawa I, Tatsumi A, Furukawa M. Myofibrosarcoma of the nasal cavity and paranasal sinus. Histopathology. 2001;39:216–7.

205. Maly A, Maly B, Eliashar R, Doviner V. Inverted papilloma-like sinonasal epithelial hyperplasia, over-shadowing underlying sinonasal fibrosarcoma: a diag-nostic pitfall. Am J Otolaryngol. 2006;27:50–3.

206. Lewis JT, Oliveira AM, Nascimento AG, Schembri-Wismayer D, Moore EA, Olsen KD, Garcia JG, Lonzo ML, Lewis JE. Low-grade sinonasal sarcoma with neural and myogenic features: a clinicopathologic analysis of 28 cases. Am J Surg Pathol. 2012;36:517–25.

207. Powers KA, Han LM, Chiu AG, Aly FZ. Low-grade sinonasal sarcoma with neural and myogenic fea-tures – diagnostic challenge and pathogenic insight. Oral Surg Oral Med Oral Pathol Oral Radiol. 2015;119:e265–9.

208. Wang X, Bledsoe KL, Graham RP, Asmann YW, Viswanathan DS, Lewis JE, Lewis JT, Chou MM, Yaszemski MJ, Jen J, Westendorf JJ, Oliveira AM. Recurrent PAX3-MAML3 fusion in biphenotypic sino-nasal sarcoma. Nat Genet. 2014;46:666–8.

209. Huang SC, Ghossein RA, Bishop JA, Zhang L, Chen TC, Huang HY, Antonescu CR. Novel PAX3-NCOA1 fusions in biphenotypic sinonasal sarcoma with focal rhabdo-myoblastic differentiation. Am J Surg Pathol. 2016;40(1):51–9.

210. Wong WJ, Lauria A, Hornick JL, Xiao S, Fletcher JA, Marino-Enriquez A. Alternate PAX3-FOXO1 oncogenic fusion in biphenotypic sinonasal sarcoma. Genes Chromosomes Cancer. 2015. doi:10.1002/gcc.22295.

Nasopharynx and Skull Base

Abstract

How many times have the terms "sinonasal" and "nasopharyngeal" been incorrectly interchanged on requisition sheets? This chapter offers more examples that emphasize the importance of anatomic and clinicoradiographic correlation in arriving at a correct diagnosis. A "hairy polyp" may appear quite unimpressive until you realize it's not a dermal lesion. A biopsy from an ectopic pituitary adenoma or macroadenoma may lead you down the incorrect path of sinonasal neuroendocrine carcinoma, a biopsy from a craniopharyngioma may have you thinking about an ameloblastoma, an ecchordosis physaliphora can mimic chordoma. In this cost conscious era where pathologists need be more time efficient, and use fewer immunohistochemical resources, less anatomic and clinical information is not an option.

Keywords

Tornwaldt's cyst · Hairy polyps · Nasopharyngeal angiofibroma · Salivary gland anlage tumor · Craniopharyngioma · Chordoma · Ecchordosis physaliphora · Nasopharyngeal carcinoma · EBV · Nasopharyngeal papillary adenocarcinoma

Glossary

Torus tubarius (tubal elevation, torus) Ridge in the posterior nasopharynx representing projection of the cartilaginous portion of the Eustacian tube.

Fossa of Rosenmüller (pharyngeal recess) Depression of the lateral nonmuscular pharyngeal wall posterior to the torus

Luschka's bursa (pharyngeal bursa, nasopharyngeal bursa, Tornwaldt's bursa) Cystic notocord remnant which may persist in the posterior nasopharynx, at the inferior aspect of the adenoids.

Rathke's pouch (Rathke's cleft cyst) Remnant of the ectodermal invagination of the stomadeum which forms the anterior pituitary gland.

Craniopharyngeal canal (hypopharyngeal duct) Remnant of embryological connection between the nasopharynx and third ventricle, which may persist in the sphenoid bone

Suprasellar Above the sella turcica

Sella turcica (Turkish saddle) Depression in sphenoid bone which houses the pituitary gland.

Clivus (Latin: slope) Shallow skullbase depression posterior to the sphenoid sinuses. The pons is dorsal to the clivus.

Pontine cistern (Prepontine cistern) Subarachnoid cistern at the ventral aspect of the pons.

Key Points

- Hairy polyp is a choristoma composed of ectodermal and mesodermal tissues
- Teratoma is composed of tissues from three germ layers; neonatal teratomas tend to be benign
- Rare female nasopharyngeal angiofibromas are usually "non-juvenile" and extra-nasopharyngeal
- 90% of craniopharyngiomas are adamantinomatous and develop in the first two decades of life
- Ectopic pituitary adenomas commonly fill the sphenoid; the sella turcica can be intact. Ectopic or macroadenomas have the potential for misdiagnosis as neuroendocrine carcinoma.
- Ecchordosis physaliphora (EP) can best be distinguished from chordoma radiographically: EP has no destructive growth pattern, no soft tissue component, and is nonenhancing with gadolinium.
- EBER ISH can be invaluable in the work-up of metastatic cervical carcinoma of unknown primary, nasopharyngeal biopsies, and adenoidal hyperplasia in post-transplant patients.

5.1   Anatomy and Histology

The nasopharynx represents the most superior compartment of the pharynx. The soft palate defines its inferior border, whereas the floor of the sphenoid sinus demarcates its superior margin. It is bordered by the posterior choanae, (anteriorly) lateral, and posterior nasopharyngeal walls (◘ Figs. 5.1 and 5.2). The adenoids (pharyngeal tonsils, tubal tonsils) represent the superior extension of Waldeyer's ring and are situated on the nasopharyngeal roof, and posterior and posteriolateral walls. The Eustachian tubes equalize middle

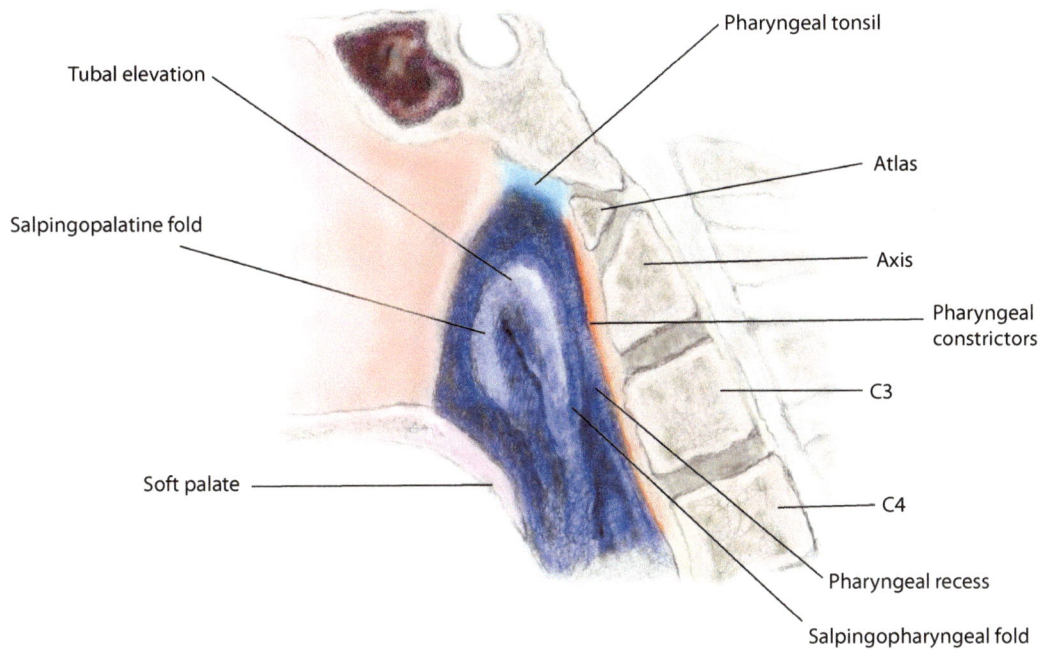

Tubal elevation

Salpingopalatine fold

Soft palate

Pharyngeal tonsil

Atlas

Axis

Pharyngeal constrictors

C3

C4

Pharyngeal recess

Salpingopharyngeal fold

◘ Fig. 5.1 The nasopharynx (*blue*) represents the most superior compartment of the pharynx. The Eustachian tubes open into the lateral nasopharynx via pharyngeal ostia; each are surrounded by a cartilaginous cushion termed torus tubarius (tubal elevation). The pharyngeal recess (fossa of Rosenmüller) is a deep recess behind each torus

ear pressure to barometric pressure; they open into the nasopharynx through the pharyngeal ostia. Each ostium is surrounded by a cartilaginous cushion termed torus tubarius (tubal elevation). The pharyngeal recess (**fossa of Rosenmüller**) represents a deep recess behind each torus. The salpingopalatine fold extends anteriorly from the torus tubarius and contains the levator veli palatini muscle. The salpingopharyngeal fold extends from the inferior posterior torus and contains the salpingopharyngeus muscle.

The pharyngeal bursa (**nasopharyngeal bursa, Luschka's bursa, Tornwaldt's Bursa**) is a blind sac which can persist in the posterior midline nasopharynx at the inferior aspect of the adenoids. It represents persistent communication of the anterior notochord with the nasopharyngeal roof. At 6 weeks gestation, the most cephalic portion of the notochord begins to regress and comes into contact with the primordial skull base. The notochord descends and makes contact with the endoderm of the developing pharynx. At this point, there is the potential for pharyngeal endoderm to ascend with the notochord to the level of the developing skull base [1, 2]. Persistence of this endodermal tract forms the pharyngeal bursa, and obstruction of this bursa leads to Tornwaldt's cyst.

Rathke's cleft represents an ectodermal invagination from the developing oral cavity which gives rise to the anterior pituitary gland, which begins to form at week four or five of gestation, The migratory path of Rathke's cleft (craniopharyngeal canal, hypopharyngeal duct) is distinct from the pharyngeal bursa (Tornwaldt's bursa).

Histologically, most of the nasopharynx is lined by stratified nonkeratinizing squamous epithelium. The lateral walls and roof are lined by alternating patches of squamous and ciliated respiratory epithelium separated by zones of transitional epithelium [3]. The nasopharyngeal aspect of the soft palate is lined by respiratory mucosa (◘ Fig. 5.3) The adenoidal lymphoid tissue has invaginated epithelial crypts lined by stratified squamous epithelium (◘ Fig. 5.4) These crypts appear smaller and less cystic, compared with the palatine tonsils.

The skull base forms the floor of the cranium and separates the brain from the orbit, nasal cavity, paranasal sinuses, nasopharynx, and spinal cord. The five bones which contribute to the formation of the skull base are: ethmoid, sphenoid, occipital, frontal and temporal bones. The skull base is divided into the anterior, middle, and posterior cranial fossae. The anterior cranial fossa extends from the posterior table of the frontal sinus to the roof of

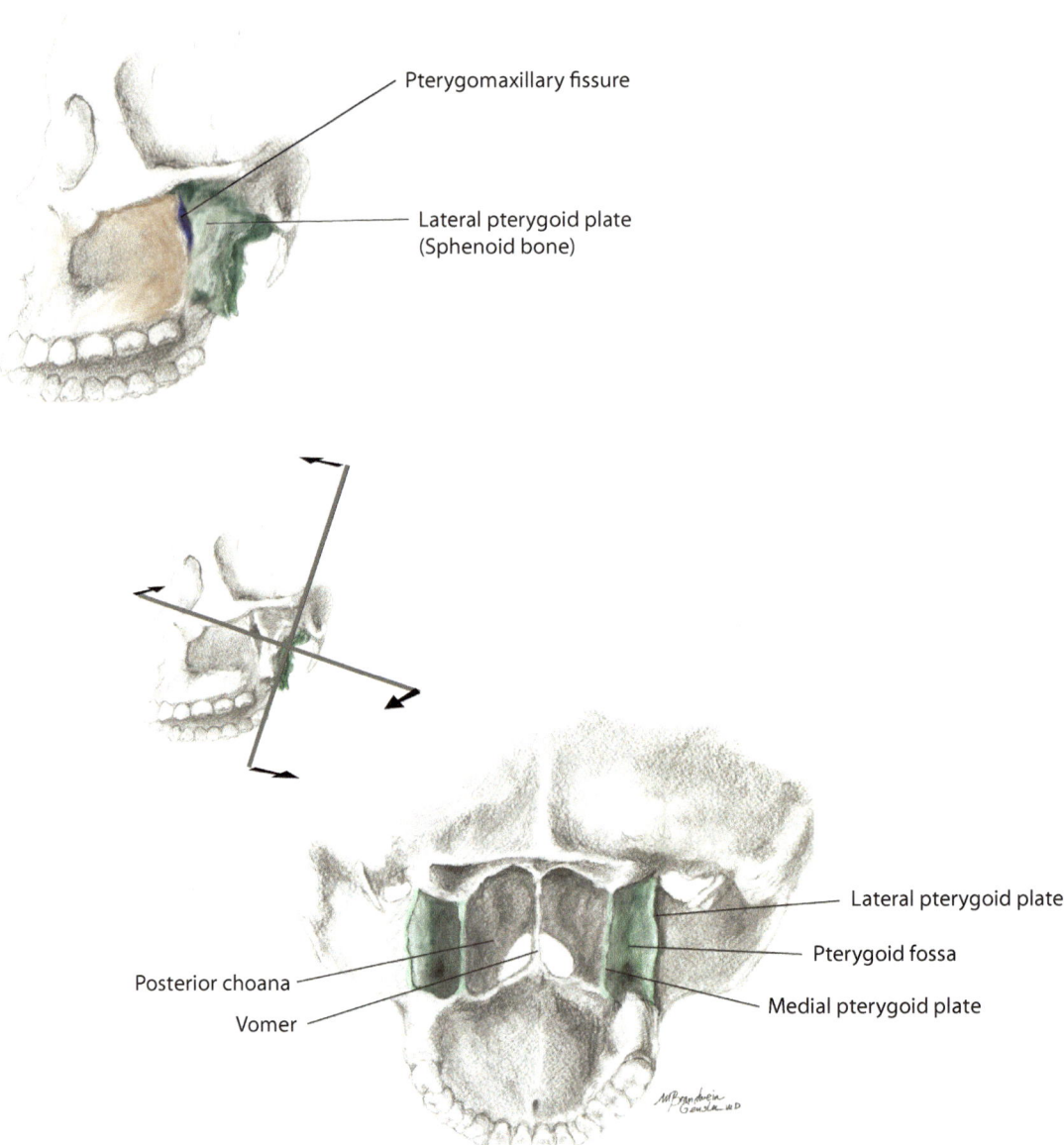

Pterygomaxillary fissure

Lateral pterygoid plate
(Sphenoid bone)

Lateral pterygoid plate

Pterygoid fossa

Posterior choana

Medial pterygoid plate

Vomer

🔲 **Fig. 5.2**   (**a**) Lateral view cranium: The pterygomaxillary fissure (*deep blue*) is the "gateway" to the pterygopalatine (sphenopalatine) fossa. The fissue is posterior to the maxilla and anterior to the lateral pterygoid plate (*green*). (**b**) Pterygoid fossa and plates (*green*), viewed posteriorly, with the cranium tipped forward. The medial pterygoid plate of the sphenoid bone comprises the medial boundary of the pterygoid fossa. The superior pharyngeal constrictor originates from the inferior third of the medial pterygoid plate. The lateral pterygoid plate comprises the lateral boundary of the pterygoid fossa and the medial boundary of the infratemporal fossa. The lateral pterygoid muscle originates from the lateral pterygoid plate

the sphenoid sinus. The cribriform plate is within the anterior cranial fossa, and is the pathway of the olfactory nerves into the superior nasal cavity. The ethmoid labyrinth is covered by the fovea ethmoidalis of the frontal bone and separates the ethmoidal cells from the anterior cranial fossa. The middle cranial fossa is bordered anteriorly by the greater wing of the sphenoid and posteriorly by the clivus, which is formed by the sphenoid and occipital bones. The sphenoid body makes up the central middle fossa

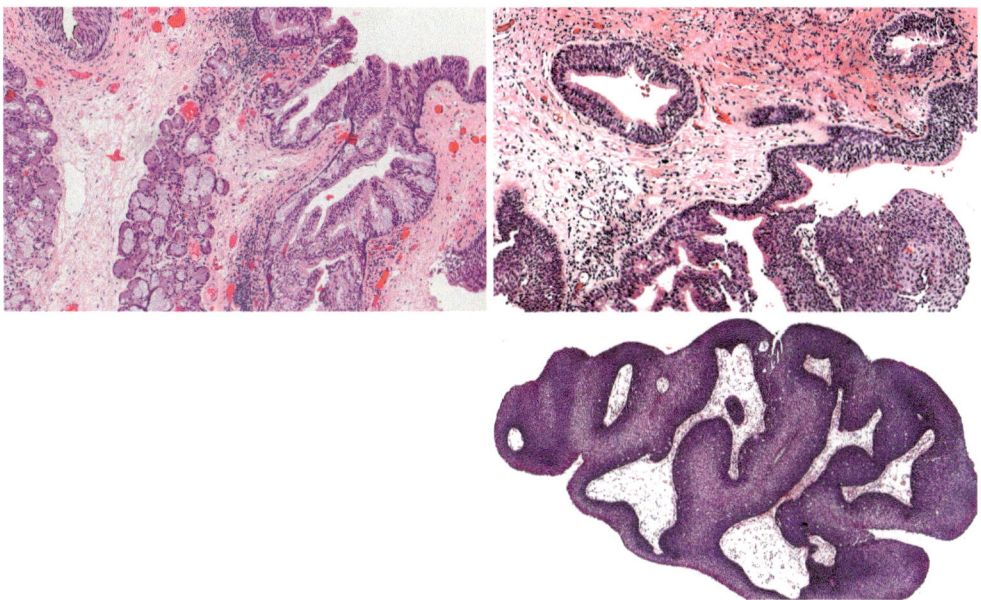

◨ **Fig. 5.3** The nasopharyngeal aspect of the soft palate is covered by respiratory mucosa. Here is an exophytic squamous papilloma arising from the nasopharyngeal aspect of the soft palate

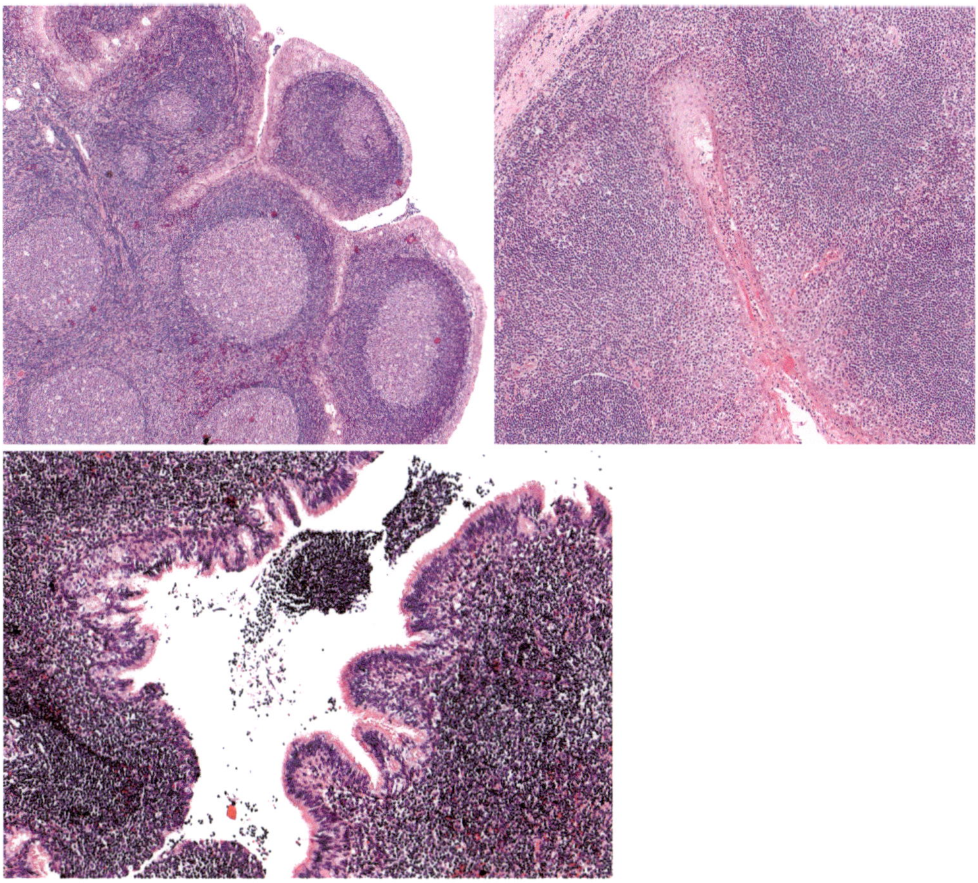

◨ **Fig. 5.4** The pharyngeal tonsil is lined by stratified columnar ciliated epithelium, which invaginates into shallow crypts

and is home to the sella turcica. The optic chiasm is situated anterior to the pituitary infundibulum, directly inferior the sella diaphragm. The posterior skull base consists primarily of the occipital bone, and parts of the sphenoid and temporal bones.

5.2   Tornwaldt's Cyst and Other Cysts

Nasopharyngeal cysts are very rare and usually asymptomatic.

Tornwaldt's cyst represents a cystic expansion of the **pharyngeal bursa,** which may persist in the posterior midline nasopharynx at the inferior aspect of the adenoids [4] (◘ Fig. 5.5) This bursa represents the communication of anterior notochord with the nasopharyngeal roof.

Rathke's cleft cyst represents a cystic expansion within the nasopharynx from persistant **craniopharyngeal canal** (hypopharyngeal duct). This duct/canal represents an embryological connection from the sellar floor through the midline sphenoid body to the nasopharynx. Failure to involute leaves a communication between the floor of the sella with the nasopharynx.

The Eustacian tubes are formed from the first and second branchial arches. The second branchial cleft

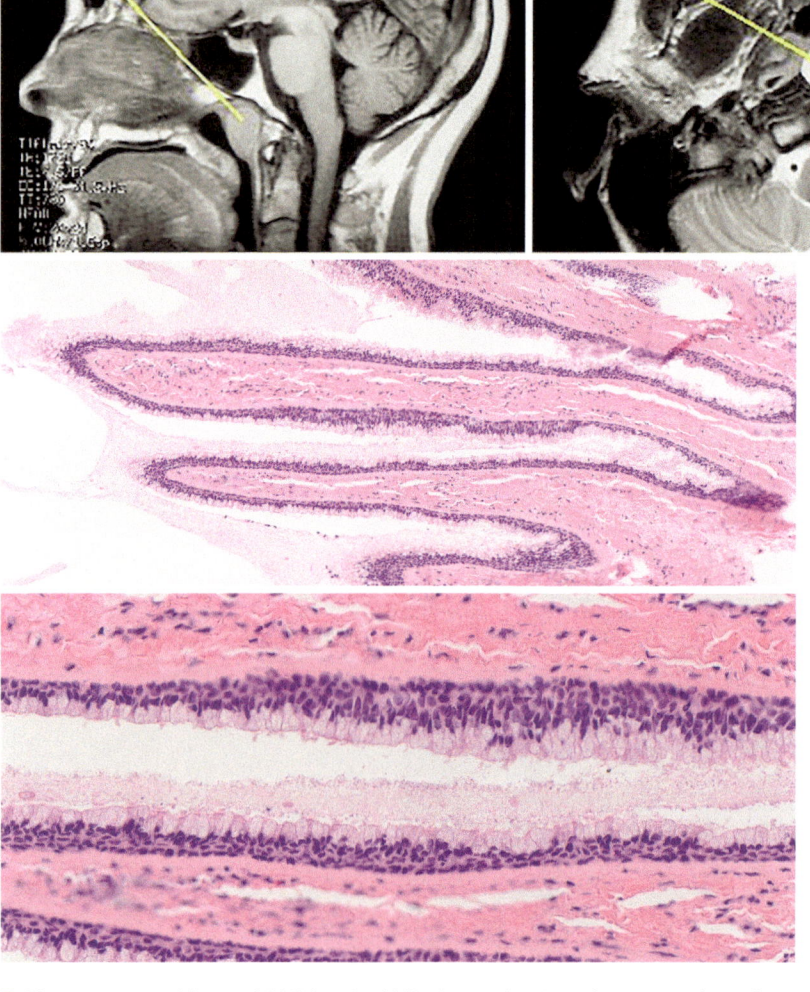

◘ **Fig. 5.5**   Tornwaldt cyst: (**a**) Mid-sagittal MR picture showing a large pear-shaped structure in the nasopharyngeal vault. (**b**) The cyst is bright on T2 weighted axial MR (Courtesy of www.ghorayeb.com). The cyst is lined by respiratory epithelium

most commonly gives rise to branchial cleft cysts, these are associated with the sternocleidomastoid muscle. Rarely though, branchial cleft cysts may occur in the lateral nasopharynx, and are distinguished from other cysts in that they are not midline.

5.3 Hairy Polyps and Teratomas

Hairy polyp (dermoid) is a choristoma which arises from the palate and extends into the nasopharynx. They are usually diagnosed at birth or shortly thereafter. A strong female predominance is noted. Babies may present with nasal dis-

charge, problems feeding, and failure to thrive. Hairy polyps are composed of mature, organized ectodermal and mesodermal tissues, but no endodermal elements [5–12]. The novice should be aware that quite a number of hairy polyps (dermoids) are misclassified in publications as nasopharyngeal "teratomas".

Grossly, hairy polyps are flesh colored; surface hair may be observed. Histologically, the polyp is covered by mature, organized skin with adexal structures. Abundant adipose tissue, as well as skeletal tissue and mature cartilage can be seen within (◘ Fig. 5.6) Tooth buds, bone, salivary tissue, and meningothelial elements are more rare in

◘ **Fig. 5.6** Hairy polyp: (**a**) This finger-like projection is covered by organized hair-bearing skin. (**b**) Mature cartilage and glandular tissue

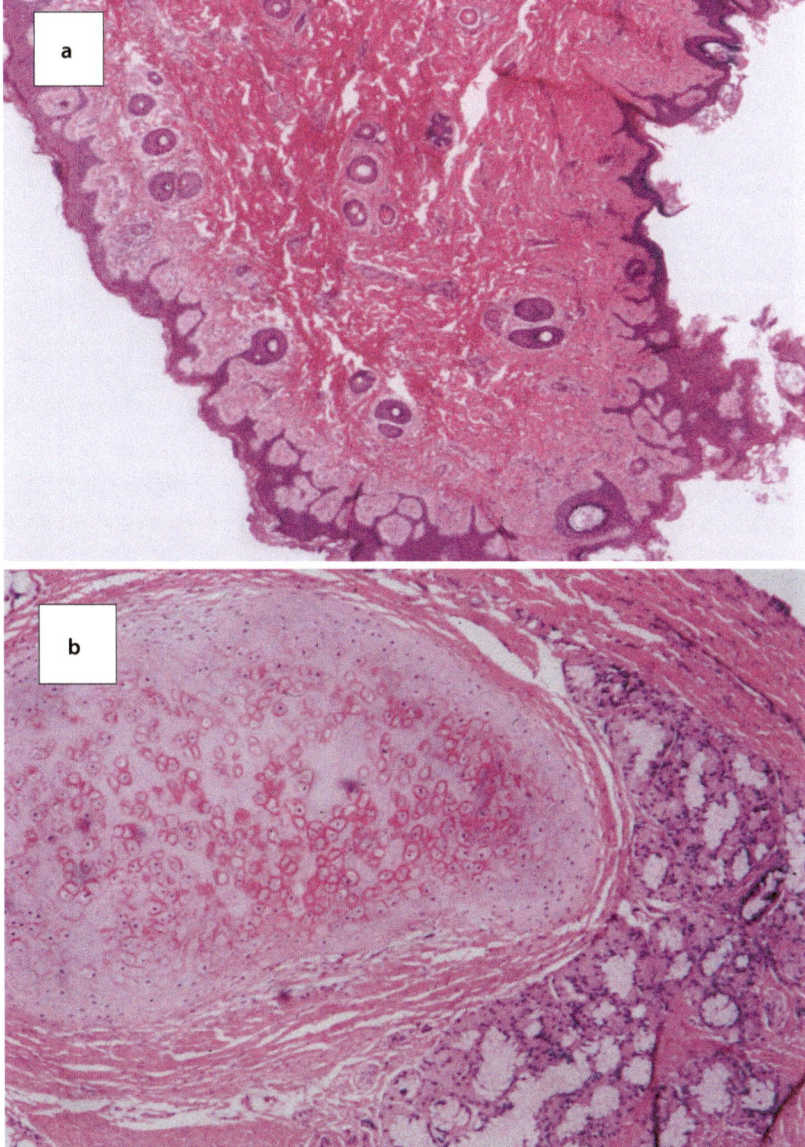

a

b

hairy polyps [12, 13]. The latter has been described as a stromal infiltrate of anastomosing pseudovascular cleft-like spaces, lined by flat to polygonal cells, with occasional multinucleated cells, **vimentin +, epithelial membrane antigen** + [13].

Excision is curative.

Teratomas are composed of *all three* germ layers (ectodermal, mesodermal and endodermal); they represent a true neoplastic process. Bonafide, pathologically documented nasopharyngeal teratomas appear to be more rare than hairy polyps [14–22]. There is no gender predisposition. Nasopharyngeal teratomas can originate in nasopharynx or from the palate and project into the pharynx. They are often associated with skull deformities such as anencephaly, hemicranias, palatal fissure. Histologically, teratomas are composed of mixed solid and cystic elements which may be mature, organized, or immature. One sees the same complement of ectodermal and mesodermal elements that are present in a hairy polyp. Additionally, brain or neurectodermal tissue are most commonly described endodermal components (◘ Fig. 5.7) Other endodermal components include liver, pancreas, respiratory and intestinal tissue. Immature mesenchymal tissue may also be seen. Neonatal teratomas from all sites tend to be benign.

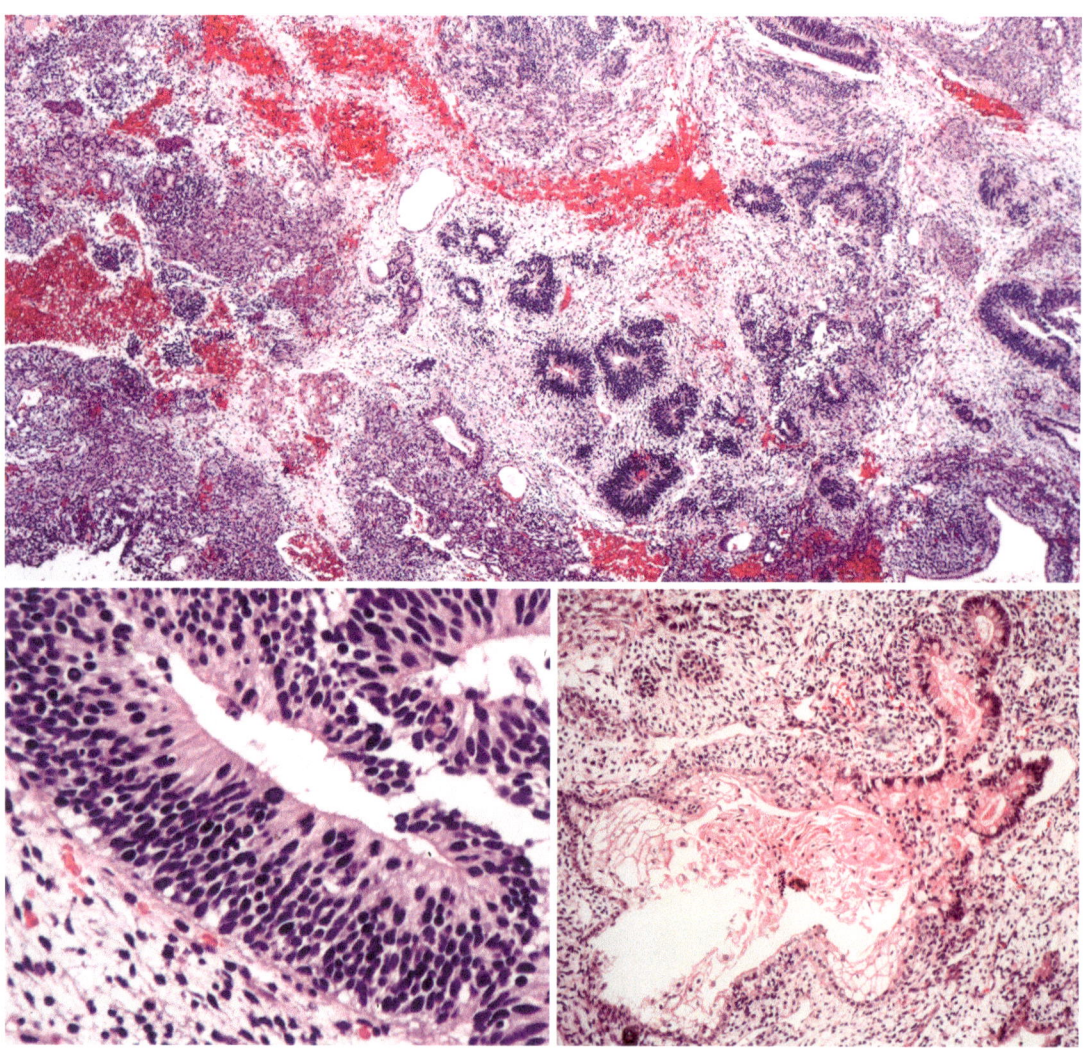

◘ **Fig. 5.7**   Teratoma: *Top:* Low-power view reveals glands embedded in immature mesenchymal matrix, alternating with more cellular undifferentiated regions. *Bottom left:* Organized glands composed of cilliated columnar cells. *Bottom right:* "Squamous differentiation here is fetal-like and glycogenated

5.4   Nasopharyngeal Angiofibroma

Nasopharyngeal angiofibromas (NAF) (juvenile nasopharyngeal angiofibromas) are extremely rare tumors with marked predilection to affect adolescent males; they account for 0.05 % of all head and neck neoplasia [19]. NAF actually originate from the superior aspect of the posterior choanae near the pterygopalatine fossa and sphenopalatine foramen and form asymmetrical tumors that prolapse into the nasopharynx. Presenting symptoms include nasal obstruction, epistaxis, facial deformity, proptosis, sinusitis, nasal discharge, serous otitis media, headache, and anosmia [21–26].

Although NAF is predominantly a male disease, occasional affected females have been reported [23, 27–35]. Publications with pathologic illustrations are even more rare [30–32]. These tumors are mostly "non-juvenile" and extra-nasopharyngeal. The male/female ratio for angiofibromas at non-nasopharynngeal sites is approximately 3/1 [35]. The most common extra-nasopharyngeal site is the maxilla; other sites include ethmoid, sphenoid, septum, and turbinates [35].

The diagnosis of NAF can be definitively established preoperatively based on the typical clinical presentation (adolescent male with epistaxis) and radiographic findings (vascular contrast-enhancing nasopharyngeal mass) (◘ Fig. 5.8) Biopsy is contra-

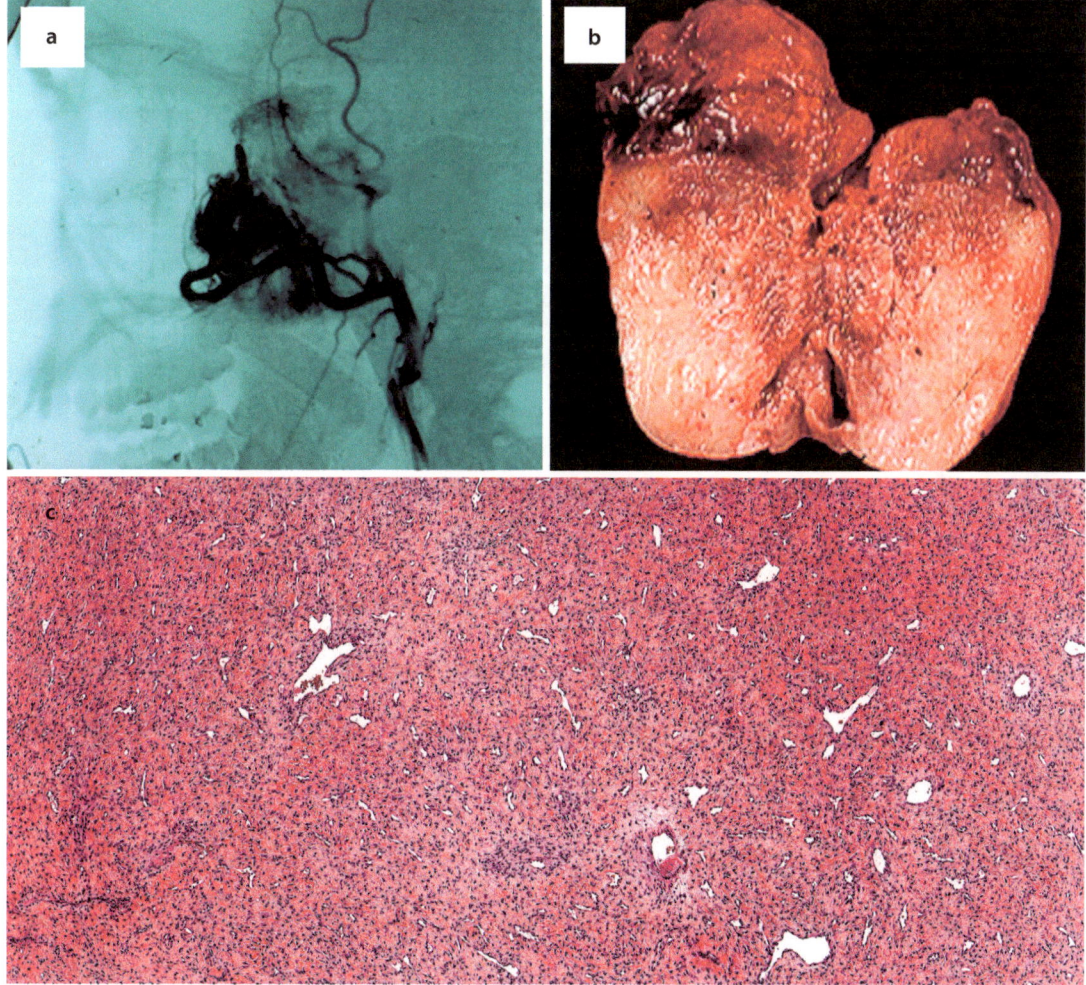

◘ **Fig. 5.8**   Juvenile nasopharyngeal angiofibroma: (**a**) Characteristic angiographic findings of hypervascular nasopharyngeal tumor. Angiography is sufficient to establish the diagnosis and staging, and allows for preoperative embolization. (**b**) Cut surface reveals a firm, spongy tumor. *Bottom*: The two components, tumor vascularity and stroma, vary in composition. Here at low-power we see numerous irregularly shaped vessels and a pink, densely cellular stroma

indicated due to the possibility of severe, uncontrollable bleeding. Extension into the pterygopalatine fossa is common (◘ Figs. 5.2 and 5.9) which widens the fossa and (pathognemonic Holman-Miller sign) [36]. MRI confirms tumor vascularity, which appears as serpiginous signal voids. Preoperative angiography with embolization is important for confirming diagnosis, staging, and treatment.

Although histologically benign, NAF has the potential for significant infiltration, the extent of which guides the surgical approach and correlates intraoperative blood loss and disease-free outcome. A number of staging systems have been published over the years; the system proposed from the University of Pittsburgh (◘ Table 5.1) incorporates post-embolization data [22]. Low-stage NAF are amenable to an endoscopic approach whereas an open approach is indicated for higher-stage NAF.

The local recurrence rate after surgery is variable (2–22 %) depending on initial stage; higher stage and contralateral arterial supply correlate with local recurrence and residual disease [21–24]. External radiation can be administered for unresectable disease [37]. Malignant progression is extremely rare, develops in the setting of multiple recurrences, and appears as progressively increasing stromal cell density and cytologic pleomorphism [38–40].

Hormonal growth factors have been long theorized as promoting NAF, given the striking propensity for post pubescent males and responsiveness to anti-androgen therapies. Y chromosome losses and X chromosome gains (including Xq11.2-q12, AR gene) are frequent [41–44]. Aberrant expression of hormonal receptors (ER-α, ER-β, AR, and PR) within NAF is variable [44–46].

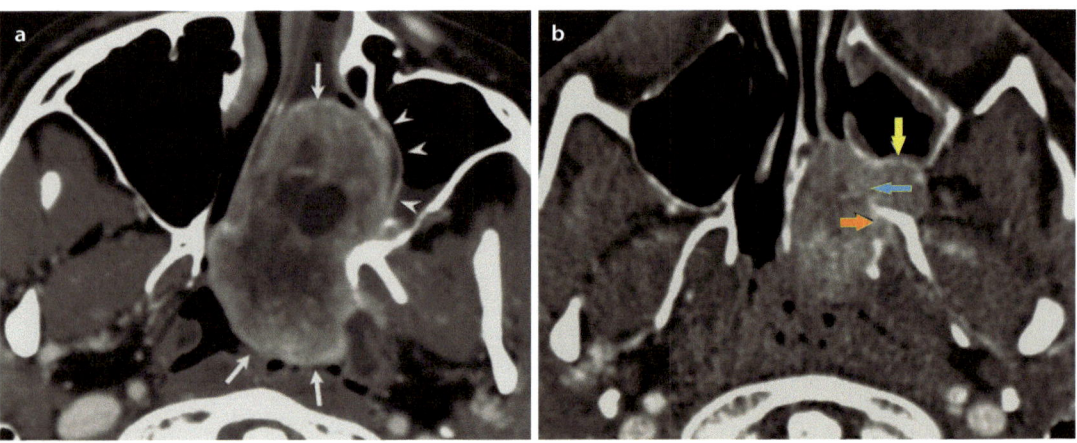

◘ **Fig. 5.9**   (**a**) Contrast enhanced axial CT showing anterior tumor growth from nasopharynx into nasal cavity with bulging into the maxilla (*arrowheads*). (**b**) Contrast enhanced axial CT showing widening of the sphenopalatine foramen (*blue arrow*), erosion of the pterygoid process (*orange arrow*), and anterior bowing of posterior maxillary wall, (*yellow arrow*) referred to as the Holman-Miller sign (Courtesy of Dr A Szymanska [36])

◘ **Table 5.1**   Initial staging of nasopharyngeal angiofibromas [22]

Stage	Description
I	Limited to nasopharynx/nasal cavity, medial pterygopalatine fossa
II	Paranasal sinuses lateral pterygopalatine fossa, antrum, ethmoid, or sphenoid, with bony destruction
III	Skull base erosion, orbital or infratemporal fossa involvement
IV	Skull base erosion, orbital or infratemporal fossa involvement. Residual vascularity after embolization, indicating intracranial circulation
V	Frank intracranial extension

Some evidence suggests a relationship between NAF, FAP (familial adenomatous polyposis), and the APC gene/β catenin pathway, which is not surprising as β catenin is known to interact with AR in other contexts [43, 47, 48, 50]. NAF is touted as being 25 times more frequent in FAP patients than age matched population, although this is still debatable [46–49]. There are isolated reports of NAF arising in FAP patients [41, 45, 48]. Germline and somatic 5q APC mutations have been detected in FAP-related NAF. [41, 48] Sporadic NAF are much more common; 75 % of them harbor activating somatic mutations in exon 3 of the β catenin gene [42]. Nuclear localization of beta-catenin protein is seen in greater than 90 % of tumours [42].

■ Histopathology

NAF is characterized by a dense mature fibrous stroma with numerous, wide, endothelial-lined blood vessels of various sizes and shapes (◘ Fig. 5.10). The vascular spaces range from slit-like, to patulous, to branched/staghorn shaped. Large vessels may have irregular or incomplete smooth muscle walls; elastic fibers usually are not present. Small vessels lack muscularis and are surrounded only by fibrous stroma. Intravascular gel-foam can be seen as a result of preoperative embolization. Stromal collagenization is variable and has a fascia-like parallel arrangement. Myxoid degeneration may be present. Stromal cells vary from mature fibroblasts with small, round, oval to stellate

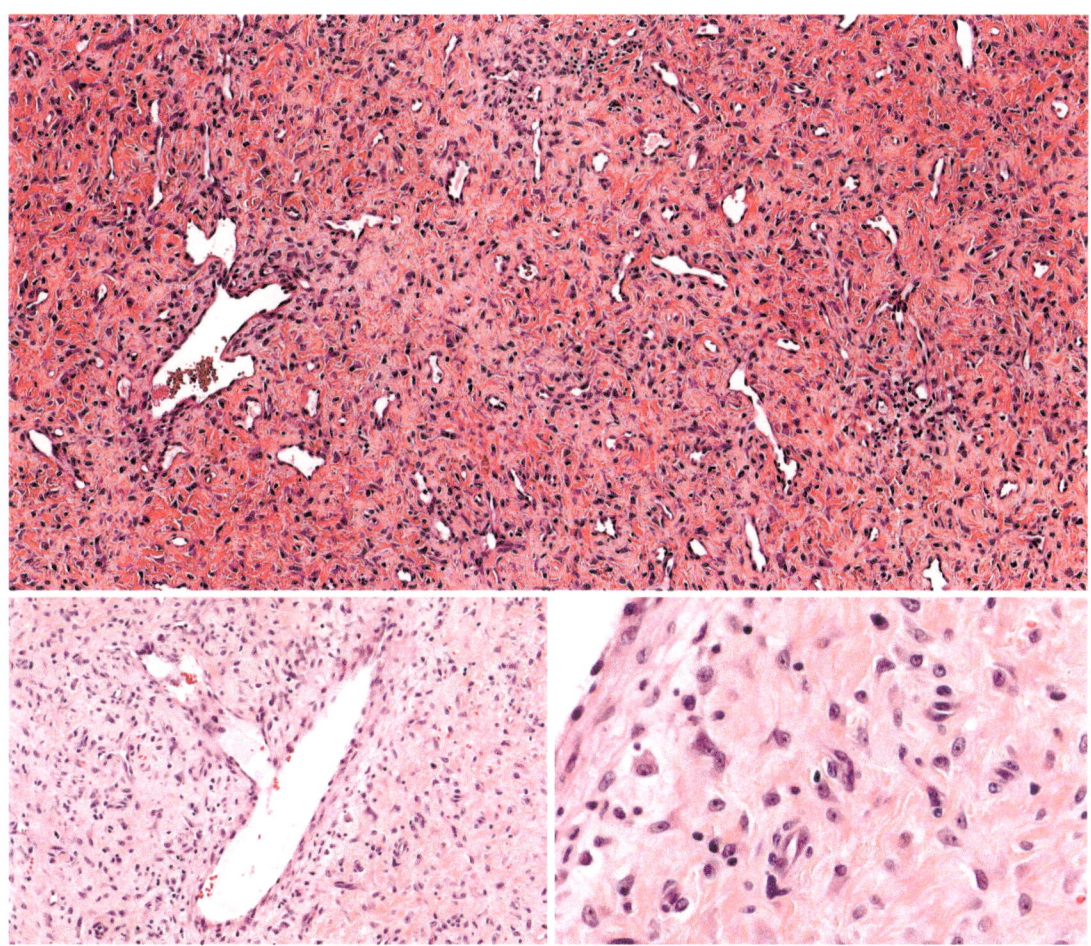

◘ **Fig. 5.10** NAF stroma is dense and collagenized. The stromal cells have spindled to triangular-shaped nuclei. The vessels have irregularly shaped lumena. Vessel walls vary from thin and nondescript to irregularly thick with variable muscle content

nuclei, to large reactive fibroblasts with regular nuclei, fine chromatin, and occasion prominent nucleoli. Stromal cells may show focally increased cellularity, but pleomorphism and mitotic activity should not be seen. Mature interspersed stromal adipose tissue ("lipomatous variant") has been described [51]. Malignant transformation is marked by increasing nuclear pleomorphism, mitotic rate, and cellular density (■ Fig. 5.11).

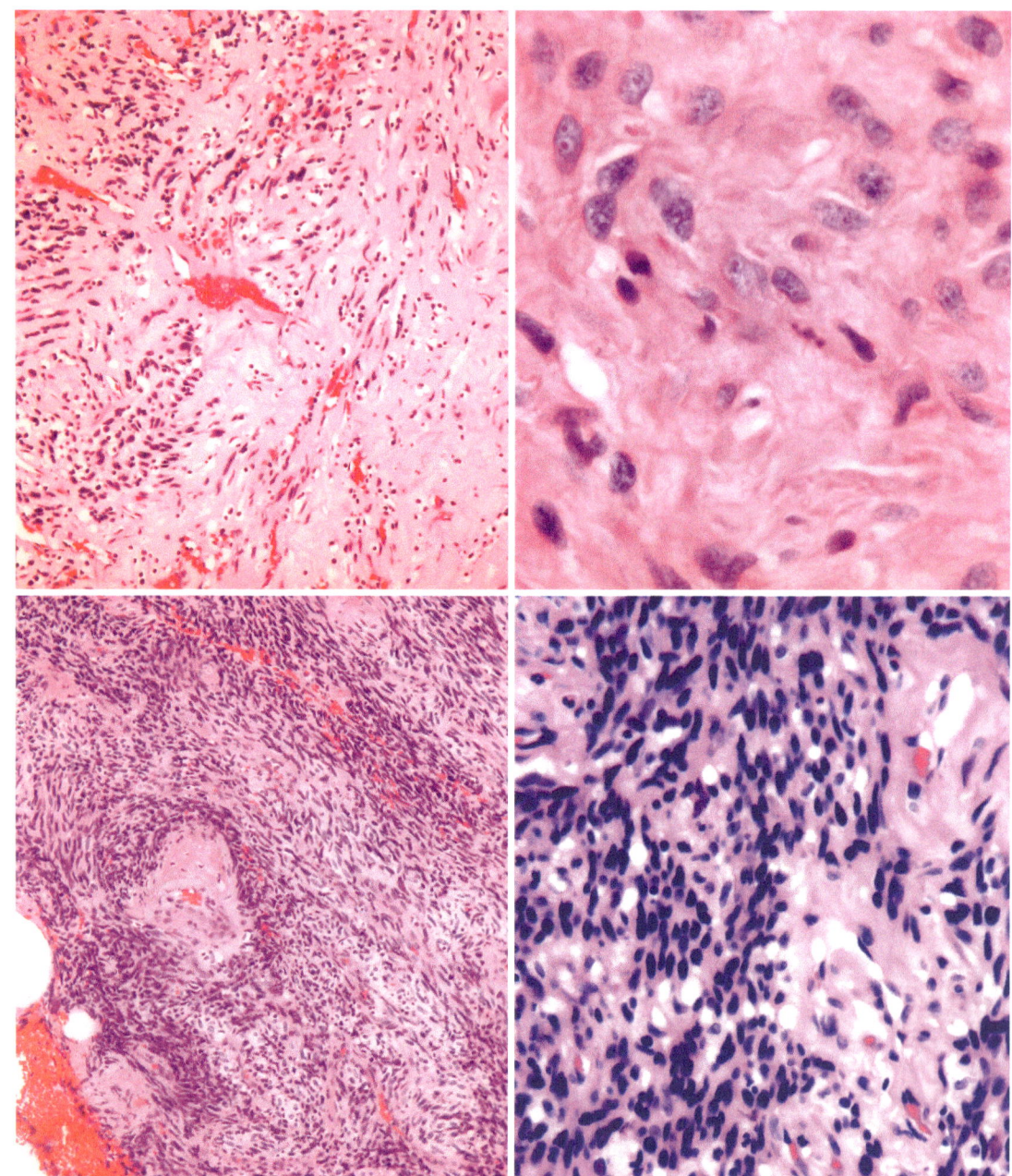

■ **Fig. 5.11**   Rare example of sarcomatous transformation in a nasopharyngeal angiofibroma with multiple recurrences. *Top* and *bottom* panels represent low- and high-power views from the first and second recurrent tumors, respectively. Malignant transformation is marked by increasing nuclear pleomorphism, mitotic rate, and cellular density

5.5 Salivary Gland Anlage Tumor (Nasopharyngeal Congenital Pleomorphic Adenoma)

The term "salivary gland anlage tumor" (SGAT) was originally coined by Dehner and colleagues and represents a polypoid nasopharyngeal tumor of neonates [52]. SGAT occurs with a pronounced male predisposition. As neonates are obligate nasal breathers, SGAT causes immediate symptoms such as nasal congestion, dyspnea, respiratory distress, and poor feeding [52–60]. These tumors are firm, pedunculated, and bosselated. They are found to be attached to the posterior nasal septum or posterior nasopharyngeal wall by a narrow pedicle. The true nature of SGAT, whether tumor or hamartoma, is unknonwn. SGAT is treated by simple excision and there have been no reported recurrences.

■ Histopathology

SGAT are biphasic tumors composed by epithelial elements embedded within mesenchymal stroma, reminiscent of pleomorphic adenomas. The epithelial elements can form cords, islands, tubules, and branching ducts (◘ Fig. 5.12). The ductal structures can reveal squamous metaplasia, keratinization, or rarely, complex papillary formations. Continuity of surface mucosa and intratumoral epithelial elements has been observed. Stromal cellularity varies from loose, myxoid-like to very dense. Dense tumor cellularity (◘ Fig. 5.13) can bring to mind malignancy, however, there is no clinical evidence of malignant potential. The densely cellular stroma is composed of short fascicles of spindle cells. The stromal nuclei are monotonous with condensed chromatin and occasional mitotic figures. Mitotic activity however can be brisk [56]. Necrosis, when present, is likely due to pedicle torsion.

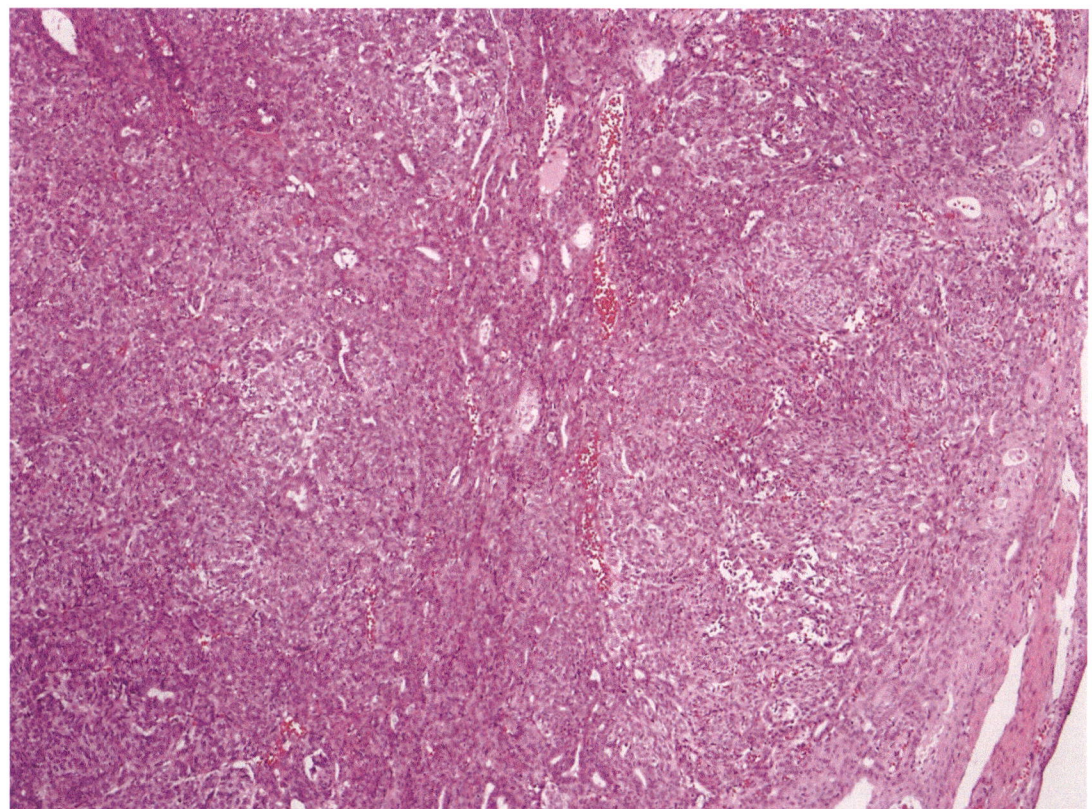

◘ **Fig. 5.12** Salivary gland anlage tumor: highly cellular biphasic neoplasm seen on low-power

◘ **Fig. 5.13** *Top:* salivary gland anlage tumor is composed of short spindled and epithelioid cells form solid cords, organoid nests, and ductoglandular structures. *Bottom:* More pronounced ductoglandular structures are seen here. They do not resemble the mature "ductal-myoepithelial unit" seen in pleomorphic adenomas

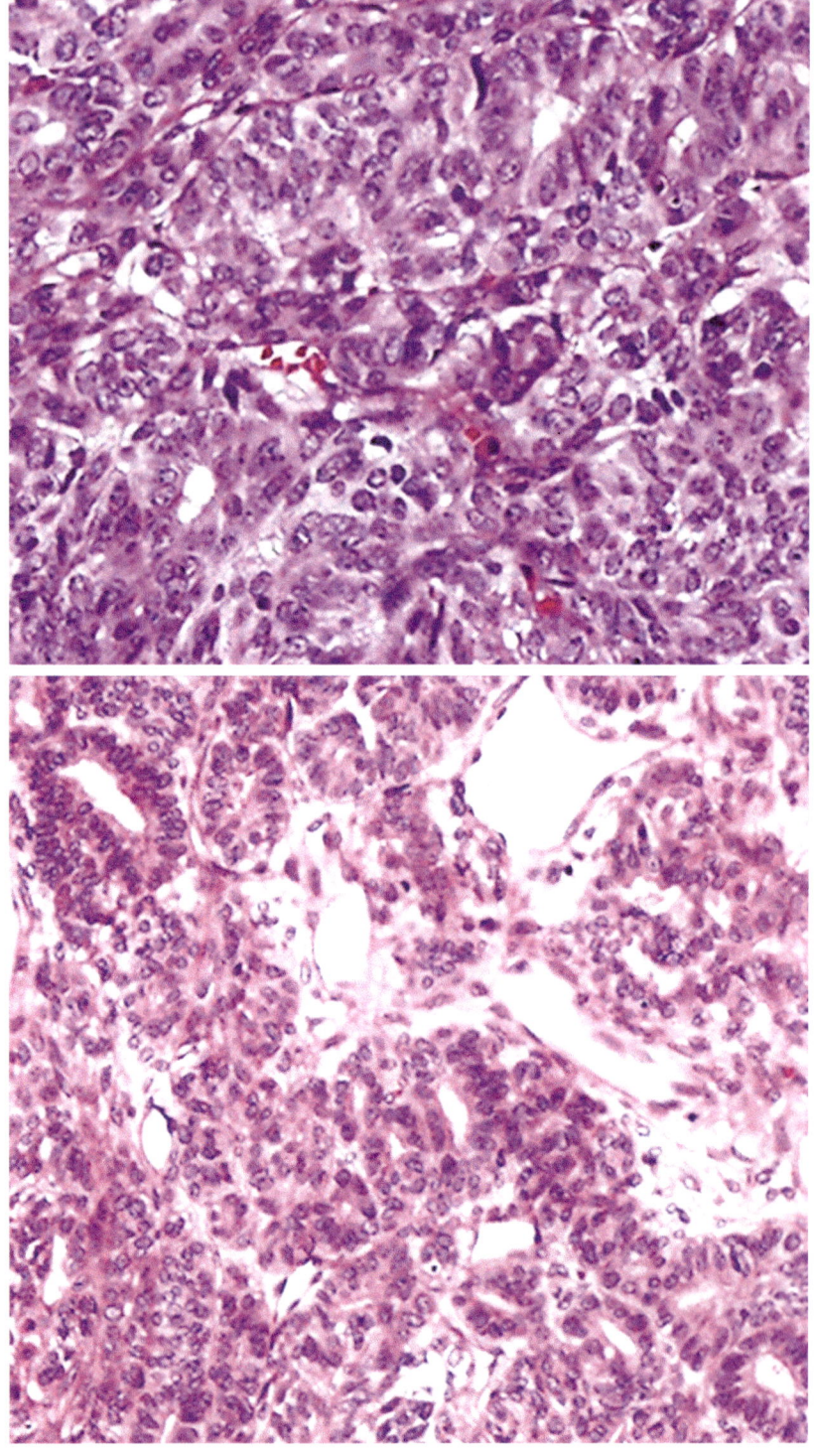

SGAT expresses epithelial and myoepithelial proteins; stromal coexpression of cytokeratin and muscle-specific actin has been demonstrated. While these tumors are reminiscent of pleomorphic adenomas, they lack mature myoepithelial differentiation (plasmacytoid cells, basement membrane material). The classic "epithelial-myoepithelial" unit of mature salivary differentiation is not seen; no cartilaginous elements have been described. The differential diagnosis in neonates is with midline congenital teratoma. SGAT lack teratomatous elements such as skin adnexal, neuronal, cartilaginous or muscular elements.

5.6 Craniopharyngioma (Rathke's Pouch Tumor)

Craniopharyngiomas are very rare, with an estimated incidence is 0.5 to 2/100,000/year [61]. They typically arise in the sellar/suprasellar region. More rarely, they can develop at sites such as nasopharynx, paranasal sinuses, and cerebellopontine angle. There is a broad patient age range with two frequency peaks: childhood, (between 5 and 14) and older adults (between 65 and 74) [62]. Craniopharyngiomas represent the most common nonglial pediatric brain tumor. Congenital tumors are extremely rare [63].

Etiologically, craniopharyngiomas are derived from precursor cells within pharyngohypophyseal duct rests which may persist along the migrational path of Rathke's pouch to the pituitary stalk [64–67] (◘ Fig. 5.14). Rare tumors can be confirmed to arise within remnant Rathke's pouch [63]. The two variants of craniopharyngiomas are adamantinomatous and papillary, which have some interesting distinctions. The adamantinomatous variant represents 90% of craniopharyngiomas; this cystic and solid tumor is seen in the first two decades of life. The papillary variant represents 10% of craniopharyngiomas and typically is seen in adults. Adamantinomatous craniopharyngiomas are associated with upregulation of the WNT/β-catenin pathway; the papillary variants have no such association. *CTNNB1* mutation is common to adamantinomatous craniopharyngioma; *CTNNB1* encodes β-catenin, a central WNT regulator. *CTNNB1* mutation inhibits β-catenin degradation and activates the WNT/β-catenin pathway; this manifests as aberrant nuclear β-catenin expression in adamantinomatous craniopharyngiomas. Papillary craniopharyngiomas lack the *CTNNB1* mutation and do not demonstrate aberrant β-catenin expression. Activation of this pathway is not the entire story; the paracrine model of craniopharyngioma development states that cluster cells with *CTNNB1* mutation support stem cells of different origin,

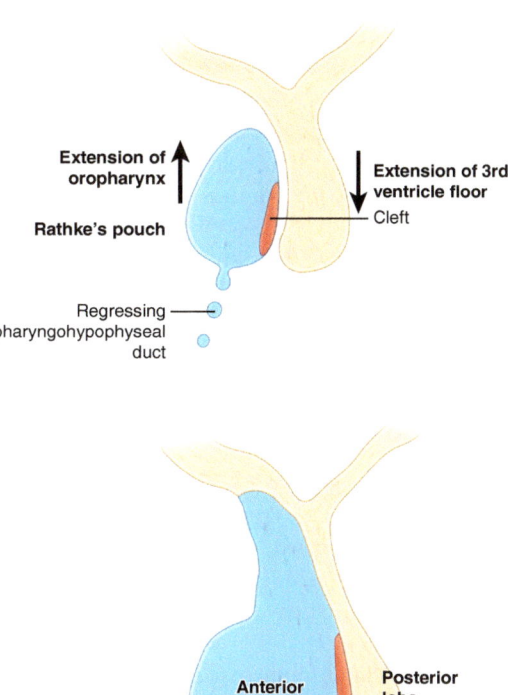

◘ **Fig. 5.14** Sagital view of pituitary development: Rathke's pouch represents an upward extension of stomadeum ectoderm which give rise to the anterior pituitary. The pharyngohypophyseal duct is the migratory route from pharynx to pituitary fossa. Downward migration from the 3rd ventricle forms the posterior pituitary

which directly give rise to craniopharyngioma [62]. Papillary craniopharyngiomas are found to harbor the BRAF V600E mutation [68].

Due to their critical anatomic location, these tumors are symptomatic and can cause one of three clinical syndromes [62, 66, 69]. Prechiasmal craniopharyngiomas represent half to two thirds of tumors, they cause optic atrophy. Patients present with progressive visual decline. Retrochiasmal craniopharyngiomas represent one third to almost one half of tumors and cause hydrocephalous. Patients complain of nausea, vomiting and double vision. Intrasellar craniopharyngiomas represent 7–17% of tumors and are classified as infradiaphragmatic or supradiagphragmatic. They cause headaches and endocrinopathies, such as panhypopituitarism, diabetes insipidis, hypogonadism, or hypothyroidism. Other presenting symptoms include seizures, and psychiatric, personality and mood changes.

Preoperative diagnosis can be established by imaging; an intrasellar/supracellular cystic tumor calcification is characteristic. Treatment is surgical (either endoscopic endonasal or stereotactic microscopic) with adjuvant radiotherapy for inadequate resections. Craniopharyngiomas are benign but recur with incomplete removal. Reported recurrence rates are 22–40 % [69–73]. Local control is improved with adjuvant radiotherapy; it is better for adults than children, and possibly better for the papillary variant compared with the adamantinomatous variant [70]. Overall survival rates at 10 years are good; mortalities are usually related to operative problems or pituitary insufficiency.

■ **Histopathology**

Adamantinomatous craniopharyngioma appears poorly circumscribed, invasive, solid, and cystic tumor; cut surface reveals a lobulated spongy tumor which exudes characterstic "motor oil fluid". Histologically, the tumor is composed of cords, nests, and lobules of epithelial tumor cells forming peripheral palisading (■ Fig. 5.15). The center of these lobules contain loose spindled tumor cells forming a stellate reticulum pattern. The cyst fluid contains cholesterol crystals, cholesterol clefts, and reactive giant cells. Necrosis and inflammation are variable. Two features are unique to adamantinomatous craniopharyngioma: "wet keratin" and calcifications. "Wet keratin" describes dense brightly eosinophilic keratin masses with anucleated ghost cells. In distinction, flaky (dry) keratin, is seen, for instance, in cholesteotoma.

Papillary craniopharyngiomas are solid, well-circumscribed tumors. Histologically, they are composed of well-differentiated stratified squamous epithelium lining fibrovascular cores which resemble squamous papillomas. Pseudopapillae can be seen. Adamantinous features (cystic spaces, machine oil, palisading, wet keratin, calcification) are absent.

Mixed adamantinous and papillary craniopharyngiomas are very rare [74]. Rare craniopharyngiomas can be confirmed to originate in Rathke's pouch by remnant cyst lining composed of simple ciliated epithelium with goblet cells that express CK8+ and CK20 + [65].

Malignant degeneration is rare and usually secondary to recurrence and radiotherapy. Malignant craniopharyngiomas are highly cellular basaloid tumors with increased nuclear\cytoplasmic ratio, mitotic activity, pleomorphism, and invasion [75].

5.7 Ectopic Pituitary Adenomas and Macroadenomas

Pituitary tumors are not usually within the realm of head and neck pathologists; they are included here as biopsies from ectopic pituitary adenomas or pituitary macroadenomas can be easily misdiagnosed. Ectopic pituitary adenomas in the setting of a normal pituitary gland (intact sella turcica) can be especially problematic as there is the potential for pathologic misdiagnosis as neuroendocrine carcinoma [76].

Most commonly, ectopic adenomas fill the sphenoid sinus [77]. Their precursors are likely derived from persistent Rathke pouch rests. From the sphenoid, they can extend into the nasal cavity or nasopharynx [78]. Pituitary macroadenomas are defined as >10 mm [79–81]. Macroadenomas can invade through the sphenoid and present for biopsy as nasal tumors, which represents another potential pitfall. Functional macroadenomas are more frequent in young patients while macroadenomas in elderly patients are more often nonfunctional. The most common functional adenoma is a prolactinoma.

■ **Histopathology**

Typically, pituitary adenoma can reveal various neuroendocrine architectural patterns such as organoid, pseudorossettes, pseudopapillae, glandular, trabecular, insular, or solid (■ Fig. 5.16). They are typically well-vascularized with variable sclerosis and hemorrhage. A grenze zone may separate the adenoma from intact respiratory mucosa. Adenoma cells can be epithelioid; occasional multinucleated tumor cells can be seen. Cellular cytoplasm can be oncocytoid, amphophilic, or granular. Nuclei have typical delicate salt and pepper chromatin. Mitoses are rare and pleomorphism is uncommon. Tumor secretions or concretions may be observed.

A number of histologic features could mimic nonpituitary malignancy. Necrosis is described in 25 % of ectopic adenomas [76]. Boney or cartilaginous invasion may be seen. Tumor cells may be non-epithelioid (plasmacytoid, spindled) and densely cellular. Preliminary immunohistochemistry on these tumors will confirm keratin and neuroendocrine marker expression (synaptophysin, chromogranin), further mimicking neuroendocrine carcinomas or olfactory neuroblastomas. Two helpful clues are 1) strong diffuse keratin

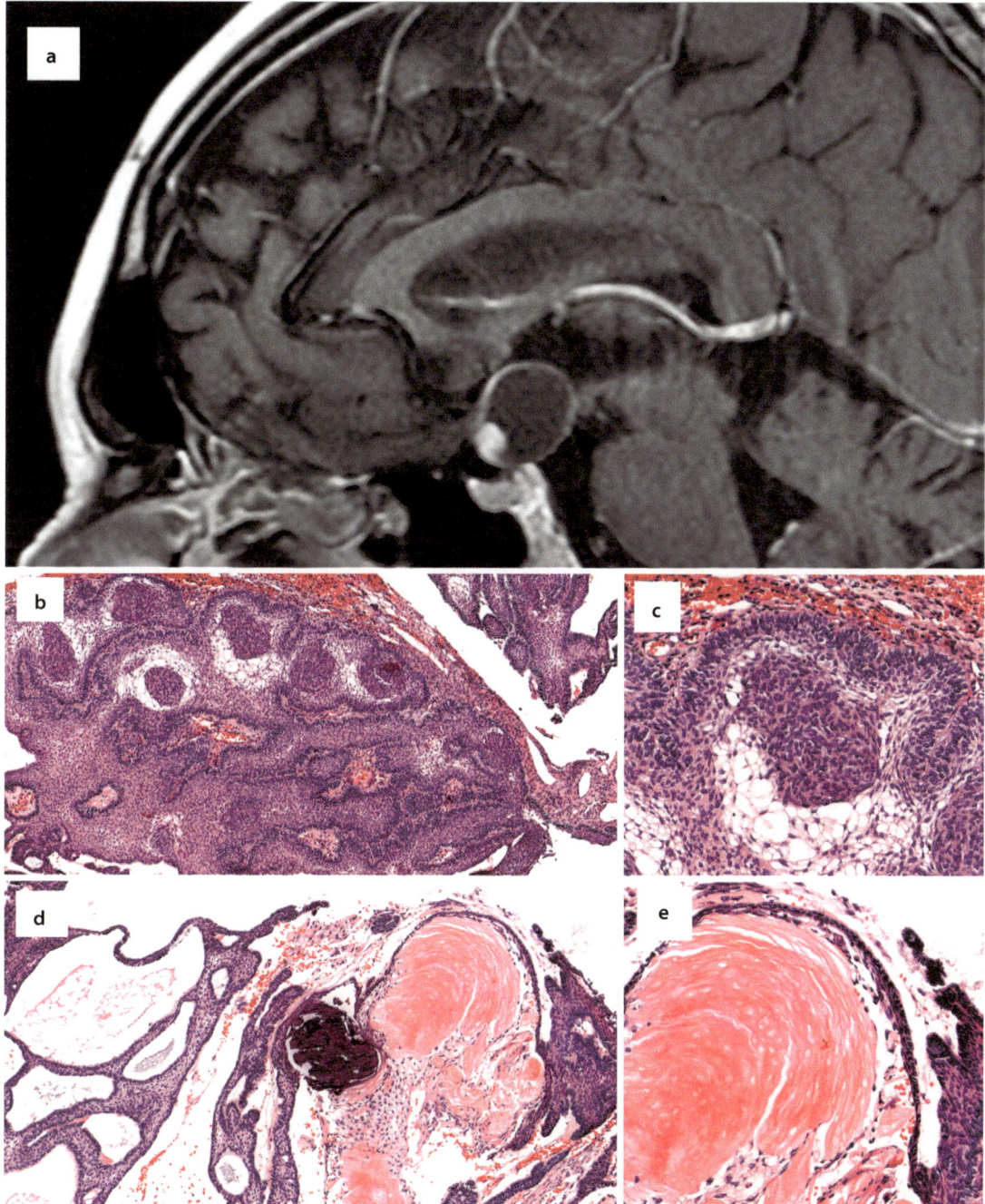

□ Fig. 5.15 Craniopharyngioma: (**a**) Sagittal post-contrast T1 weighted image demonstrates a cystic suprasellar mass. There is enhancement of the thin peripheral cyst wall and the anterior mural nodule (Courtesy Dr. Phil Chapman, University of Alabama at Birmingham). (**b**) Crangiopharyngioma forming anastomosing ribbons and cellular eddies. Stellate reticulum pattern and peripheral palisading can be observed at low-power. (**c**) Spindled squamoid cells form a dense eddy, loosely cohesive stellate reticulum, and dense peripheral palisading. (**d**) Cyst formation, "wet" keratin and calcifications. (**e**) "Wet" keratin is compact and anucleate

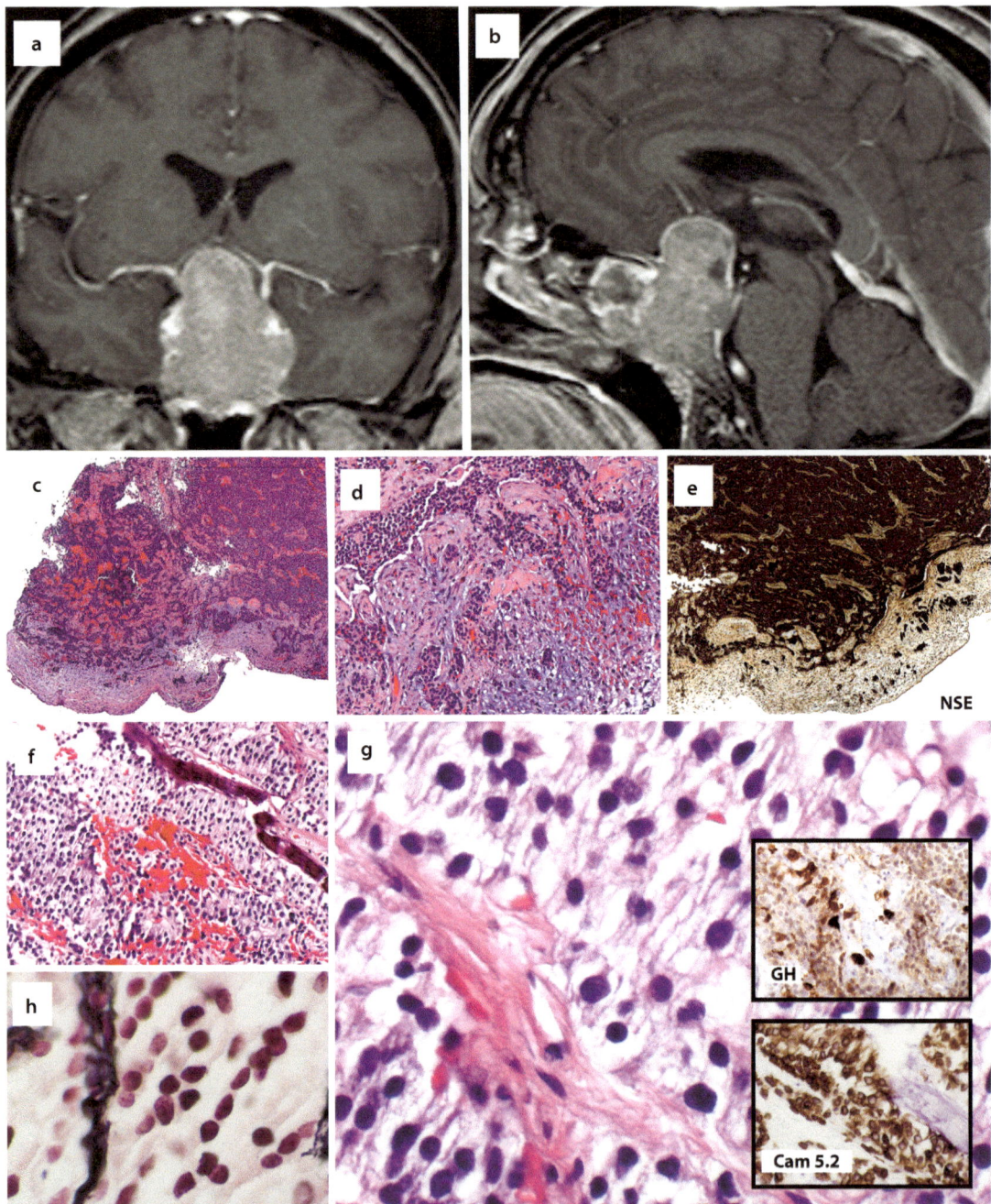

Fig. 5.16 Pituitary macroadenoma: (**a**) Coronal post-contrast MRI through sella demonstrates large sellar mass with suprasellar extension, bilateral cavernous sinus invasion, and invasion of the sphenoid sinus and clivus inferiorly. (**b**) Sagittal post-contrast MRI better demonstrates the extensive involvement of the sphenoid sinus and clivus, with minimal extension posteriorly into the retroclival epidural space (Courtesy Dr. Phil Chapman, University of Alabama at Birmingham). (**c**) Low-power view of pituitary macroadenoma. (**d**) Higher power view demonstrating tumor nests within a myxoid background. (**e**) Immunohistochemistry reveals strong neuron specific enolase expression. (**f**) Tumor with carcinoid-like nesting pattern infiltrating bone. (**g**, **h**). High-power reveals uniform dark condensed nuclei. The insets demonstrate expression of Cam5.2, and growth hormone (*GH*). This was originally diagnosed as a neuroendocrine carcinoma, well-differentiated. IHC for GH was performed on consultation

expression is at odds with the diagnosis of olfactory neuroblastomas, and 2) features of a grade II/III neuroendocrine carcinomas are absent (pleomorphism, mitotic activity). Once a pituitary origin is considered, prolactin is the most commonly expressed marker; other hormones either in multiples or individually (FSH, LH, GH, TSH, ACTH).

5.8　Chordoma and Ecchordosis Physaliphora

Chordomas are extremely rare bone tumors derived from remnant notochord with an estimated incidence of 0.08/100,000 [82–84]. There is a broad age frequency peak, from 3rd to 5th decades, and a male to female ratio of 1.6:1. Typically, half of all chordomas arise in the sacrum, one third arise in the clivus, (central mid-skull base), and the remainder originate in the cervical vertebrae and other sites. Clival chordomas are more common in younger patients and patients with familial chordomas, whereas sacral chordomas are more common in older patients [85]. Familial chordomas represent an extremely rare subgroup and are estimated to comprise 0.4 % of all chordomas [86]. Familial chordomas are associated with an autosomal dominant pattern of inheritance; nine familial cohorts have been described [87]. The transcription factor *T gene* (*brachyury* homolog), a member of the T-box group of morphogenetic genes, is important in notocord development and is uniquely overexpressed in most chordomas. Germline duplication of *T gene* (*brachyury* homolog) is common in familial chordomas, but rare in sporadic cases [87, 88].

Chordomas are slow-growing and indolent; large tumors may produce cranial nerve palsies and sellar chordomas may cause endocrinopathies. Radiographically, chordomas are destructive midline tumors with a bony epicenter; calcifications and sequestered bone fragments can be seen as well. The MRI appearance is characteristic: isointense or hypointense on T1-weighted MRI, hyperintense on T2-weighted MRI, and gadolinium enhancing (◘ Fig. 5.17). This latter point is very useful when distinguishing ecchordosis physaliphora from chordoma (see below).

Ecchordosis physaliphora which does not substantially enhance with gadolinium.

Although low-grade, chordomas are associated with a significant likelihood of local recurrence. The goal of treatment is complete surgical resection (endoscopic and/or open surgical approach), which may be limited by tumor size and location, plus adjuvant radiotherapy. Five percent of chordoma patients present with metastatic disease in the lungs, bone, skin, or brain, Survival is less affected by distant metastasis than by local recurrence, which is the most important predictor of mortality. Overall survival rates at 5, 10, and 20 years are 68, 40, and 13 %, respectively [82].

■　**Histopathology**

Gross examination reveals a soft, gelatinous tumor with lobular contours, cysts, hemorrhage, and calcifications. Chordomas are classified as either classical, atypical, chondroid, or dedifferentiated. Classical chordoma is a myxoid neoplasm with a lobular growth pattern separated by fibrous septate. The tumor cells are medium-sized with round nuclei. Tumor cell cytoplasm may be eosinophic, or abundant, clear, and vacuolated (◘ Fig. 5.18). Clear cell change and vacuolization may be observed from low-power. The unique and characteristic intracellular bubble-like vacuoles are termed physalifrous cells. Variable cytologic atypia may be seen. Tumor cellularity varies from low- to intermediate and myxoid matrix is abundant. The tumor cells are somewhat cohesive and form interconnecting cords, strands, nests, or may be distributed as single cells against the blueish myxoid background.

Atypical chordomas are characterized by greater cellularity, cytologic pleomorphism, necrosis, and epithelioid, spindled or round tumor cells. Myxoid matrix and physalifrous cells are limited. Chondroid chordomas contain hyaline cartilage-like matrix with single cells within chondroid lacunae, in addition to conventional chordoma. Dedifferentiated chordomas are characterized by undifferentiated pleomorphic sarcoma adjacent to conventional chordoma.

All chordomas typically express S100, cytokeratin, and epithelial membrane antigen. Nuclear brachyury protein expression is common in chordomas and chondroid chordomas,

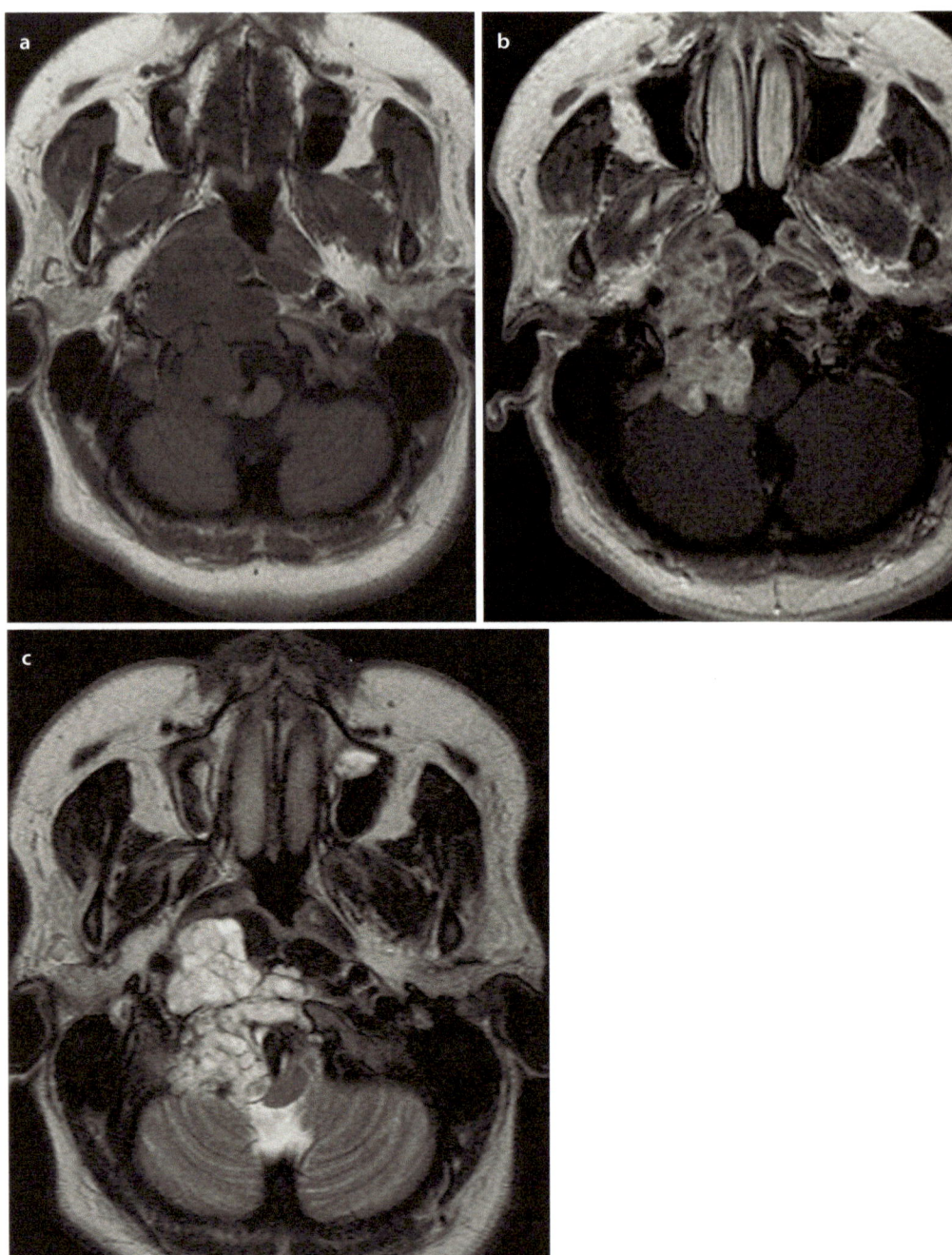

☐ Fig. 5.17   Chordoma: (**a**) Magnetic resonance imaging (MRI) T1 weighted scan shows a destructive lesion centered in the clivus, with intermediate to low signal intensity. Signal heterogeneity is present due to the various tumor densities: fluid and gelatinous mucoid substance, prior hemorrhage, necrosis. (**b**) T1 with gadolinium accentuates heterogeneous enhancement with a honeycomb appearance corresponding to low T1 signal areas within the tumour (**c**) T2 weighted scan demonstrated characteristic very high signal (Courtesy of Christopher Therasse, Northwestern University, Chicago, Allison Weyer, Erie County Medical Center)

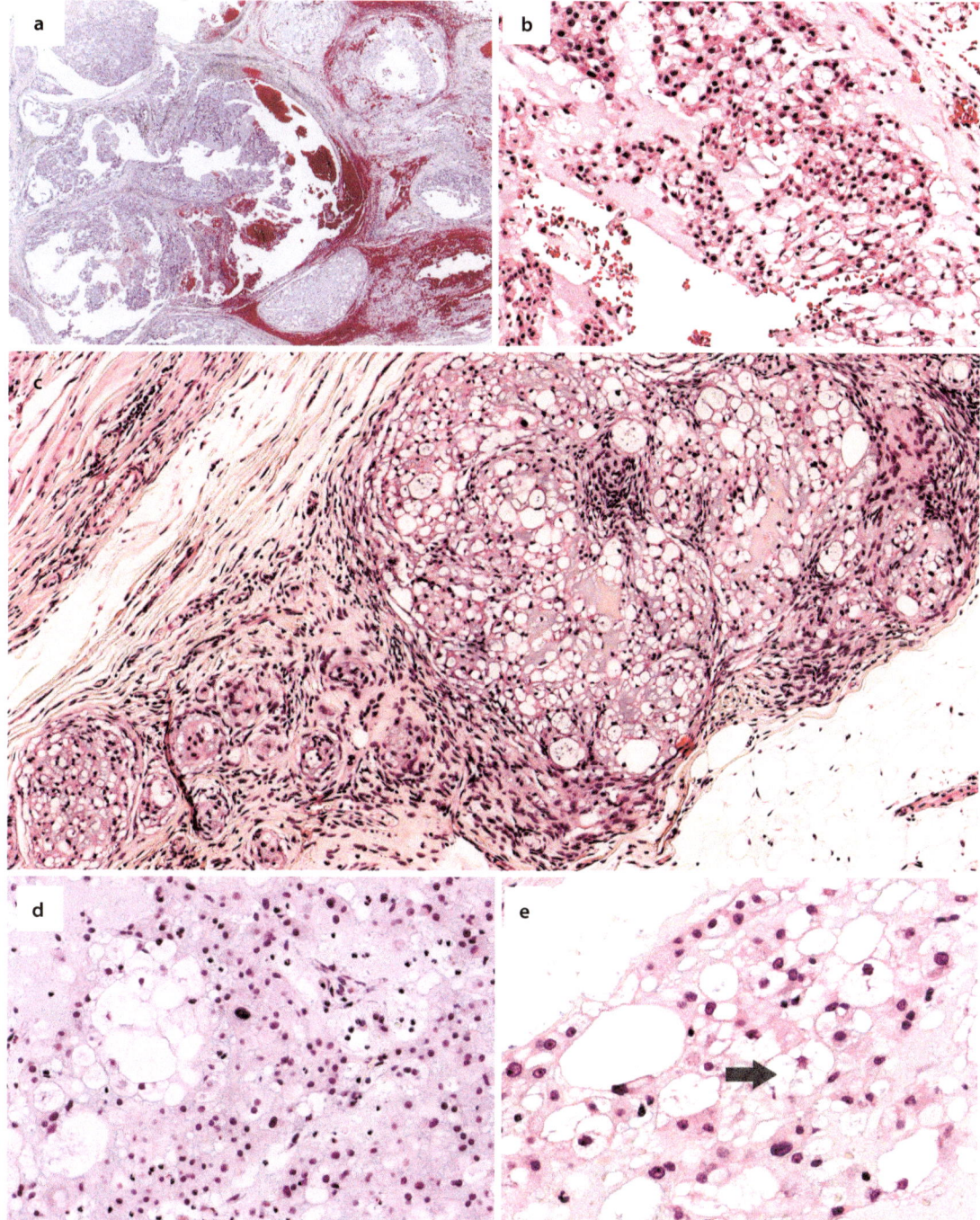

◼ **Fig. 5.18** Chordoma: (**a**) Low-power view of multiple blue-ish myxoid nodules with hemorrhage. (**b, c**) Medium-sized tumor cells with round nuclei and eosinophilic cytoplasm forming cords and nested patterns, respectively. (**d**) Characteristic clear cytoplasmic vacuoles. (**e**) *Black arrow* points to a pathogneumonic physalifrous (soap bubble) cell

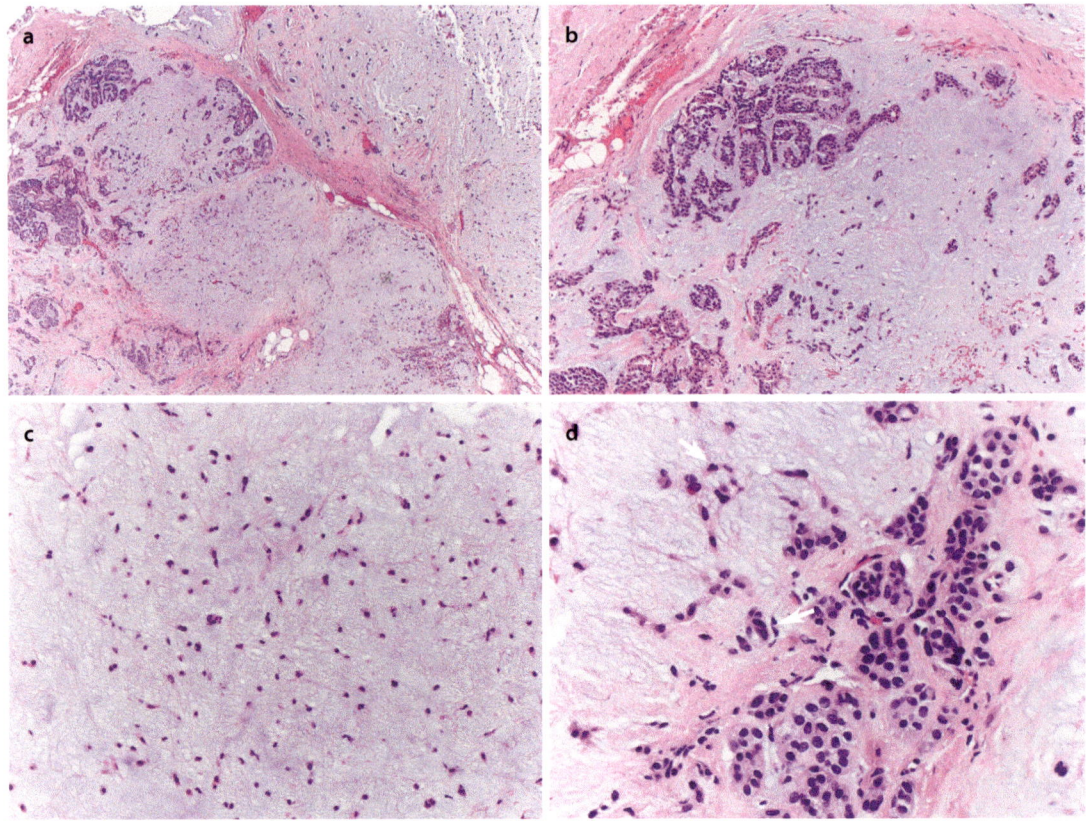

Fig. 5.19 Benign mixed tumor (pleomorphic adenoma) of skull base enters into the differential diagnosis of chordoma. (**a, b**) The lobulated growth pattern and myxoid background are reminiscent of a chordoma. Abundant clear cytoplasmic vacuoles are not present. (**c**) The individual small tumor spindle cells are myoepithelial. (**d**) Higher power: *white arrows* further highlight myoepithelial tumor cells, which are characteristic for pleomorphic adenoma and not part of chordoma

but not seen in chondrosarcomas or many other sarcomas [88, 89].

The differential diagnoses of clival chordomas include rare salivary pleomorphic adenomas which can extend to skull base (Fig. 5.19), chondrosarcomas, and **e**cchordosis physaliphora (see below).

■ Ecchordosis Physaliphora

Ecchordosis physaliphora (EP) is a rare congenital hamartoma arising from notochord remnants. Typically, they are assymptomatic incidental radiographic findings [90]. When EP evoke symptoms, patients may present with cerebrospinal fluid rhinorrhea, headache, visual changes, or pain [91]. EP are commonly located in the retroclival prepontine region (prepontine cystern) and attached to the dorsal clivus by a pedicle or pro-

trusion that may be associated with a bony defect. Radiographically, classical EP has a cystic intraclival component which is hypointense on T1-weighted MRI and hyperintense on T2-weighted MRI. Most EP do not demonstrate substantial gadolinium enhancement, which is a distinguishing feature from chordoma.

Histologically, EP can be indistinguishable from chordoma with a lobular growth pattern; lesional cells have eosinophilic and vacuolated cytoplasm, and physalifrous cells may be seen [91, 92]. The immunohistochemical profile is identical to chordoma (Fig. 5.20). EP can best be distinguished from chordoma radiographically. EP has no destructive growth pattern, no soft tissue component, and is nonenhancing with gadolinium.

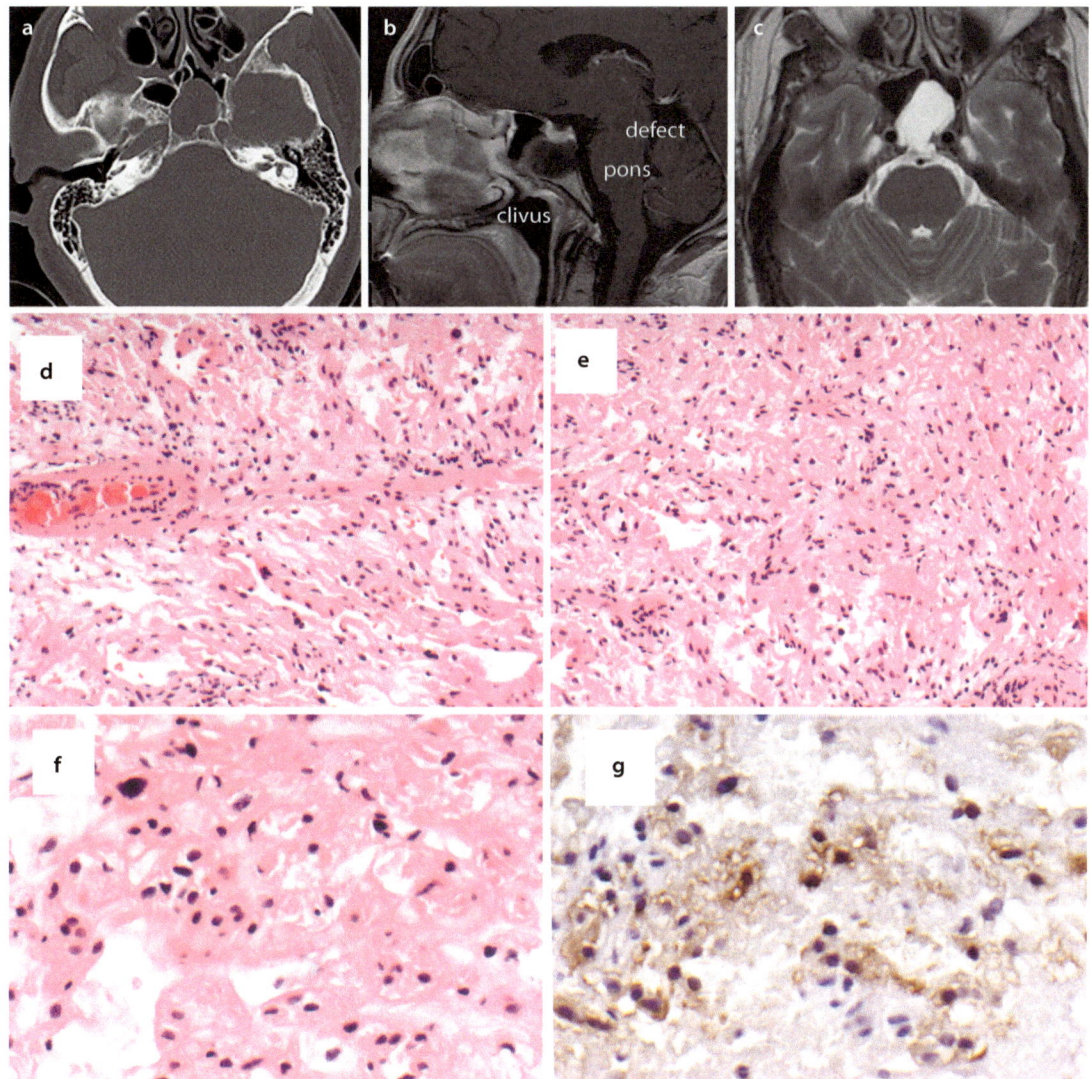

Fig. 5.20 Ecchordosis Physaliphora: (**a**) Magnetic resonance imaging (MRI) T1 weighted scan shows a hypointense expansile prepontine clival lesion. (**b**) Bony defect can be appreciated in the dorsal clivus (*arrow*). (**c**) The lesion is hyperintense on T2 weighted scan. There is no gadolinium enhancement. (**d**, **e**) At low power, small to medium-sized bland cells with round, oval and spindled nuclei are seen within an eosinophilic matrix. (**f**) Some cytoplasmic clearing is seen. However, compare this with ◙ Fig. 5.18. Basophilic matrix and prominent cytoplasmic bubbly vacuoles are absent. (**g**) This tissue expressed S100 (pictured), cytokeratin and EMA

5.9 Nasopharyngeal Carcinoma

Almost 90,000 new nasopharyngeal carcinomas (NPC) were diagnosed worldwide in 2012 [92]. Geographically, East Asia, especially southeast China (Guangxi, Hunan, Fujian, and Guangdong, Hong Kong) have the highest incidences, representing the perfect epidemiological storm of genetic susceptibility, EBV reactivation, and exposure to promoters [92–94].

There is a striking male predominance and a wide age range at diagnosis. The peak incidence in high-risk populations is the 4^{rth} and 5th decades; there is an additional incidence peak during early adolescence in high- and intermediate-risk populations. The early incidence peak in high-risk

Southern Chinese is due to early introduction of traditional preserved foods to babies.

Epstein Barr virus (EBV) is important in the etiology of NPC and is leveraged for population screening, prognostication, disease monitoring, and pathologic diagnosis. The vast majority of endemic Asian NPC (75–99 %) are nonkeratinizing and EBV+. In the US, 75 % of NPC are keratinizing and more common in Caucasians, whereas 25 % are nonkeratinizing and more common in Asian Americans [95].

EBV clonality is determined by the episomal tandem repeat (TR) sequences. Normally, a variable number of TR repeats are incorporated into the virion as it circularizes. Electrophosis of digested DNA hybridized with a TR probe will reveal multiple sized fragments indicative of EBV heterogeneity. Finding a single dominant band by the same process indicates TR homogeneity and therefore clonal EBV, which denotes a causative relationship. Clonal EBV is found in most endemic, nonkeratinizing NPCs including precursor lesions [96, 97]. By contrast, nonendemic, keratinizing NPC are generally EBV negative [98, 99].

EBV DNA load measured from nasopharyngeal swabs in high-risk populations (elevated serum IgA to EBV viral capside antigen (VCA)) can be used as a sensitive screening tool for initial diagnosis [100]. Serum EBV DNA load directly correlates with stage at diagnosis; high DNA load at diagnosis, or detectable DNA post treatment is associated with relapse and poor outcome [101–103].

The transmigration of infected B-cells through the epithelial crypts of Waldeyer's ring infects pharyngeal epithelium via cell-to-cell transfer of CR2 bound EBV on B cell membranes to epithelial apical membranes, assisted by EBV gp350 [104]. Primary epithelial infection is predominantly lytic (productive). Free virus can then infect adjacent exposed basolateral epithelial membranes via BNRF-2 (EBV early antigen) and integrin $\alpha5\beta1$. EBV infection alone is insufficient for epithelial immortalization or transformation and requires pre-existing and subsequent genetic events such as p16 silencing, telemorase activation, and MAPK signaling [105]. p16 promoter methylation is significantly more common in NPC compared to control subjects [106]. On the other hand, *p53* is usually wild-type. Aberrant NFκβ, WNT, and PI3K–AKT signaling pathways are common in NPC, which impact downstream angiogenesis, cell proliferation, and apoptosis

pathways; notably LMP1 and LMP2 can activate the PI3K–AKT pathway [107, 108].

The familial case clustering long documented among the Chinese speaks for genetic susceptibility. Comprehensive meta-analyses have identified the HLA haplotype HLA-A*0207, as well as other consistent genetic polymorphisms (*RAD51L1, XRCC1, MDM2, TP53, MMP1, MMP2, and* CYP2E1) as potential genetic risk factors for NPC [109, 110].

A number of environmental promoters are well known to have significant causative roles. Traditional preserved salted fish, fruits, vegetables, eggs, beans, and meats are associated with increased NPC risk [111–116]. Ho first suggested the relationship between Cantonese salted fish intake and carcinogenesis in 1971 [94]. Tankas, boat-dwelling fishermen and families, consume more salted fish and have a significantly higher incidence of NPC, compared to land dwellers. Salted fish is a cheap dietary staple in Southern China, but not in Northern China, where the incidence of NPC is much lower. Traditionally, fish is salted, rather than cooked, since fuel is expensive. Salted fish is commonly the first solid food given to weaned babies; ingestion of salted fish during childhood greatly increases the risk of developing NPC. Salted Cantonese type fish contain volatile mutagenic nitrosamines, which relate to the manner of fish preparation. Rather than gut and clean the fish after being caught, they are salted ungutted and whole, and undergo partial putrification referred to as "soft meat". The bacteria in the fish gut reduces the nitrates in sea salt to mutagenic nitrosamines.

Folk medicines and herbal drugs from the *Euphorbiaceae* and *Thymelaeaceae* families of plants are common in Southern China and the central Africa (Burkett's lymphoma belt) are also associated with increased risk of NPC [117–121]. Examples of these plants include *Euphorbia lathyris, Croton tiglium, Croton megalocarpus, Croton macrostachyus, Jatropha curcas*, and *Aleurites fordii*; these plants contain diterpene esters (such as phorbol esters), which can reactivate latent EBV in Raji cells. Croton oil contains 12-0-tetradecanoyl-phorbol-13-acetate (TPA) and is a classic example of a tumor initiator. Tung oil is derived from *Aleurites fordii*, and 85 % of the world's tung oil is produced in Southern China. Tung oil is ubiquitous as a waterproofing agent, (valued by boat dwellers), in wood polish, and in bases for oil paints, varnishes and inks. Inhalation of pollen and contaminated soil dust can also exert a promoting effect;

soil extracts from around *Aleurites fordii* (tung oil trees) can also reactivate latent EBV in Raji cells. Lastly, and not surprisingly, cigarette smoking is associated with a dose-dependent, increased relative risk for developing NPC [122].

The symptoms and findings for NPC patients on presentation can relate either to a nasopharyngeal mass, (epistaxis, obstruction, nasal discharge), Eustachian tube dysfunction, (tinnitus, unilateral serous otitis media, unilateral conductive hearing loss), skull base infiltration, (headache, diplopia, facial pain or palsy, sensory hearing loss, involvement of the facial nerve and/or abducens nerve) (◘ Fig. 5.21). Trotter's triad refers to the classic diagnostic triad of palatal fullness, deafness and trigeminal neuralgia. Some patients may present with cervical metastases from an "unknown" primary. Demonstrating EBER in the metastatic carcinoma in this setting is invaluable. At times, the nasopharyngeal mucosa may appear intact despite an infiltrating submucosal carcinoma. In this context, the fossa of Rosenmuller is especially targeted for "blind" nasopharyngeal biopsies.

The therapeutic mainstay is primary radiotherapy to the nasopharynx and necks for Stage I disease (◘ Table 5.2). Blanchard and colleagues recently published a comprehensive meta-analysis including published and unpublished clinical trials of over 5000 NPC patients; 89 % had Stage III/IV disease and 96 % were classified as WHO II/III (see below) [123]. They concluded that the addition of concurrent chemotherapy to radiotherapy significantly improved locoregional control, progression free survival, distant control, and disease-specific survival for patients with high-stage disease. In general, tumor stage is a significant prognosticator, and positive lymph nodes can predict propensity for distant metastasis, which typically involves the lungs, liver and bone. The overall survival at 5 years for Stage I, II, III and IV NPC has been reported at 89–97 %, 64–70 %, 53–54 %, 37–41 % respectively. Disease-related mortality is usually due to tumor invasion of skull base, cranium, and middle or posterior cranial fossa.

■ **Histopathology**

Historically, the World Health Organization (WHO) classified NPC as WHO I (keratinizing SCC), WHO II (transitional type carcinoma or nonkeratinizing SCC) and WHO III (undifferentiated carcinoma); WHO I NPC had been consid-

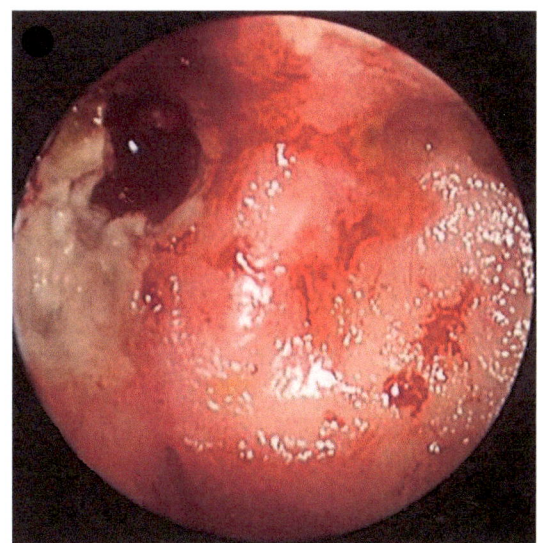

◘ **Fig. 5.21** Recurrent nasopharyngeal carcinoma within the depths of Rosenmuller's fossa, right nasopharynx. Note debris, bleeding and concave defect, as well as radiation induced mucosal changes in the posterior nasopharynx (Courtesy of Dr. Richard V. Smith, Montefiore Medical Center, Bronx, NY)

ered less radiosensitive that WHO II/III NPC. However, histology was not found to be an independent prognosticator and the value of this schema became debatable. Currently, NPC are classified as either nonkeratinizing (NK-NPC) or keratinizing (K-NPC).

NK-NPC demonstrates a variety of growth patterns with a variable degree of lymphocytic infiltrate. NK-NPC may form discreet islands, broad bands, and anastomosing ribbons, (transitional type pattern). Cell junctions (intercellular bridges) may be either obvious, or absent (syncytial growth pattern). NK-NPC may also have a "dendritic" appearance, as cell junctions are visible and "stretched out" due to infiltrating lymphocytes. NK-NPC may also be singly dispersed as small islands or single cells within a lymphoid stroma, which may easily be undetected. The tumor cells types can appear undifferentiated, basaloid, epithelioid (cuboidal or columnar) or spindled (◘ Fig. 5.22). "Undifferentiated" NPC (formerly referred to as WHO III or "lymphoepithelioma") is characterized by large, nonkeratinizing tumor cells with high nuclear/cytoplasmic ratio, vesicular nuclei, and large amphophilic nucleoli, resembling immunoblasts and form small islands or infiltrate as individual tumors cells within a dense lymphoid background (◘ Fig. 5.23).

■ **Table 5.2**	8th AJCC staging for NPC
T Category	**T Criteria**
T1	Tumor confined to nasopharynx, or extension to oropharynx and/or nasal cavity without parapharyngeal involvement
T2	Tumor with extension to parapharyngeal space, *and/or adjacent soft tissue involvement (medial pterygoid, lateral pterygoid, pre-vertebral muscles)*[a]
T3	Tumor with infiltration of bony structures at skull base, cervical vertebra, pterygoid structures, and/or paranasal sinuses
T4	Tumor with intracranial extension, involvement of cranial nerves, hypopharynx, orbit, parotid gland and/or extensive soft tissue infiltration beyond the lateral surface of the lateral pterygoid muscle
N Category	**N Criteria**
NX	Regional lymph nodes cannot be assessed
N0	No regional lymph node metastasis
N1	Unilateral metastasis in cervical lymph node(s) and/or unilateral or bilateral metastasis in retropharyngeal lymph node(s), ≤6 cm, *above the caudal border of cricoid cartilage*[a]
N2	Bilateral metastasis in cervical lymph node(s), ≤6 cm, *above the caudal border of cricoid cartilage*[a]
N3	Unilateral or bilateral metastasis in cervical lymph node(s), >6 cm, *and/or extension below the caudal border of cricoid cartilage*[a]
M Category	**M Criteria**
M0	No distant metastasis
M1	Distant metastasis

Anatomic stage and prognostic groups

If T...	and N...	and M...	then Stage
CIS	0	0	**0**
1	0	0	**1**
1	1	0	**2**
2	0, 1		
1,2	2	0	**3**
3	0,1,2		
4	0,1,2	0	**4A**
Any T	*3*[a]		
Any T[a]	*Any N*[a]	1	**4B**

Reproduced with permission from AJCC cancer staging manual 8th edition, 2016
[a]Italics represent changes from the 7th AJCC staging schema

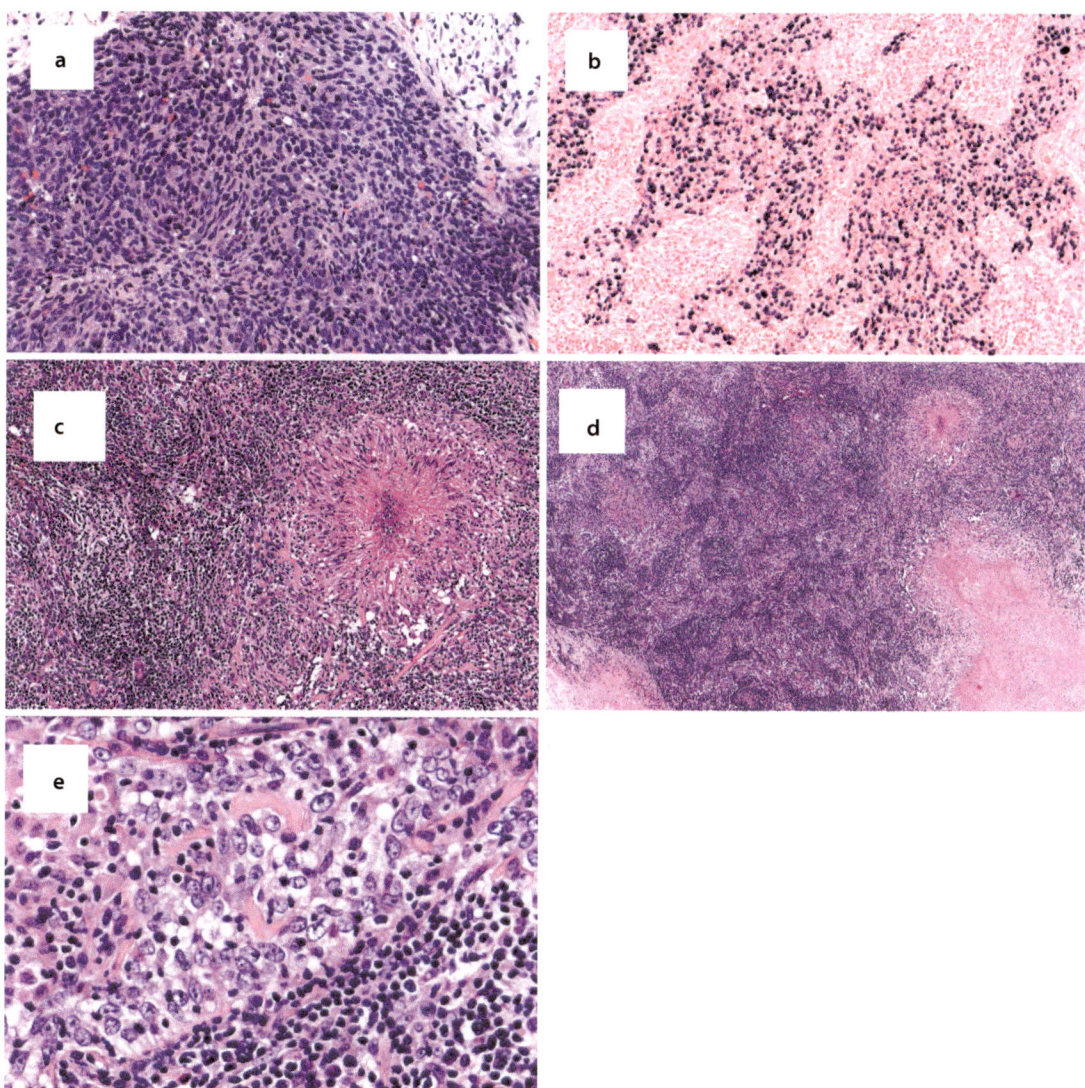

◘ Fig. 5.22 (**a**) Nasopharyngeal carcinoma (NPC) composed of basaloid spindled tumor cells. (**b**) Diffuse EBV signaling by *in-situ* hybridization for EBER. (**c, d**) A biopsy from the nasopharynx with necrotizing granuloma. A very wise person once said to me, "The worst situation for a pathologist is to make one diagnosis, and then close his/her mind to other possibilities. Some people will make a diagnosis, and then stop looking". Look at the strands of cells at the periphery of this granuloma. (**e**) Same case, higher power. These strands, in fact, are NPC! (Courtesy of Dr Beverly Wang, University of California, Irvine Medical Center)

The basaloid cell type has high nuclear/cytoplasmic ratio and dark chromatin. The epithelioid cell type has pink cytoplasm but no overt keratinization. The nucleus is usually undifferentiated, vesicular, with large amphophilic nucleoli. IHC for cytokeratins and *in-situ* hybridization for EBER can both be extremely helpful for the detection of primary or metastatic nonkeratinizing NPC (◘ Fig. 5.24), especially in the case of individually infiltrating/metastasizing tumor cells.

Keratinizing NPC is defined by the presence of intercellular bridges and keratinization, and is identical to usual keratinizing upper aerodigestive tract SCC.

in a biopsy may be akin to finding a needle in a haystack. The *curved arrow* (center) points to a rare carcinoma cell (*inset*) in this field

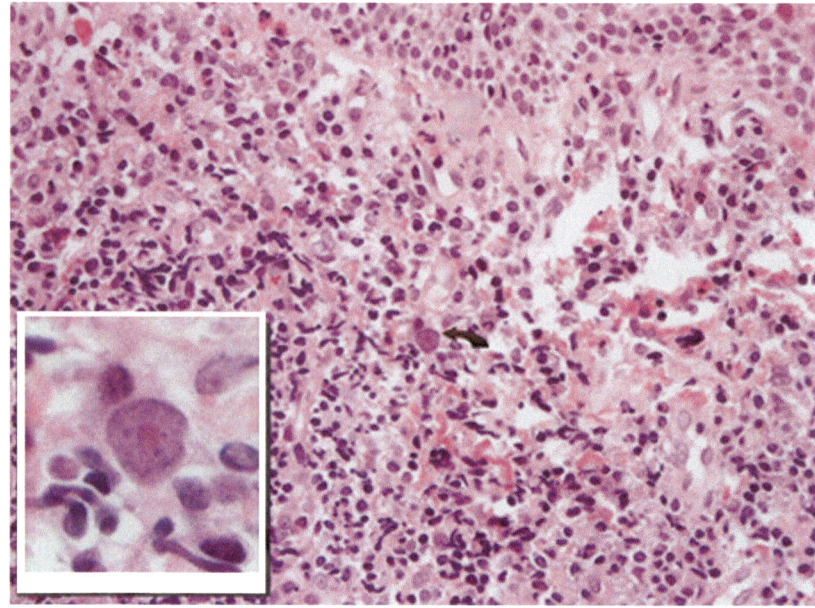

■ **Fig. 5.24**   *Top:* Metastatic nonkeratinizing carcinoma to a cervical lymph node, with a syncitial pattern and large and prominent nucleoli. This is one typical NPC phenotype. IHC for p16 and ISH for EBER should be performed for metastatic cervical disease with unknown primary site. *Bottom:* Demonstrating EBER in this context is invaluable, dramatically shifting staging, treatment, and follow-up protocols

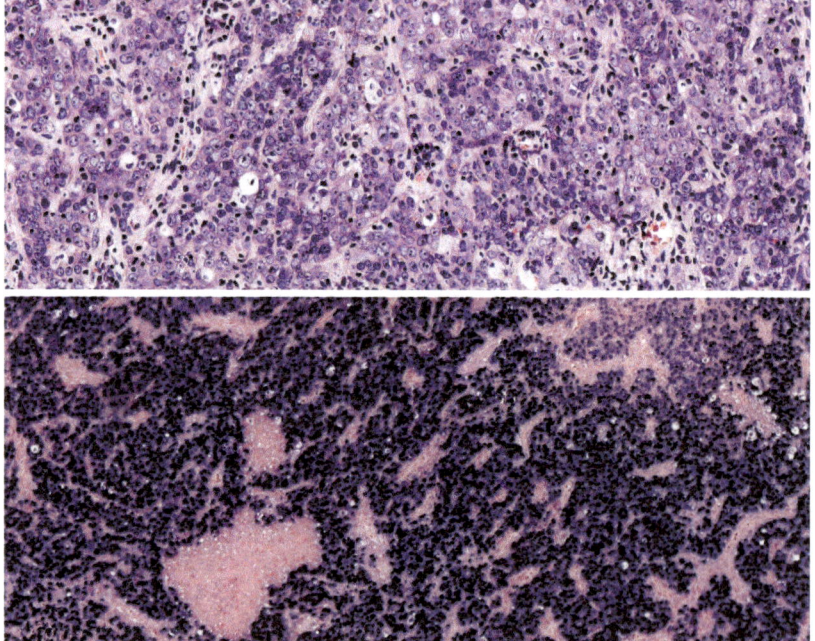

5.10   Post Transplant Lymphoproliferative Disease – Adenoids

Post-transplant lymphoproliferative disease (PTLD) is an uncommon and potentially fatal complication of organ transplantation. Risk of developing PTLD is increased in EBV-naïve recipients (more commonly children) and increased immunosuppression intensity (cardiac, pulmonary, and intestinal transplant recipients compared to renal transplant recipients). PTLD are classified as (1) Early lesions (plasmacytic, infectious monomucleosis-like, florid follicular hyperplasia), (2) Polymorphic (mixed B and T cells, polyclonal), (3) Monomorphic (B-cell,

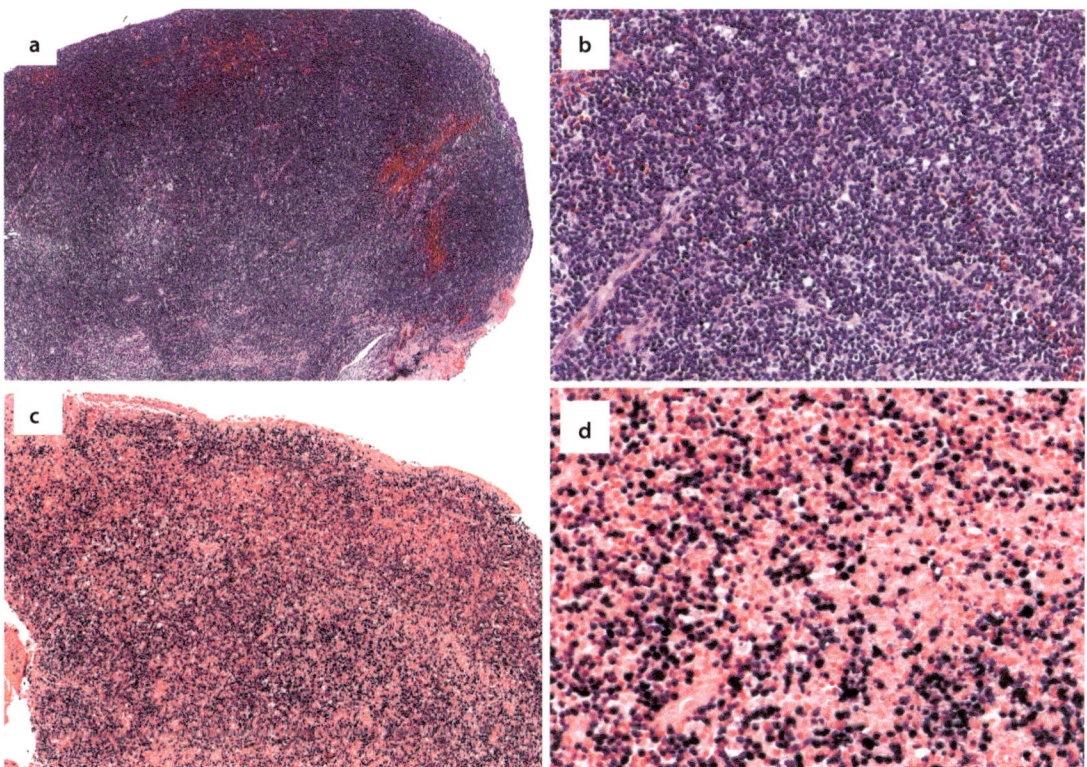

◘ Fig. 5.25 Polymorphic Post-transplant Lymphoproliferative Disease: (**a, b**) Low- and intermediate power view of adenoids from a lung transplant recipient; the architecture is diffusely effaced. A polymorphous infiltrate is seen at high-power. (**c, d**) *In-situ* hybridization for EBER reveals abnormal diffuse staining

T-cell), or (4) Classical Hodgkin's lymphomas. Early lesions most often involve the tonsils and adenoids (Waldeyer's ring) and represent benign hyperplasias; they actually bystep designation as "PTLD" [124–126]. These early lesions may or may not be EBV-related [127]. Polymorphic and monomorphic PTLD of the tonsils and adenoids are less common than early lesions.

■ **Histopathology**

Early lesions demonstrate follicular hyperplasia, and expansion of interfollicular regions, with preservation of follicular architecture. The follicles retain polarization of the mantle zone. The interfollicular regions can be plasma cell rich with Russell bodies. There is a variable degree of increased EBER expression which may be localized to interfollicular regions. The histology of early lesions that are unrelated to EBV is similar, but ISH for EBER is negative.

Polymorphic PTLD is characterized by diffuse effacement of follicular architecture and a polymor-

phous, polyclonal lymphocytic infiltrate. Atypical lymphocytes may be observed. ISH for EBER reveals strong, diffuse expression (◘ Fig. 5.25). Monomorphic PTLD represents lymphoma; the most common type is diffuse large B cell, followed by Burkitt's lymphoma (MYC+); T-cell lymphomas are uncommon. PTLD classical Hodgkin's lymphoma (CD30+/CD15+) are extremely rare [128, 129].

5.11 Thyroid-Like Low-Grade Nasopharyngeal Papillary Adenocarcinoma

Generally, primary adenocarcinomas arising from the nasopharynx are extremely unusual. Thyroid-like low-grade nasopharyngeal papillary adenocarcinoma is a rare and distinct tumor defined by light-microscopic resemblance to papillary thyroid carcinoma and expression of TTF1 transcription factor. Wenig and colleagues described nine patients, ages 11–64, with exophytic neoplasia arising from the posterior, lateral, or superior nasopharyngeal walls [130]. These tumors were noted to have optically clear nuclear features of papillary thyroid carcinoma, but lacked thyroglobulin expression. Subsequent reports of nuclear TTF-1 expression [131–135] allows for the definitive distinction of this tumor from other entities (e.g., intestinal type adenocarcynoma and salivary polymorphous adenocarcinoma) (■ Table 5.3).

Thyroid-like low-grade nasopharyngeal papillary adenocarcinoma are amenable to conserva-tive endoscopic resection. Importantly, local recurrence or metastatic disease has not been reported to date.

■ Histopathology

Transition of the overlying mucosa to tumor for-mation can be observed. Complex, interconnected papillations with distinct fibrovascular cores are seen and psammoma bodies may be observed (■ Fig. 5.26). "Colloid-free" follicular-glandular

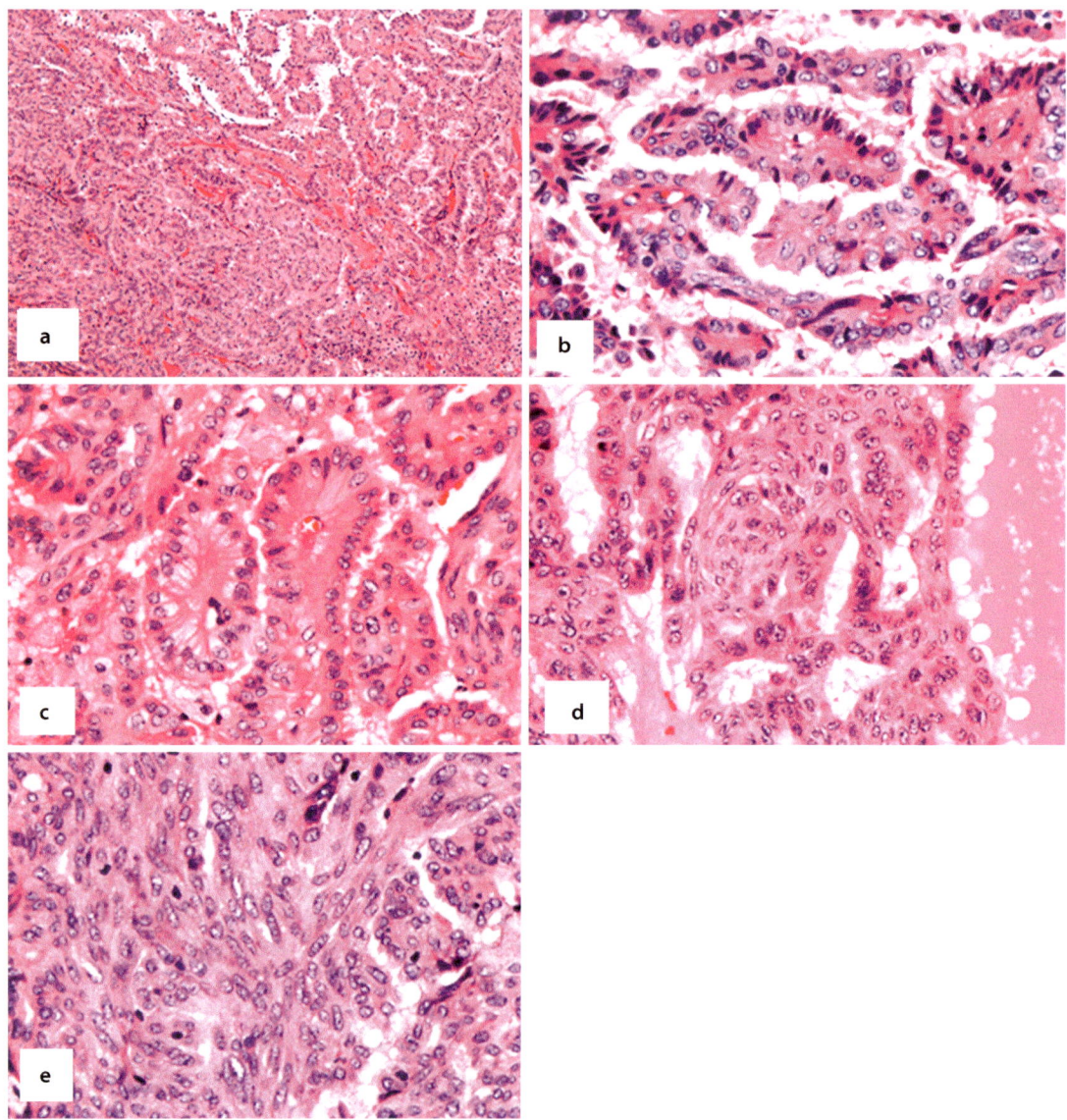

■ **Fig. 5.26** Low-Grade Nasopharyngeal Papillary Adenocarcinoma: (**a**) Solid and papillary areas. (**b**, **c**) The tumor is composed of columnar cells with overlapping oval cleared nuclei forming papillae, thus resembling papillary thyroid carcinoma. (**d**) Thyroid follicle-structures (*right*) and morula (*center*). (**e**) Epithelioid and spindled tumor cells. Low-grade nasopharyngeal papillary adenocarcinoma expresses TTF-1 but not thyroglobulin (Courtesy of Dr. B Wenig, Mount Sinai Medical Center, New York, New York)

◘ Table 5.3 Thyroid-like low-grade nasopharyngeal papillary adenocarcinoma: IHC

	TTF-1	Thyroglobulin	CK7	CK20	CDX2
Thyroid-like low-grade nasopharyngeal papillary adenocarcinoma	Yes	No	Yes	No	No
Salivary polymorphous adenocarcinoma	No	No	Yes	No	No
Intestinal-type adenocarcinoma	No	No	Yes	Yes	Yes
Metastatic papillary thyroid carcinoma	Yes	Yes	Yes	No	No

formation with crowded back-to-back glands are seen. Solid areas, whorls, and morulas can be present. Tumor infiltration into surrounding tissues has been observed, but not perineural or lymphovascular invasion. The tumor nuclei are oval, overlapping, with optically cleared chromatin, and mild to moderate degree of pleomorphism. Nuclear grooves and holes and holes are lacking.

Self Study

1. Which statement regarding Fig. 5.27 is most likely to be correct?
   (a) This is a nasopharyngeal biopsy from a young Chinese American woman. Skullbase CT and MR should be performed.
   (b) This is a nasopharyngeal biopsy from a young American Caucasian woman, status post lung transplant for cystic fibrosis. The next step would involve decreasing her immunosuppression.
   (c) This is a nasopharyngeal biopsy from a 15-year old African American male with obstructive sleep apnea.
   (d) This is a nasopharyngeal biopsy from a 15-year old Caucasian American female recently diagnosed with classical Hodgkin's disease. Where is Thomas Hodgkin buried?

2. Which statement regarding Fig. 5.28 is most likely to be correct?
   (a) This is a nasopharyngeal biopsy from a 15-year old Caucasian American male; IHC is for TTF-1.
   (b) This is a nasopharyngeal biopsy from a 15-year old male who complained of epistaxis and nasal obstruction. Holman-Miller sign is present radiographically.
   (c) This is a nasopharyngeal biopsy from a 50-year old male Caucasian American carpenter; serum EBV DNA is elevated.
   (d) This is a nasopharyngeal biopsy from a 70-year old Chinese male; IHC is for Cam 5.2

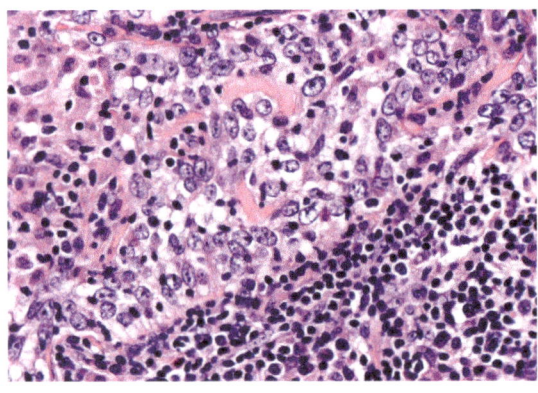
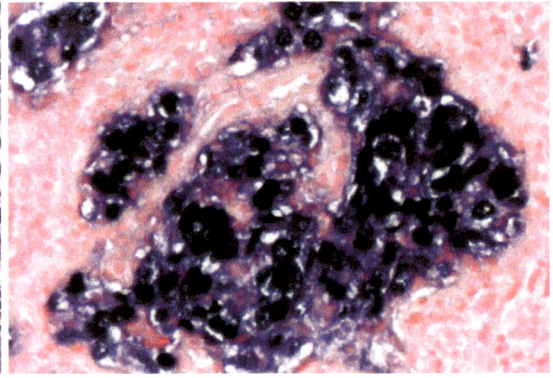

■ **Fig. 5.27**   Self study

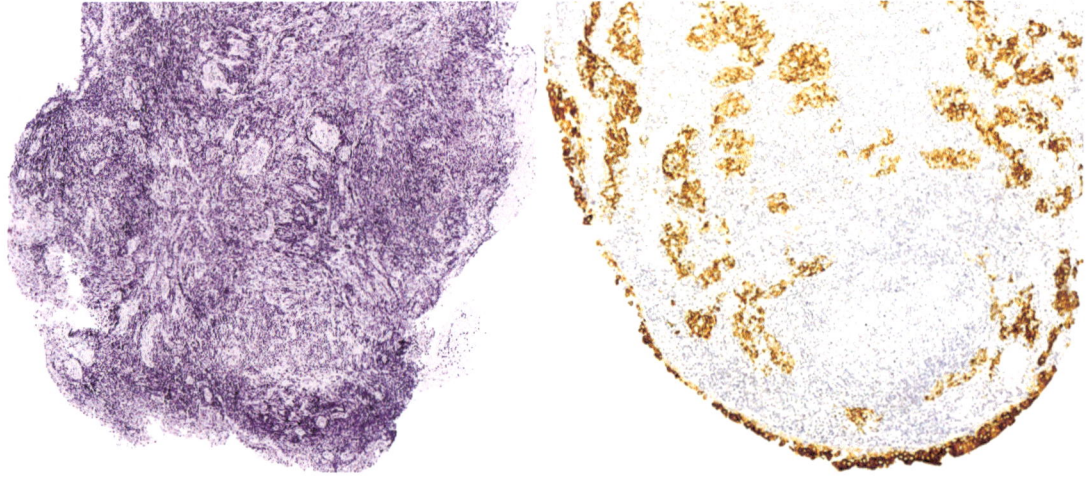

■ **Fig. 5.28**   Self study

3. Which statement regarding 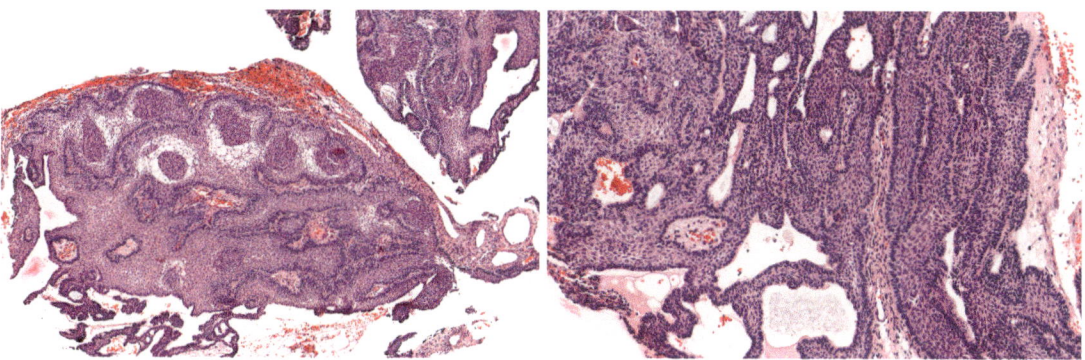 Fig. 5.29 is most likely to be correct?
   (a) *CTNNB1* mutation and aberrant β-catenin expression are common.
   (b) "Wet keratin" and calcifications distinguished one variant, which commonly harbor the BRAF V600E mutation.
   (c) This tumor arises from Tornwaldt's bursa.
   (d) Standard of care consists of primary radiotherapy.

Fig. 5.29   Self study

Answers

1. Which statement regarding ▣ Fig. 5.27 is most likely to be correct?

   This is a nonkeratinizing nasopharyngeal carcinoma (NK-NPC) (left). The right image is of ISH for EBER.

   (a) This is a nasopharyngeal biopsy from a young Chinese American woman. Skullbase CT and MR should be performed. *Yes.* The carcinoma cells (left) have an immunoblast-like appearance. The relatively sharp demarcation from adjacent lymphocytes, on light microscopy and EBER ISH (right) speaks for their epithelial origin. The incidence of NPC in first generation Chinese Americans is less than in endemic regions, yet higher than Caucasian Americans.

   (b) This is a nasopharyngeal biopsy from a young American Caucasian woman, status post lung transplant for cystic fibrosis. The next step would involve decreasing her immunosuppression. *No* – A lymphoproliferative process is ruled out by the above features.

   (c) This is a nasopharyngeal biopsy from a 15-year old African American male with obstructive sleep apnea. *No* – Normal adenoidal crypt epithelial cells have smaller nuclei and are more mature. Any EBER signals, if present, would be confined to a few lymphocytes.

   (d) This is a nasopharyngeal biopsy from a 15-year old Caucasian American female recently diagnosed with classical Hodgkin's disease. Where is Thomas Hodgkin buried? Thomas Hodgkin, a preeminent pathologist, was also the personal physician of Sir Moses Montefiore. He died of dysentery while accompanying Montefiore on one of his many trips to Israel, and is buried in Jaffa.

2. Which statement regarding ▣ Fig. 5.28 is most likely to be correct?

   This is another NK-NPC, and the IHC is for keratin.

   (a) This is a nasopharyngeal biopsy from a 15-year old Caucasian American male;

IHC is for TTF-1. *No*–Thyroid-like low-grade nasopharyngeal papillary adenocarcinoma form predominantly exophytic tumors. TTF-1 will be expressed in nuclei; you might be able to appreciate that this image demonstrates cytoplasmic staining.

   (b) This is a nasopharyngeal biopsy from a 15-year old male who complained of epistaxis and nasal obstruction. Holman-Miller sign is present radiographically. *No* – The Holman-Miller sign (bowing of the posterior antral wall anteriorly) is pathogneumonic for nasopharyngeal angiofibroma.

   (c) This is a nasopharyngeal biopsy from a 50-year old male Caucasian American carpenter; serum EBV DNA is elevated. *No* – NPC in US Caucasians is more likely to be keratinizing and unrelated to EBV.

   (d) This is a nasopharyngeal biopsy from a 70-year old Chinese male; IHC is for Cam 5.2.–**Yes**

3. Which statement regarding ▣ Fig. 5.29 is most likely to be correct?

   This is an adamantinomatous craniopharyngioma, which is usually associated aberrant activation of the WNT/β-catenin pathway

   (a) *CTNNB1* mutation and aberrant β-catenin expression are common. *Yes*

   (b) "Wet keratin" and calcifications distinguished one variant, which commonly harbor the BRAF V600E mutation. *No.* Wet keratin" and calcifications distinguish the adamantinomatous variant from the papillary variant; the latter commonly harbors the BRAF V600E mutation.

   (c) This tumor arises from Tornwaldt's bursa. *No.* It arises along the migrational path of Rathke's pouch.

   (d) Standard of care consists of primary radiotherapy. *No.* Adamantinomatous craniopharyngioma is associated with a significant rate of local recurrence. Standard of care is primary surgery (either endoscopic endonasal or stereotactic microscopic) with adjuvant radiotherapy for inadequate resections.

References

1. Babić MS. Relationship between notochord and the bursa pharyngea in early human development. Cell Differ Dev. 1990;32:125–30.
2. Ikushima I, Korogi Y, Makita O, Komohara Y, Kawano H, Yamura M, Arikawa K, Takahashi M. MR imaging of Tornwaldt's cysts. AJR Am J Roentgenol. 1999;172:1663–5.
3. Ali MY. Histology of the human nasopharyngeal mucosa. J Anat. 1965;99:657–72.
4. Marom T, Russo E, Ben Salem D, Roth Y. Nasopharyngeal cysts. Int J Pediatr Otorhinolaryngol. 2009;73:1063–70.
5. Heller D, Brandwein M, Klein M, Biller H. Hairy polyp. Am J Rhinol. 1989;3:5–8.
6. Ibrahim N, Wooles NR, Elloy M, Da Forno P. A hairy situation. BMJ Case Rep. 2015;2015. pii: bcr2015209825. doi:10.1136/bcr-2015-209825.
7. Dutta M, Roy S, Ghatak S. Nasopharyngeal choristoma (hairy polyps) an overview and current update on presentation, management, origin and related controversies. Eur Arch Otorhinolaryngol. 2015;272:1047–59.
8. Manica D, Neto CS, Schweiger C, Cortina M, Kuhl G. Dermoid of the nasopharynx causing neonatal respiratory distress. Int Arch Otorhinolaryngol. 2013;17:407–8.
9. Maeda Y, Suenaga H, Sugiyama M, Saijo H, Hoshi K, Mori Y, Takato T. Clinical presentation of epignathus teratoma with cleft palate; and duplication of cranial base, tongue, mandible, and pituitary gland. J Craniofac Surg. 2013;24:1486–91.
10. Parajuli R, Thapa S, Maharjan S. Mature nasopharyngeal teratoma in a child. Case Rep Otolaryngol. 2015;2015:515474. doi:10.1155/2015/515474.
11. Tariq MU, Din NU, Bashir MR. Hairy polyp, a clinicopathologic study of four cases. Head Neck Pathol. 2013;7:232–5.
12. He J, Wang Y, Zhu H, Qiu W, He Y. Nasopharyngeal teratoma associated with cleft palate in newborn: report of 2 cases. Oral Surg Oral Med Oral Pathol Oral Radiol Endod. 2010;109:211–6.
13. Olivares-Pakzad BA, Tazelaar HD, Dehner LP, Kasperbauer JL, Bite U. Oropharyngeal hairy polyp with meningothelial elements. Oral Surg Oral Med Oral Pathol Oral Radiol Endod. 1995;79:462–8.
14. Hossein A, Mohammad A. Huge teratoma of the nasopharynx. Am J Otolaryngol. 2007;28:177–9.
15. Ozturk A, Gunay GK, Akin MA, Arslan F, Tekelioglu F, Coban D. Multiple intraoral teratoma in a newborn infant: epignathus. Fetal Pediatr Pathol. 2012;31:210–6.
16. Maartens IA, Wassenberg T, Halbertsma FJ, Marres HA, Andriessen P. Neonatal airway obstruction caused by rapidly growing nasopharyngeal teratoma. Acta Paediatr. 2009;98:1852–4.
17. Sreetharan SS, Prepageran N. Benign teratoma of the nasal cavity. Med J Malaysia. 2004;59:678–9.
18. Saha SP, Hobson E, Joss S. Nasopharyngeal teratoma associated with a complex congenital cardiac anomaly. Clin Dysmorphol. 2007;16:113–4.
19. Lim CM, Ho CS, Pang KP, Ng SB, Goh HK. Nasopharyngeal teratoma in an adult. Ear Nose Throat J. 2005;84:550–1.
20. Ulger Z, Egemen A, Karapinar B, Veral A, Apaydin F. A very rare cause of recurrent apnea: congenital nasopharyngeal teratoma. Turk J Pediatr. 2005;47:266–9.
21. Andrews JC, Fisch U, Valavanis A, Aeppli U, Makek MS. The surgical management of extensive nasopharyngeal angiofibromas with the infratemporal fossa approach. Laryngoscope. 1989;99:429–37.
22. Snyderman CH, Pant H, Carrau RL, Gardner P. A new endoscopic staging system for angiofibromas. Arch Otolaryngol Head Neck Surg. 2010;136:588–94.
23. López F, Suárez V, Costales M, Suárez C, Llorente JL. Treatment of juvenile angiofibromas: 18-year experience of a single tertiary centre in Spain. Rhinology. 2012;50:95–103.
24. Chan KH, Gao D, Fernandez PG, Kingdom TT, Kumpe DA. Juvenile nasopharyngeal angiofibroma: vascular determinates for operative complications and tumor recurrence. Laryngoscope. 2014;124:672–7.
25. Fyrmpas G, Konstantinidis I, Constantinidis J. Endoscopic treatment of juvenile nasopharyngeal angiofibromas: our experience and review of the literature. Eur Arch Otorhinolaryngol. 2012;269:523–9.
26. Mattei TA, Nogueira GF, Ramina R. Juvenile nasopharyngeal angiofibroma with intracranial extension. Otolaryngol Head Neck Surg. 2011;145:498–504.
27. Boghani Z, Husain Q, Kanumuri VV, Khan MN, Sangvhi S, Liu JK, Eloy JA. Juvenile nasopharyngeal angiofibroma: a systematic review and comparison of endoscopic, endoscopic-assisted, and open resection in 1047 cases. Laryngoscope. 2013;123:859–69.
28. Perić A, Sotirović J, Cerović S, Zivić L. Immunohistochemistry in diagnosis of extranasopharyngeal angiofibroma originating from nasal cavity: case presentation and review of the literature. Acta Medica (Hradec Kralove). 2013;56(4):133–41.
29. Salimov A, Ozer S. A rare location of angiofibroma in the inferior turbinate in young woman. Int Arch Otorhinolaryngol. 2015;19(2):187–90.
30. Perić A, Baletić N, Cerović S, Vukomanović-Durdević B. Middle turbinate angiofibroma in an elderly woman. Vojnosanit Pregl. 2009;66(7):583–6.
31. Szymańska A, Korobowicz E, Gołabek W. A rare case of nasopharyngeal angiofibroma in an elderly female. Eur Arch Otorhinolaryngol. 2006;263:657–60.
32. Mohindra S, Grover G, Bal AK. Extranasopharyngeal angiofibroma of the nasal septum: a case report. Ear Nose Throat J. 2009;88:E17–9.
33. Patrocínio JA, Patrocínio LG, Borba BH, Bonatti Bde S, Guimarães AH. Nasopharyngeal angiofibroma in an elderly woman. Am J Otolaryngol. 2005;26:198–200.
34. Akbas Y, Anadolu Y. Extranasopharyngeal angiofibroma of the head and neck in women. Am J Otolaryngol. 2003;24:413–6.
35. Windfuhr JP, Remmert S. Extranasopharyngeal angiofibroma: etiology, incidence and management. Acta Otolaryngol. 2004;124:880–9.

36. Szymańska A, Szymański M, Czekajska-Chehab E, Szczerbo-Trojanowska M. Invasive growth patterns of juvenile nasopharyngeal angiofibroma: radiological imaging and clinical implications. Acta Radiol. 2014;55:725–31.

37. Chakraborty S, Ghoshal S, Patil VM, Oinam AS, Sharma SC. Conformal radiotherapy in the treatment of advanced juvenile nasopharyngeal angiofibroma with intracranial extension: an institutional experience. Int J Radiat Oncol Biol Phys. 2011;80:1398–404.

38. Donald PJ. Sarcomatous degeneration in a nasopharyngeal angiofibroma. Otolaryngol Head Neck Surg. 1979;87:42–6.

39. Makek MS, Andrews JC, Fisch U. Malignant transformation of a nasopharyngeal angiofibroma. Laryngoscope. 1989;99:1088–92.

40. Spagnolo DV, Papadimitriou JM, Archer M. Postirradiation malignant fibrous histiocytoma arising in juvenile nasopharyngeal angiofibroma and producing alpha-1-antitrypsin. Histopathology. 1984;8:339–52.

41. Schick B, Rippel C, Brunner C, Jung V, Plinkert PK, Urbschat S. Numerical sex chromosome aberrations in juvenile angiofibromas: genetic evidence for an androgen-dependent tumor? Oncol Rep. 2003;10:1251–5.

42. Abraham SC, Montgomery EA, Giardiello FM, Wu TT. Frequent beta-catenin mutations in juvenile nasopharyngeal angiofibromas. Am J Pathol. 2001;158:1073–8.

43. Ponti G, Losi L, Pellacani G, Rossi GB, Presutti L, Mattioli F, Villari D, Wannesson L, Alicandri Ciufelli M, Izzo P, De Rosa M, Marone P, Seidenari S. Wnt pathway, angiogenetic and hormonal markers in sporadic and familial adenomatous polyposis-associated juvenile nasopharyngeal angiofibromas (JNA). Appl Immunohistochem Mol Morphol. 2008;16:173–8.

44. Silveira SM, Custódio Domingues MA, Butugan O, Brentani MM, Rogatto SR. Tumor microenvironmental genomic alterations in juvenile nasopharyngeal angiofibroma. Head Neck. 2012;34:485–92.

45. Montag AG, Tretiakova M, Richardson M. Steroid hormone receptor expression in nasopharyngeal angiofibromas. Consistent expression of estrogen receptor beta. Am J Clin Pathol. 2006;125:832–7.

46. Liu Z, Wang J, Wang H, Wang D, Hu L, Liu Q, Sun X. Hormonal receptors and vascular endothelial growth factor in juvenile nasopharyngeal angiofibroma: immunohistochemical and tissue microarray analysis. Acta Otolaryngol. 2015;135:51–7.

47. Giardiello FM, Hamilton SR, Krush AJ, Offerhaus JA, Booker SV, Petersen GM. Nasopharyngeal angiofibroma in patients with familial adenomatous polyposis. Gastroenterology. 1993;105:1550–2.

48. Ferouz AS, Mohr RM, Paul P. Juvenile nasopharyngeal angiofibroma and familial adenomatous polyposis: an association? Otolaryngol Head Neck Surg. 1995;113:435–9.

49. Klockars T, Renkonen S, Leivo I, Hagström J, Mäkitie AA. Juvenile nasopharyngeal angiofibroma: no evidence for inheritance or association with familial adenomatous polyposis. Fam Cancer. 2010;9:401–3.

50. Valanzano R, Curia MC, Aceto G, Veschi S, De Lellis L, Catalano T, La Rocca G, Battista P, Cama A, Tonelli F, Mariani-Costantini R. Genetic evidence that juvenile nasopharyngeal angiofibroma is an integral FAP tumour. Gut. 2005;54:1046–7.

51. Guo G, Paulino AFG. Lipomatous variant of nasopharyngeal angiofibroma. A case report. Arch Otolaryngol Head Neck Surg. 2002;128:448–50.

52. Dehner LP, Valbuena L, Perez-Atayde A, et al. Salivary gland anlage tumor ("congenital pleomorphic adenoma"). a clinicopathologic, immunohistochemical and ultrastructural study of nine cases. Am J Surg Pathol. 1994;18:25–36.

53. Har-El G, Zirkin HY, Tovi F, Sidi J. Congenital pleomorphic adenoma of the nasopharynx (report of a case). J Laryngol Otol. 1985;99:1281–7.

54. Boccon-Gibod LA, Grangeponte MC, Boucheron S, Josset PP, Roger G, Berthier-Falissard ML. Salivary gland anlage tumor of the nasopharynx: a clinicopathologic and immunohistochemical study of three cases. Pediatr Pathol Lab Med. 1996;16:973–83.

55. Cohen EG, Yoder M, Thomas RM, Salerno D, Isaacson G. Congenital salivary gland anlage tumor of the nasopharynx. Pediatrics. 2003;112:e66–9.

56. Herrman BW, Dehner LP, Lieu JEC. Congenital salivary gland anlage tumor: a case report and review of the literature. Int J Ped Otorhinnolaryng. 2005;69:149–56.

57. Mogensen MA, Lin AC, Chang KW, Berry GJ, Barnes PD, Fischbein NJ. Salivary gland anlage tumor in a neonate presenting with respiratory distress: radiographic and pathologic correlation. Am J Neuroradiol. 2009;30:1022–3.

58. Tinsa F, Boussetta K, Bousnina S, Menif K, Nouira F, Haouet S, Sahtout S. Congenital salivary gland anlage tumor of the nasopharynx. Fetal Pediatr Pathol. 2010;29:323–9.

59. Gauchotte G, Coffinet L, Schmitt E, Bressenot A, Hennequin V, Champigneulle J, Vignaud JM. Salivary gland anlage tumor: a clinicopathological study of two cases. Fetal Pediatr Pathol. 2011;30:116–23.

60. Marien A, Maris M, Verbeke S, Creytens D, Verlooy J, Van Reempts P, Boudewyns A. An unusual tumour causing neonatal respiratory distress. B-ENT. 2012;8:149–51.

61. Stamm AC, Vellutini E, Balsalobre L. Craniopharyngioma. Otolaryngol Clin North Am. 2011;44:937–52.

62. Martinez-Barbera JP. 60 years of neuroendocrinology: biology of human craniopharyngioma: lessons from mouse models. J Endocrinol. 2015;226:T161–72.

63. Kostadinov S, Hanley CL, Lertsburapa T, O'Brien B, He M. Fetal craniopharyngioma: management, postmortem diagnosis, and literature review of an intracranial tumor detected in utero. Pediatr Dev Pathol. 2014;17:409–12.

64. Wang KC, Hong SH, Kim SK, Cho BK. Origin of craniopharyngiomas: implication on the growth pattern. Childs Nerv Syst. 2005;21:628–34.

65. Alomari AK, Kelley BJ, Damisah E, Marks A, Hui P, DiLuna M, Vortmeyer A. Craniopharyngioma arising in a Rathke's cleft cyst: case report. J Neurosurg Pediatr. 2015;15:250–4.

66. Fernandez-Miranda JC, Gardner PA, Snyderman CH, Devaney KO, Strojan P, Suárez C, Genden EM, Rinaldo A, Ferlito A. Craniopharyngioma: a pathologic, clinical, and surgical review. Head Neck. 2012;34:1036–44.

67. Larkin SJ, Ansorge O. Pathology and pathogenesis of craniopharyngiomas. Pituitary. 2013;16:9–17.

68. Larkin SJ, Preda V, Karavitaki N, Grossman A, Ansorge O. BRAF V600E mutations are characteristic for papillary craniopharyngioma and may coexist with CTNNB1-mutated adamantinomatous craniopharyngioma. Acta Neuropathol. 2014;127:927–9.

69. Rosenfeld A, Arrington D, Miller J, Olson M, Gieseking A, Etzl M, Harel B, Schembri A, Kaplan A. A review of childhood and adolescent craniopharyngiomas with particular attention to hypothalamic obesity. Pediatr Neurol. 2014;50:4–10.

70. Šteňo J, Bízik I, Šteňo A, Matejčík V. Recurrent craniopharyngiomas in children and adults: long-term recurrence rate and management. Acta Neurochir. 2014;156:113–22.

71. Koutourousiou M, Gardner PA, Fernandez-Miranda JC, Tyler-Kabara EC, Wang EW, Snyderman CH. Endoscopic endonasal surgery for craniopharyngiomas: surgical outcome in 64 patients. J Neurosurg. 2013;119:1194–207.

72. Winkfield KM, Tsai HK, Yao X, Larson E, Neuberg D, Pomeroy SL, Ullrich NJ, Cohen LE, Kieran MW, Scott RM, Goumnerova LC, Marcus KJ. Long-term clinical outcomes following treatment of childhood craniopharyngioma. Pediatr Blood Cancer. 2011;56:1120–6.

73. Mortini P, Losa M, Pozzobon G, Barzaghi R, Riva M, Acerno S, Angius D, Weber G, Chiumello G, Giovanelli M. Neurosurgical treatment of craniopharyngioma in adults and children: early and long-term results in a large case series. J Neurosurg. 2011;114:1350–9.

74. Okada T, Fujitsu K, Ichikawa T, Mukaihara S, Miyahara K, Kaku S, Uryuu Y, Niino H, Yagishita S, Shiina T. Coexistence of adamantinomatous and squamous-papillary type craniopharyngioma: case report and discussion of etiology and pathology. Neuropathology. 2012;32:171–3.

75. Wang W, Chen XD, Bai HM, Liao QL, Dai XJ, Peng DY, Cao HX. Malignant transformation of craniopharyngioma with detailed follow-up. Neuropathology. 2015;35:50–5.

76. Thompson LD, Seethala RR, Müller S. Ectopic sphenoid sinus pituitary adenoma ESSPA) with normal anterior pituitary gland: a clinicopathologic and immunophenotypic study of 32 cases with a comprehensive review of the English literature. Head Neck Pathol. 2012;6:75–100.

77. Johnston PC, Kennedy L, Weil RJ, Hamrahian AH. Ectopic ACTH-secreting pituitary adenomas within the sphenoid sinus. Endocrine. 2014;47:717–24.

78. Ali R, Noma U, Jansen M, Smyth D. Ectopic pituitary adenoma presenting as a midline nasopharyngeal mass. Ir J Med Sci. 2010;179:593–5.

79. Silva Junior NA, Reis F, Miura LK, Vieira GH, Queiroz LS, Garmes HM, Benetti-Pinto CL. Pituitary macroadenoma presenting as a nasal tumor: case report. Sao Paulo Med J. 2014;132:377–81.

80. Öngürü Ö, Düz B, Şimşek H, Günal A, Gönül E. Pituitary macroadenomas (>3 cm) in young adulthood: pathologic and proliferative characteristics. Neurol Neurochir Pol. 2015;49:212–6.

81. Ravichandran TP, Bakshi R, Heffner RR, Gibbons KJ, Bates VE, Durante DJ, Kinkel WR. Aggressive giant pituitary adenoma presenting as a nasopharyngeal mass: magnetic resonance imaging and pathologic findings. J Neurooncol. 1999;41:71–5.

82. Walcott BP, Nahed BV, Mohyeldin A, Coumans JV, Kahle KT, Ferreira MJ. Chordoma: current concepts, management, and future directions. Lancet Oncol. 2012;13:e69–76.

83. Fernandez-Miranda JC, Gardner PA, Snyderman CH, Devaney KO, Mendenhall WM, Suárez C, Rinaldo A, Ferlito A. Clival chordomas: a pathological, surgical, andradiotherapeutic review. Head Neck. 2014;36:892–906.

84. Jones PS, Aghi MK, Muzikansky A, Shih HA, Barker 2nd FG, Curry Jr WT. Outcomes and patterns of care in adult skull base chordomas from the surveillance, epidemiology, and End results (SEER) database. J Clin Neurosci. 2014;21:1490–6.

85. Ridenour 3rd RV, Ahrens WA, Folpe AL, Miller DV. Clinical and histopathologic features of chordomas in children and young adults. Pediatr Dev Pathol. 2010;13:9–17.

86. Wang KE, Wu Z, Tian K, Wang L, Hao S, Zhang L, Zhang J. Familial chordoma: a case report and review of the literature. Oncol Lett. 2015;10:2937–40.

87. Kelley MJ, Shi J, Ballew B, Hyland PL, Li WQ, Rotunno M, Alcorta DA, Liebsch NJ, Mitchell J, Bass S, Roberson D, Boland J, Cullen M, He J, Burdette L, Yeager M, Chanock SJ, Parry DM, Goldstein AM, Yang XR. Characterization of T gene sequence variants and germline duplications in familial and sporadic chordoma. Hum Genet. 2014;133:1289–97.

88. Miettinen M, Wang Z, Lasota J, Heery C, Schlom J, Palena C. Nuclear brachyury expression is consistent in chordoma, common in germ cell tumors and small cell carcinomas, and rare in other carcinomas and sarcomas: an immunohistochemical study of 5229 cases. Am J Surg Pathol. 2015;39:1305–12.

89. Oakley GJ, Fuhrer K, Seethala RR. Brachyury, SOX-9, and podoplanin, new markers in the skull base chordoma vs chondrosarcoma differential: a tissue microarray-based comparative analysis. Mod Pathol. 2008;21:1461–9.

90. Chihara C, Korogi Y, Kakeda S, Nishimura J, Murakami Y, Moriya J, Ohnari N. Ecchordosis physaliphora and its variants: proposed new classification based on high-resolution fast MR imaging employing steady-state acquisition. Eur Radiol. 2013;23:2854–60.

91. Krisht KM, Palmer CA, Osborn AG, Couldwell WT. Giant ecchordosis physaliphora in an adolescent girl: case report. J Neurosurg Pediatr. 2013;12:328–33.

92. Oh JK, Weiderpass E. Infection and cancer: global distribution and burden of diseases. Ann Glob Health. 2014;80:384–92.

93. Petersson F. Nasopharyngeal carcinoma: a review. Semin Diagn Pathol. 2015;32:54–73.

94. Ho JH. Some epidemiologic observations on cancer in Hong Kong. Natl Cancer Inst Monogr. 1979;53:35–47.

95. Marks JE, Phillips JL, Menck HR. The national cancer data base report on the relationship of race and national origin to the histology of nasopharyngeal carcinoma. Cancer. 1998;83:582–8.

96. Pathmanathan R, Prasad U, Sadler R, Flynn K, Raab-Traub N. Clonal proliferations of cells infected with Epstein-Barr virus in preinvasive lesions related to nasopharyngeal carcinoma. N Engl J Med. 1995;333:693–8.

97. Raab-Traub N. Epstein-Barr virus in the pathogenesis of NPC. Semin Cancer Biol. 2002;12:431–41.

98. Niedobitek G, Hansmann ML, Herbst H, Young LS, Dienemann D, Hartmann CA, Finn T, Pitteroff S, Welt A, Anagnostopoulos I, et al. Epstein-Barr virus and carcinomas: undifferentiated carcinomas but not squamous cell carcinomas of the nasopharynx are regularly associated with the virus. J Pathol. 1991;165:17–24.

99. Pathmanathan R, Prasad U, Chandrika G, Sadler R, Flynn K, Raab-Traub N. Undifferentiated, nonkeratinizing, and squamous cell carcinoma of the nasopharynx. Variants of Epstein-Barr virus-infected neoplasia. Am J Pathol. 1995;146:1355–67.

100. Chen Y, Zhao W, Lin L, Xiao X, Zhou X, Ming H, Huang T, Liao J, Li Y, Zeng X, Huang G, Ye W, Zhang Z. Nasopharyngeal Epstein-Barr virus load: an efficient supplementary method for population-based nasopharyngeal carcinoma screening. PLoS One. 2015;10:e0132669.

101. Sun P, Chen C, Cheng YK, Zeng ZJ, Chen XL, Liu LZ, Gu MF. Serologic biomarkers of Epstein-Barr virus correlate with TNM classification according to the seventh edition of the UICC/AJCC staging system for nasopharyngeal carcinoma. Eur Arch Otorhinolaryngol. 2014;271:2545–54.

102. Yip TT, Ngan RK, Fong AH, Law SC. Application of circulating plasma/serum EBV DNA in the clinical management of nasopharyngeal carcinoma. Oral Oncol. 2014;50:527–38.

103. Chan JY, Wong ST. The role of plasma Epstein-Barr virus DNA in the management of recurrent nasopharyngeal carcinoma. Laryngoscope. 2014;124:126–30.

104. Tsao SW, Tsang CM, Pang PS, Zhang G, Chen H, Lo KW. The biology of EBV infection in human epithelial cells. Semin Cancer Biol. 2012;22:137–43.

105. Yip YL, Pang PS, Deng W, Tsang CM, Zeng M, Hau PM, Man C, Jin Y, Yuen AP, Tsao SW. Efficient immortalization of primary nasopharyngeal epithelial cells for EBV infection study. PLoS One. 2013;8:e78395.

106. Shao Y, Jiang H, Wu X, Luo Y, Tang W. p16 promoter hypermethylation is associated with increased risk of nasopharyngeal carcinoma. Mol Clin Oncol. 2014;2:1121–4.

107. Tsao SW, Tsang CM, To KF, Lo KW. The role of Epstein-Barr virus in epithelial malignancies. J Pathol. 2015;235:323–33.

108. Chou J, Lin YC, Kim J, You L, Xu Z, He B, Jablons DM. Nasopharyngeal carcinoma--review of the molecular mechanisms of tumorigenesis. Head Neck. 2008;30:946–63.

109. Hildesheim A, Wang CP. Genetic predisposition factors and nasopharyngeal carcinoma risk: a review of epidemiological association studies, 2000–2011: Rosetta stone for NPC: genetics, viral infection, and other environmental factors. Semin Cancer Biol. 2012;22:107–16.

110. Yang J, Li L, Yin X, Wu F, Shen J, Peng Y, Liu Y, Sun Y, Lu H, Zhang Y. The association between gene polymorphisms and risk of nasopharyngeal carcinoma. Med Oncol. 2015;32:398.

111. Fong YY, Walse EO'F. Carcinogenic nitrosamines in Cantonese salt-dried fish. Lancet. 1971;ii:1032.

112. Fong YY, Chan WC. Bacterial production of Di-methyl nitrosamine in salted fish. Nature. 1973;243:421–2.

113. Jia WH, Luo XY, Feng BJ, Ruan HL, Bei JX, Liu WS, Qin HD, Feng QS, Chen LZ, Yao SY, Zeng YX. Traditional Cantonese diet and nasopharyngeal carcinoma risk: a large-scale case–control study in Guangdong. China BMC Cancer. 2010;10:446.

114. Ren ZF, Liu WS, Qin HD, Xu YF, Yu DD, Feng QS, Chen LZ, Shu XO, Zeng YX, Jia WH. Effect of family history of cancers and environmental factors on risk of nasopharyngeal carcinoma in Guangdong. China Cancer Epidemiol. 2010;34:419–24.

115. Ward MH, Pan WH, Cheng YJ, Li FH, Brinton LA, Chen CJ, Hsu MM, Chen IH, Levine PH, Yang CS, Hildesheim A. Dietary exposure to nitrite and nitrosamines and risk of nasopharyngeal carcinoma in Taiwan. Int J Cancer. 2000;86:603–9.

116. Geser A, Charnay N, Day NE, de-The G, Ho HC. Environmental factors in the etiology of nasopharyngeal carcinoma: report on a case–control study in Hong Kong. IARC Sci Publ. 1978;20:213–29.

117. Hildesheim A, West S, DeVeyra E, De Guzman MF, Jurado A, Jones C, Imai J, Hinuma Y. Herbal medicine use, EBV and risk of nasopharyngeal carcinoma. Cancer Res. 1992;52:3048–51.

118. Clifford P, Beecher JL. Nasopharyngeal cancer in Kenya. Clinical and environmental aspects. Brit J Canc. 1964;18:25–43.

119. Ito Y, Ohigashi H, Koshimizu K, Yi Z. Epstein-Barr virus-activating principle in the ether extracts of soils collected from under plants which contain active diterpene esters. Cancer Lett. 1983;19:113–7.

120. Ito Y, Tokuda H, Ohigashi H, Koshimizu K. Distribution and characterization of environmental promoter substances as assayed by synergistic Epstein-Barr virus-activating system. Princess Takamatsu Symp. 1983;14:125–37.

121. Zeng Y, Miao XC, Jaio B, et al. EBV activation in Raji cells with ether extracts of soil from different areas in china. Cancer Lett. 1984;23:53–9.

122. Lin JH, Jiang CQ, Ho SY, Zhang WS, Mai ZM, Xu L, Cm, Lam TH. Smoking and nasopharyngeal carcinoma mortality: a cohort study of 101,823 adults in Guangzhou. China BMC Cancer. 2015;15:906.

123. Blanchard P, Lee A, Marguet S, Leclercq J, Ng WT, Ma J, Chan AT, Huang PY, Benhamou E, Zhu G, Chua DT, Chen Y, Mai HQ, Kwong DL, Cheah SL, Moon J, Tung Y, Chi KH, Fountzilas G, Zhang L, Hui EP, Lu TX, Bourhis J, Pignon JP; MAC-NPC collaborative group. Chemotherapy and radiotherapy in nasopharyngeal carcinoma: an update of the MAC-NPC meta-analysis. Lancet Oncol. 2015;16:645–55.

124. Khedmat H, Taheri S. Post-transplantation lymphoproliferative disorders localizing in the adenotonsillar region: report from the PTLD.Int survey. Ann Transplant. 2011;16:109–16.

125. Akbas A, Tiede C, Lemound J, Maecker-Kolhoff B, Kreipe H, Hussein K. Post-transplant lymphoproliferative disorders with naso- and oropharyngeal manifestation. Transpl Int. 2015;28:1299–307.

126. Nelson BP, Wolniak KL, Evens A, Chenn A, Maddalozzo J, Proytcheva M. Early posttransplant lymphoproliferative disease: clinicopathologic features and correlation with mTOR signaling pathway activation. Am J Clin Pathol. 2012;138:568–78.

127. Williamson RA, Huang RY, Shapiro NL. Adenotonsillar histopathology after organ transplantation. Otolaryngol Head Neck Surg. 2001;125:231–40.

128. Swerdlow SH, Webber SA, Chadburn A, Ferry JA. Posttransplant lymphoproliferative disorder. In: Swerdlow SH, Campo E, Harris NL, et al., editors. WHO classification of tumours of haematopoietic and lymphoid tissues. 4th ed. Lyon: IRAC; 2008. p. 343–51.

129. Gheorghe G, Albano EA, Porter CC, McGavran L, Wei Q, Meltesen L, Danielson SM, Liang X. Posttransplant Hodgkin lymphoma preceded by polymorphic posttransplant lymphoproliferative disorder: report of a pediatric case and review of the literature. J Pediatr Hematol Oncol. 2007;29:112–6.

130. Wenig BM, Hyams VJ, Heffner DK. Nasopharyngeal papillary adenocarcinoma. A clinicopathologic study of a low-grade carcinoma. Am J Surg Pathol. 1988;12:946–53.

131. Carrizo F, Luna MA. Thyroid transcription factor-1 expression in thyroid-like nasopharyngeal papillary adenocarcinoma: report of 2 cases. Ann Diagn Pathol. 2005;9:189–92.

132. Oishi N, Kondo T, Nakazawa T, Mochizuki K, Kasai K, Inoue T, Yamamoto T, Watanabe H, Hatsushika K, Masuyama K, Katoh R. Thyroid-like low-grade nasopharyngeal papillary adenocarcinoma: case report and literature review. Pathol Res Pract. 2014;210:1142–5.

133. Wu PY, Huang CC, Chen HK, Chien CY. Adult thyroid-like low-grade nasopharyngeal papillary adenocarcinoma with thyroid transcription factor-1 expression. Otolaryngol Head Neck Surg. 2007;137:837–8.

134. Ohe C, Sakaida N, Tadokoro C, Fukui H, Asako M, Tomoda K, Uemura Y. Thyroid-like low-grade nasopharyngeal papillary adenocarcinoma: report of two cases. Pathol Int. 2010;60:107–11.

135. Fu CH, Chang KP, Ueng SH, Wu CC, Hao SP. Primary thyroid-like papillary adenocarcinoma of the nasopharynx. Auris Nasus Larynx. 2008. doi:10.1016/j.anl.2007.10.009.

Index